ADDITIONAL PRAISE FOR *RECIPES FOR LIFE AFTER WEIGHT-LOSS SURGERY, REVISED & UPDATED:*

"Ms. Furtado is a leading national and international expert in dietary issues relating to weight-loss surgery and played a key role in the formulation of the dietary guidelines currently recommended by the American Society for Metabolic and Bariatric Surgery. Her dietary insights and suggested recipes are based on over ten years of clinical experience counseling and caring for patients after surgical weight loss. This new book is clearly a must-have not only for patients after bariatric surgery, but also for health care providers and dieticians helping to manage these patients after surgery."

—THOMAS MAGNUSON, M.D., chair, Department of Surgery, Johns Hopkins Bayview Medical Center and director, Johns Hopkins Center for Bariatric Surgery

"Margaret Furtado [is] one of the most highly acclaimed nutritionists in bariatrics. Follow the dietary guidelines she recommends in this book and enjoy the many delicious recipes at each stage of your postoperative progression to health and weight-loss success."

—CYNTHIA BUFFINGTON, PH.D., director of research and education, Metabolic Medicine and Surgery Institute, Florida Hospital Celebration (Florida) Health

"An essential read for anyone who is dedicated to optimizing weight loss."

—HIEN T. NGUYEN, M.D., bariatric surgeon, Johns Hopkins Center for Bariatric Surgery

"Whether you are considering bariatric surgery or are post-op, this is a must-read! Margaret is my go-to resource for bariatric nutrition, and her book can bring this wealth of knowledge to you."

—KIMBERLY E. STEELE, M.D., bariatric surgeon, Johns Hopkins Center for Bariatric Surgery

"Margaret Furtado has compassionately and professionally helped bariatric surgical patients at three majorbariatric surgical programs, that being: Tufts Medical Center, Massachusetts General Hospital, and Johns Hopkins Center for Bariatric Surgery. Margaret's greatest accomplishment is creating this amazing book for surgical patients, which allows them to enjoy eating while maintaining the dietary restrictions. The book should be a requirement for all patients contemplating surgery."

—SCOTT A. SHIKORA, M.D., F.A.C.S., division chief, general and bariatric surgery, Tufts Medical Center, Boston, Massachusetts

"Margaret Furtado's door is always open to the constant stream of weight-loss surgery patients, colleagues, and students who seek her expertise in nutrition. She is tireless in her dedication to the field of nutrition and especially to the practice of bariatrics."

—CYNTHIA FINLEY, R.D., L.D.N., clinical dietitian specialist, Johns Hopkins Center for Bariatric Surgery

First published in the USA in 2006 by
Fair Winds Press, a member of
Quayside Publishing Group
100 Cummings Ctr, Suite 406-L
Beverly, MA 01915
www.fairwindspress.com

16 15 14 13 12   1 2 3 4 5

ISBN: 978-1-59233-496-4
Digital edition published in 2012
eISBN: 978-1-61058-182-0

Library of Congress Cataloging-in-Publication Data available

Cover design by Kathie Alexander
Book design by Yee Design
Photography by Steve Galvin except Bill Bettencourt on pages 6, 9, 10, 79, 118, 128,
158, and 219

Printed and bound in Singapore

This book is not intended to replace the services of a physician. Any application of
the recommendations set forth in the following pages is at the reader's discretion.
The reader should consult with his or her own physician or specialist concerning
the recommendations in this book.

RECIPES FOR LIFE AFTER WEIGHT-LOSS SURGERY

REVISED & UPDATED

DELICIOUS DISHES FOR NOURISHING THE NEW YOU

MARGARET M. FURTADO, M.S., R.D., L.D.N.

LYNETTE SHULTZ, L.R.C.P., R.T.

CHEF JOSEPH EWING, B.S.

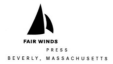

FAIR WINDS
PRESS
BEVERLY, MASSACHUSETTS

Contents

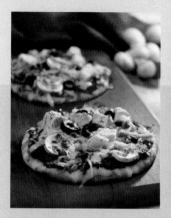 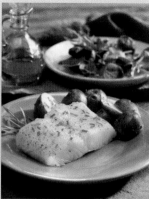 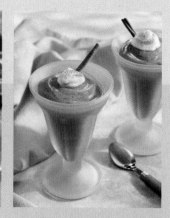

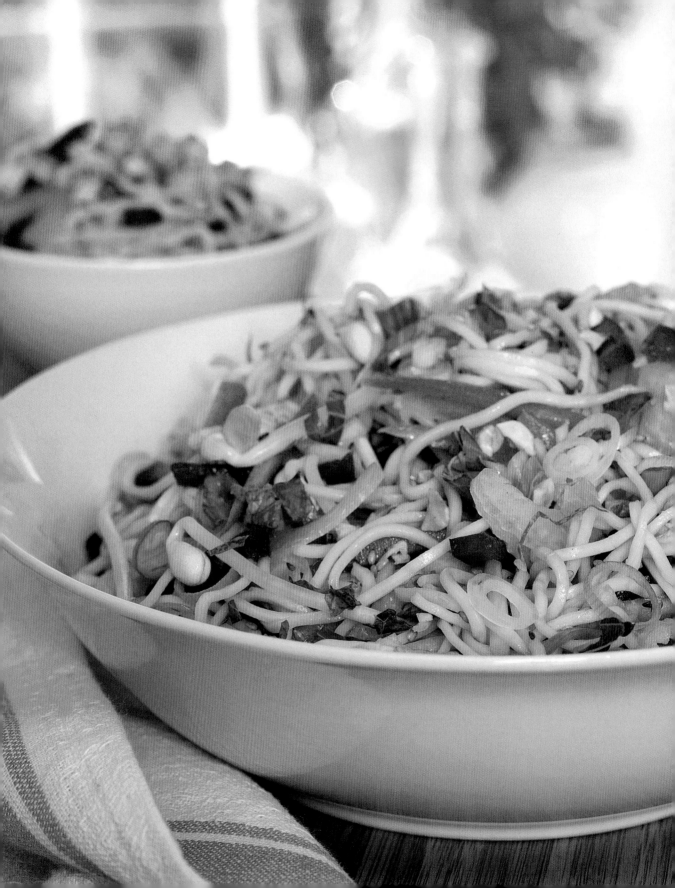

Foreword

There have been explosive increases in both the incidence of severe obesity and bariatric surgery in the last decade. (Bariatric surgical procedures have increased more than 600 percent.) These phenomena are experienced worldwide. This massive expansion in an operative procedure in such a short time period is unprecedented in the history of medicine. It is estimated that more than 200,000 Americans (and another 200,000 adults worldwide) undergo a bariatric operation each year. This dramatic increase in operative cases is in part a testament to the safety and efficacy of the currently performed surgical procedures, including the Roux-en-Y gastric bypass, laparoscopic adjustable gastric band, and the biliopancreatic diversion (with or without duodenal switch).

Although the operative procedures are relatively safe, patients must dramatically alter their eating habits to accommodate and cooperate with the surgery to achieve meaningful and sustainable weight loss. All of the current procedures profoundly change one's eating. In all cases, patients must eat smaller portion sizes, as well as more nutritious choices to overcome the potential nutritional deficiencies that could result from the nutrient restriction, malabsorption, or food preference alterations caused by surgery. While significant eating habit changes are a reality of life for the postoperative (also called postop) bariatric patient, a major goal of the surgery is to enable the morbidly obese patient to feel "more normal," not abnormal. However, dietary changes such as these can have adverse behavioral effects and enhance the perception that the obese individual is permanently a "patient."

Recipes for Life after Weight-Loss Surgery: Delicious Dishes for Nourishing the New You, written by Margaret Furtado, a dietitian with extensive experience nutritionally caring for bariatric surgical patients, is a wonderful and novel book that attempts to support the tenet that patients should feel like normal people after surgery. This book contains hundreds of recipes for delicious dishes that cover an array of tastes for all meal times. In addition, the meals are appropriate for bariatric surgery, covering the nutritional requirements for these patients. Each recipe includes the required ingredients, preparation instructions, and nutritional breakdown.

While *Recipes for Life after Weight-Loss Surgery* does not address all of the postoperative problems many patients face after surgery, it does cure the concerns about the boring or "medical-like" diets that patients often find themselves following after surgery. This book should be a staple for all bariatric surgical patients.

Scott A. Shikora, M.D, F.A.C.S.
Chief, Division of Bariatric Surgery
Tufts-New England Medical Center
Boston, Massachusetts

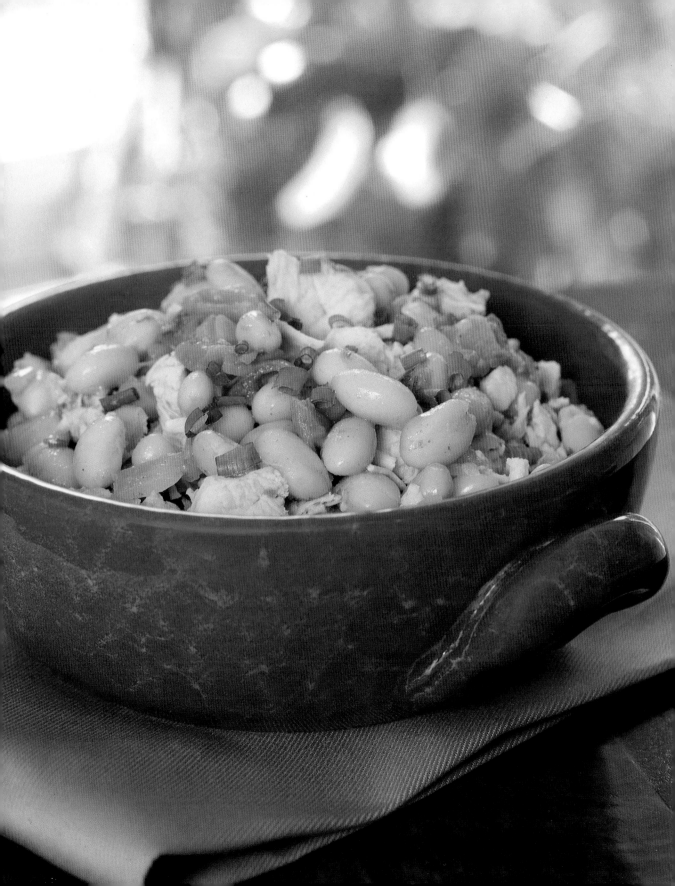

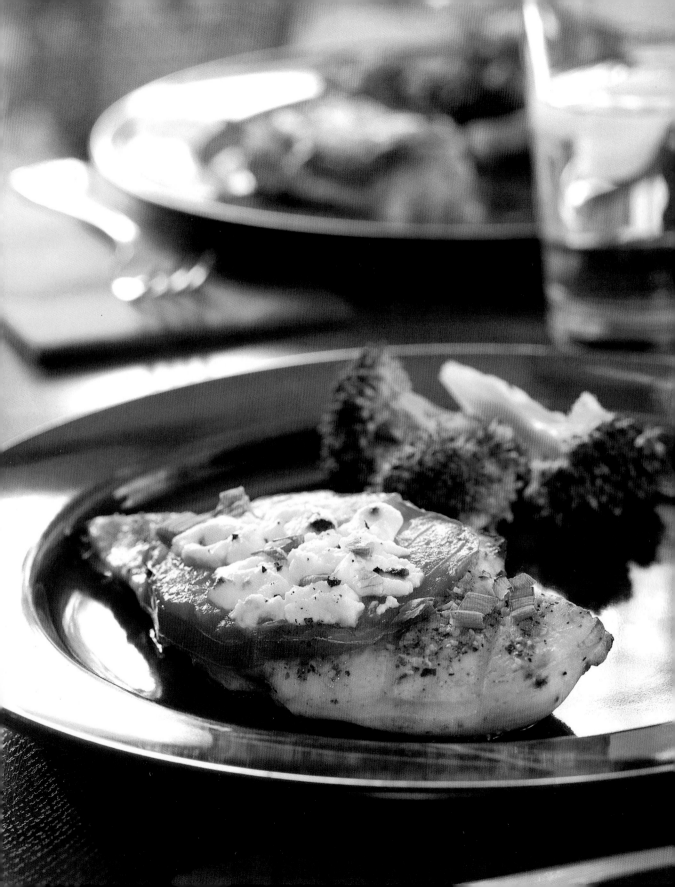

Introduction

Congratulations! You've made a very important decision to improve your health by having weight-loss surgery. Now it's time to use good nutrition to maximize not only your weight loss, but your health, vitality, and renewed sense of well-being. I'm happy to share my extensive nutrition background and expertise in weight-loss surgery with you, and I am thrilled you've chosen *Recipes for Life after Weight-Loss Surgery* to help guide you in this exciting new period in your life! Let's get started!

The guidelines outlined in the following pages are general instructions and suggestions that I typically provide to my bariatric surgery patients based upon years of experience and input from three different bariatric surgery centers of excellence I've had the privilege of working at. This new edition of *Recipes for Life after Weight-Loss Surgery* features an amazing and well-trained chef, Joseph Ewing, B.S., with whom I had the pleasure to work on my second book. Joe is also a nutritionist—and soon to be a registered dietitian, like me—so he lends a great touch to the updated version of this book!

Also in this edition, I've included nutritional guidelines for a newly available and increasingly popular bariatric surgery called the vertical sleeve gastrectomy (VSG), commonly referred to as "the sleeve." I'm delighted to contribute my expertise here for the benefit of those who are either pursuing or already have had this excellent procedure; this information will also be handy for your loved ones and supporters.

The specific nutrition recommendations—such as calories, protein, vitamins, and minerals—are based upon the most recent research studies. However, because bariatric, or weight-loss, surgery is still a fairly new field, there may be variability among medical institutions and/or bariatric surgery teams, in terms of nutritional recommendations. Please check with your hospital's staff, including your dietitian, for your particular nutritional instructions.

The information provided in this section is general, rather than the exact diet I provide to my patients, because this book is meant to focus on our healthy recipes after your weight-loss surgery. I offer just an overview of clinical nutrition guidelines, such as foods that you may want to avoid because of common intolerances and foods you may want to eat because of vitamins and minerals that may be deficient after your surgery.

Below each recipe title, you will see a texture category—Full Liquids, Puree, Mechanical Soft, or Regular—to help you decide when it might be appropriate to try that particular recipe. I've omitted the "weeks out" recommendation after each procedure, which was in the original version of this book, and replaced it with this classification of textures. I felt it would make the book easier to follow and would not contradict the suggested time frames provided by your surgical team for texture trials. I trust this will help streamline things for you and make it that much easier to navigate the "nutritional waters" after the oftentimes overwhelming initial weeks following your weight-loss surgery.

You should always keep in mind that your individual surgical center, as well as your individual tolerances, are key in terms of when you are ready to advance your diet and the foods your body can tolerate. Please listen to your body, as well as your surgical team members, and slowly add new foods as recommended, one new food at a time to better ascertain which food(s) your body is able to digest well. Keep in mind that these are merely suggestions and check with your center's dietitian and team for your specific diet guidelines.

Each recipe has been carefully analyzed for its nutritional content. After each recipe, you'll find the number of calories; grams of protein and carbohydrates; total fat, saturated fat, sugars, and fiber; and milligrams of cholesterol and sodium, for each serving. The nutritional analysis includes all ingredients in the recipe, except ingredients that are optional or garnishes, or the recipes for the rubs.

As you read these guidelines, and later on the recipes, please keep in mind that everyone is different and the recommendations in this book are just suggestions. You should always refer to your doctor and weight-loss surgery team for individual guidance regarding your diet, vitamins, etc. For example, your center might recommend that you puree all of your solid foods in a blender the first weeks or even a month or more after your weight-loss surgery. Many surgical centers have different philosophies regarding advancing the diet. As you get to the recipes in this book, you will notice that each is labeled with different textures, which will correspond with what stage you are at in your diet after surgery. The texture labels in the book are Full Liquids, Puree, Mechanical Soft, and regular (listed here in order from easiest tolerated to more advanced). As your diet progresses, you can choose recipes with textures that your doctor and dietitian have allowed as well as the food textures below that level (i.e., if you can tolerate a Mechanical Soft texture, you can also try the recipes labeled "Puree" and "Full Liquids." Please follow your center's diet instructions. You might need to wait a month or two before trying some of our recipes, but you'll get there when you're ready!

As you try the recipes, listen to your body and avoid foods that seem to be ill-tolerated (such as those that cause vomiting or chest pain). On the other hand, although many of my weight-loss surgery patients don't tolerate certain foods—such as doughy breads, rolls, pasta, and rice—you may find that you have no problem with them at all. However, the guidelines are based upon a solid nutritional foundation and general feedback from my weight-loss surgery patients regarding foods they often find hard to tolerate and those that seem to cause no problems at all. The recipes in this book were chosen based upon what most of my patients said they could tolerate. For example, I didn't think many weight-loss surgery patients could tolerate muffins, and I often discourage the doughy, high-calorie variety you might find at your local coffee shop. However, after requests from some of my surgical patients and a conference with my chef friend and coauthor, Lynette, nondoughy, healthy, tasty muffin recipes were born!

Tolerance for foods and eating after weight-loss surgery varies from one person to another, regardless of which weight-loss surgery they had. Please don't feel anxious or concerned if you find you cannot tolerate foods with which most people have no problem. We are all unique, and therefore only you can decide what feels right in your body.

Healthy Diet Guidelines for All Weight-Loss Surgeries

Before I review the nutrition guidelines following surgery, it's important to discuss the components of a healthy diet and how it relates to your diet. The word "diet" often has some negative connotations, but here it simply refers to your new healthy eating plan. As you'll see from our recipes, healthy eating can be delicious and easy!

Fluids

It may be easy to overlook, but dehydration or suboptimal fluid intake is the most frequent commonality among patients that I see after weight-loss surgery. This is not surprising since much of the population only drinks fluids when they're thirsty, which means they're already at least a little dehydrated. I often advise my weight-loss surgery patients to aim for at least 48 ounces of total fluid per day, but preferably at least 64 ounces per day. Even then, I recommend gauging urine color (if dark yellow or concentrated, you probably need to drink more fluid). Also, if you feel dizzy when you stand or sit, or you pinch the skin on your knuckle and it takes longer to "bounce back" than it usually does, you probably need more fluid.

It's very important to drink fluids, especially after weight-loss surgery, to help flush out toxins and to help your body run efficiently overall. Every time you ingest protein, your kidneys need water to flush out the toxins from the protein.

Water is the fluid I most highly recommend to patients to drink. However, I sometimes hear from patients that water tastes "heavy" or "metallic" right after weight-loss surgery. If this is the case, adding lemon, lime, or diluting your favorite calorie-free (non-carbonated) beverage with the water may help. If it doesn't, then drink unsweetened or artificially sweetened teas or other drinks (non carbonated).

Juice can be dehydrating, and may even cause dumping syndrome (the sweaty, shaky, awful feeling some gastric bypass surgery patients get after eating sweets after surgery) if you drink them quickly and they're more concentrated. It's best to avoid juices altogether for weight loss, as well as overall tolerance. I don't advise more than 4 ounces of any kind of juice per day (especially not grape or cranberry juice, unless they're diet juices), since juice beverages are typically high in sugar and calories.

Caffeinated drinks like regular coffee and tea are typically discouraged, especially right after surgery, since caffeine is a diuretic and getting enough fluid in after surgery is difficult for a lot of people. Decaffeinated coffee or tea are fine, as long as you're not adding cream or sugar (skim milk or artificial sweeteners are okay).

Carbonated beverages are also generally discouraged because they tend to cause gas and bloating, which are already an issue for many people (at least for a brief period after surgery). In addition, there is a school of thought among some surgeons and other clinicians that continuous pressure from carbonated beverages could widen the connection from the new stomach pouch to the middle part of the small intestine (among gastric bypass patients), and this could lessen the feeling of fullness, which could cause weight regain, or lessen overall weight loss.

Alcohol after weight-loss surgery is generally discouraged, especially within the first six months, since it is a diuretic. Check with your doctor regarding alcohol; he or she will likely recommend that you have only a very small amount (if any).

In some of our recipes, you will find wine in the ingredient list, since it's often used for flavor. Even though the alcohol evaporates during the cooking process, substitutions for alcohol have been provided. The flavor should be just as good, and the peace of mind of not worrying about having alcohol in the house will be priceless.

Possible challenges with fluids. Over the years, I've often heard from my patients that, other than the metallic taste, water "sits heavy" or "won't go down." What seems to help them, at least 99 percent of the time, is putting water or other liquids, including protein drinks, in the freezer. I've had patients go from only 20 ounces of fluid per day to more than 60 ounces by making just this change. Why would this work? Well, from chemistry refresher courses I recently took, ice is less dense than water—hence, why it floats—so the lower density of the ice helps it to go down better. Sugar-free popsicles might help, too, but I recommend adding them toward the end of the day rather than the beginning so that they won't take your appetite or, if you had gastric bypass surgery, room in your pouch.

If, however, you're constantly craving ice or waking up to chew on ice, talk to your surgical team immediately, because chronic or very strong ice cravings could very well be a red flag for iron deficiency, the most common issue long-term after gastric bypass surgery. (Studies reveal that 20 years after gastric bypass surgery, 50 percent of both men and nonmenstruating women may be low in iron.) Please keep in mind that dehydration is among the most common immediate issues after weight-loss surgery. If your urine is more apple juice–color than straw-color, speak to your surgical team, including your dietitian, right away. You don't want to end up back in the hospital one week after your surgery because you couldn't get enough fluids in!

Protein

Protein will always be important in your diet, both before and after your weight-loss surgery. Your surgical center will provide you with specific guidelines for protein intake, but I generally recommend a minimum of 60–80 grams of protein per day (before and after your surgery), and higher amounts if you've had BPD surgery (up to 120 grams of protein per day may be needed). As you'll see in the clinical nutrition guidelines in chapter 1, protein is very important for proper healing after surgery, as well as for life-long health. If you're not taking in enough protein, it could, in the long run, cause serious health problems, such as edema, or fluid build-up in the bodily tissue. Other protein deficiency-related health problems include anemia, as well as hair loss (which is often linked to rapid weight loss rather than nutritional deficiencies, but could be worsened by low protein in the diet).

In the first weeks or months after surgery, your diet may be 40 to 50 percent protein due to lower food intake overall, and the inability to eat much at one time. This higher percentage of protein early on after your weight-loss surgery is recommended in order to help you meet your body's protein needs.

Foods high in protein include egg whites, meat, chicken, fish, tofu, and dairy products. As you'll read in the following chapters, meat and chicken, especially if dry or tough, may not go down well, so you will want to make sure these foods are moist and diced rather than grilled. Some people also have a problem with lactose intolerance after gastric bypass surgery, so if you experience this (gas, bloating, and diarrhea are possible signs), try substituting low-sugar soy milk or take a lactase enzyme pill with the milk products to help your body digest the milk sugar. Probiotics ("healthy bacteria"), such as acidophilus, might also help with lactose intolerance, since it may help your body better digest lactose, or milk sugar. Speak to your doctor or dietitian about whether probiotics may be for you after your surgery. There's so much research going on right now with probiotics, including the possibility of improving vitamin B$_{12}$ levels, as well as helping with constipation and overall gastrointestinal upset. Some research suggests these healthy bacteria might even help you maintain a healthy weight!

Carbohydrates

In this day of low-carb dieting, "carbohydrates" is almost a dirty word when it comes to diets. However, it's important for weight-loss surgery patients to incorporate healthy carbohydrates into their diets, both before and after surgery. Healthy carbs include 100 percent whole wheat bread (thin slices or toast are better tolerated than thick slices), brown rice, whole wheat pasta, and fresh fruit and vegetables. However, right after your weight loss surgery, you are typically not allowed to have these foods, since they're not well tolerated right away. Be sure to stick with foods recommended by your doctor during this time.

I generally recommend that most people include at least 40 percent of carbohydrates in their total caloric intake, both prior to surgery and for a few months after surgery, to provide energy. Carbohydrates are the premiere sources of energy for the brain and the body in general, so if you're not ingesting enough carbohydrates in the months after your surgery, you may very well find that your energy is lacking, to say the least. In this revised edition, I've included sample menus, for use both early postop and several months down the road, with suggested carbohydrate (and protein) levels to help your body function at its best. Don't be afraid of carbs! As I tell my patients: These days, the word "carb" is a dreaded, four-letter word. But carbohydrates help you get energy and they can help your body "spare" protein to ensure that the protein you take in is actually used for your muscles and to help you heal. My carbohydrate recommendations for my patients are 70 grams by 3 months out, 100 grams by 6 months out, and the Recommended Daily Allowance (RDA) of 130 grams by 1 year out. From my clinical experience, I'm convinced that patients who are able to reach these carbohydrate "milestones" have more energy, are better able to oxidize fat (the research confirms this), and, anecdotally, seem not only to lose more weight but have an easier time adapting to a maintenance diet of a healthy balance of fruits, vegetables, protein, and good fats.

Sugars

You'll notice in the recipes that I've included "sugars" information. Every 4 grams of "sugars" represents 1 teaspoon (or 1 packet) of sugar.

There are varying schools of thought, but dumping syndrome may increase if you're consuming foods or beverages high in simple sugars. The term "sugars" on a nutrition label refers to simple sugars. Even if you never "dump" or had the banding surgery, which does not involve dumping risk, it's still not a bad idea to watch the sugars in your diet. I've restricted the recipes to about 15 grams of sugars or less (no more than 4 teaspoons of sugar) for general health. Your surgical center may allow you more sugar than this, but I think you'll find the recipes just as delicious without the extra sugar.

Fats

In order to have a balanced, healthy diet, try to limit fats in your diet to no more than 30 percent of your total calories. Ideally, most of the fat in your diet will come from "heart-healthy" fats, such as olive, macadamia, and peanut oils. These fats will help decrease total cholesterol and low-density lipoproteins (LDLs). Heart-healthy fats may also have a role in increasing the good cholesterol, or high-density lipoproteins (HDLs). However, please keep in mind that even healthy fats are higher in calories compared to carbohydrates and proteins. In moderation, healthy fats can be part of a healthy, balanced diet, but try to keep the overall calories from fat no greater than 30 percent, even if they're healthy fats.

The least healthy fats of all are the trans fatty acids, followed by the saturated fats. Trans fats are typically found in processed foods, such as french fries, peanut butter, crackers, and margarine. Such fats are extremely unhealthy and raise levels of bad cholesterol, so try to avoid them. (Trans fats are formed by a process known as hydrogenation, which turns the fat into a solid and is used by food manufacturers to extend the shelf life of their products.) When you look at a food label's ingredients, trans fat can be spotted by the term "partially hydrogenated."

Saturated fats are hard at room temperature, and include stick butter and margarine, bacon, and fatty cuts of meat. Saturated fats are also included in the nutrition information, so please read all labels. After a while, you'll be a pro at deciphering which foods are the best health bargains, and to which ones you just want to say "no."

A Word about Calories

I can't tell you how often my patients ask me, "But Margaret, how many calories should I be eating?" While I respect that they want to look at calories, and may have counted calories all their lives, I try deemphasizing calories and instead focus on the proper nourishing of their bodies. For example, a healthy level of protein is 60 to 80 grams per day for most patients. Healthy levels of carbohydrates are those I noted on page 17. As for fat, if you're using online food logs that calculate fat grams, strive for somewhere between 20 and 50 grams of fat per day, depending, of course, on how far out from surgery you are and how much total food per day is appropriate for your body and level of physical activity.

Don't worry if you're not eating more than 500 or so calories in the first weeks, or even months, after your surgery. Studies show the "average" bariatric surgery patient doesn't consume more than 500 to 700 calories a day within the first few months of surgery. Your body will take what it needs from your fat reserves (sorry that there isn't a more eloquent way to put this!) and you'll be okay, as long as you get fluids, healthy carbohydrates (e.g., fruits, veggies, whole grains), your protein goal, and some healthy fats (as stated above). Of course, taking your vitamin/mineral supplements is also key to properly nourishing your body after your weight-loss procedure. Talk to your dietitian about supplements of calcium, and, if applicable, vitamin B$_{12}$, iron, and (if you've had duodenal switch surgery) fat-soluble vitamins.

Remember, this is a new, healthy way of nourishing your body. Of course, if you find your weight is headed up fast, perhaps due to "dietary indiscretions," I highly recommend keeping careful food logs (paper or online), and bring the logs when you see your dietitian or surgical team member to better decipher why you're gaining weight. Some weight gain (5 pounds or so, on average) from your lowest weight after surgery is common and to be expected, but more than that, or rapid weight gain, should be brought to the immediate attention of your surgical team.

This deemphasis on calories is why you won't see listed the caloric content of most of our new meal plans. Rest assured, they're adequate for most people at the particular time points noted. If your center suggests a particular calorie level for you, however, it's not wrong, since every center does things differently. Calories are just not what I like to focus on.

Fiber

If you look at a food label, you'll see that fiber is actually included under carbohydrates in the nutrition information. However, by definition, humans do not possess the enzyme necessary to use fiber for calories or energy, which explains the recent trend to exclude fiber from the carbohydrate content of foods.

There are two kinds of fiber: soluble and insoluble. They are both important in the diet but perform different functions. How can you tell which fiber is soluble or insoluble? If you peel an apple and place the peel in a glass of water and stir it around, nothing happens (it doesn't dissolve in the water). This is an example of insoluble fiber. In general, bran and the skins and peels of fruits and vegetables contain insoluble fiber, which helps with constipation because it speeds the food through your gastrointestinal tract. If you take the pulp of an apple, on the other hand, and submerge it in water, you'll find it dissolves. This is an example of soluble fiber (e.g., applesauce). Soluble fiber may help with lowering cholesterol in some cases (e.g., oatmeal), and may also help if you're having diarrhea, because it is a natural stool binder.

The American Cancer Society recommends that 25 to 30 grams of fiber be included in our daily diet to potentially lower the risk for colon cancer, and possibly other cancers as well. Fiber also tends to help us feel fuller because it slows down the rate of blood sugar release and stomach emptying.

If you recently had weight-loss surgery, your center may recommend that you not include fiber in your diet during the first weeks or even months after your surgery to ensure that your new stomach and connection are working properly. Even if you did not have surgery that affects absorption (e.g., gastric banding), your surgical center may ask you not to include fiber in your diet for a while, especially after an adjustment or fill, since the narrowing from your pouch to the lower part of your stomach may be much more narrow, and too much fiber too soon may cause intolerance issues. As always, please check with your surgical center for specific dietary recommendations.

Vitamin and Minerals

Many surgical centers will do blood tests prior to your weight-loss surgery to ensure that you're in the best possible health before going into the operating room. It's not uncommon for people to have some vitamin and mineral deficiencies, so don't be alarmed if your doctor tells you that these deficiencies need to be corrected preceding surgery. I have found several studies citing Vitamin D deficiency or issues with iron, anemia, or Vitamin B_{12} before surgery.

It's important to take the prescription your doctor gives you to be in as good nutritional shape as possible before your life-changing weight-loss surgery. After surgery, it will be imperative to take your vitamins (with minerals) and calcium with Vitamin D, as well as any other supplements or medications prescribed for you.

If you are told that you have a vitamin or mineral deficiency after your surgery (and you've been taking all the supplements your doctor has ordered), don't be too hard on yourself. Studies show that even people who follow a healthy diet and take their recommended supplements following their surgery may have some deficiencies, so it might be that you need some additional supplementation. If not corrected right away, a Vitamin B_{12} deficiency may cause numbness or tingling in your fingers and memory loss. If not corrected for several weeks or months, it may even cause irreparable neurological damage. Thiamin, another B vitamin (vitamin B_1, to be exact), is *very* dangerous if it gets low, since the plummet can happen very rapidly, and, in rare cases, can result in death! Please keep in mind this is highly uncommon, but if you have chronic vomiting and/or have new onset of burning and/or numbness in your feet, contact your center immediately since complications due to a thiamin deficiency can progress very quickly, and you certainly want to catch it before it results in something serious. My patients who have reported new onset of burning in their feet have told me that within one day they weren't able to feel their ankles. After IV thiamin treatment, they were almost as good as new the next day. Catching it quickly is key!

Don't be alarmed, dear readers. These deficiencies are fairly rare, especially if you follow your center's recommended course of dietary supplementation, eat right, and have your blood tests done at time points advised by your surgical center. Remember, the vitamin/mineral regimen is for a lifetime, not just for the immediate weeks or months after surgery. If you don't like the vitamin you're taking, talk to your surgical team, including your dietitian, to find an alternative. Keep in mind that solid vitamins/minerals and calcium may get stuck or may not be as well absorbed as chewable, liquid, or powder varieties. Time-released or enteric coated vitamins, supplements, and medications also may be poorly absorbed, especially after a procedure like gastric bypass surgery. So, the benefits of repairing your deficiencies are well worth it.

CHAPTER 1

The Early Postoperative Nutritional Guide

In this chapter, I'll talk about gastric bypass surgery, gastric banding surgery, and biliopancreatic diversion, with or without a duodenal switch. Each type of surgery has slightly different nutritional requirements. Let's talk about each in turn.

Gastric Bypass Surgery

Congratulations on your gastric bypass (GBP) surgery!

Gastric bypass surgery reduces the size of your stomach so that it holds about 1 ounce instead of the usual 1 quart, making it the size of your thumb instead of the size of a football. This smaller stomach is then typically reconnected to the second part of the small intestine (the jejunum). Gastric bypass surgery can help speed up your weight loss by making it harder to eat much food at one time, and it also increases satisfaction after meals, especially in the early postoperative (also called postop) period. This slower eating helps increase the feeling of fullness and satisfaction for many gastric bypass patients, although in the first few months after this surgery you may not have any appetite at all (a good thing, many of my patients find!). This may be one of the only times in your life when you have to remind yourself to eat. This may be because of the temporary decrease of hunger hormones in the stomach because of the nature of the surgery. Some people really enjoy this honeymoon period when they feel the freedom from the incessant hunger they may have felt before the GBP surgery. Others find it hard to get all the protein necessary to heal, and they may use high-protein supplements (low in sugar and fat) to help achieve proper nutrition.

If you find yourself in the honeymoon period after your gastric bypass surgery, ensure you eat a minimum of three meals per day to help you meet your body's needs. Don't worry about not feeling hungry; enjoy this honeymoon. As long as you're drinking enough fluid and eating enough protein, you should be doing fine.

Appetite

Over time, the stomach pouch outlet (the passageway or connection from the new stomach pouch to the middle part of the small intestine) will stretch until it can hold 4 to 8 ounces, or approximately $1/2$ to 1 cup, at one sitting. This helps to get more protein in at one time, but it may also result in an increased appetite and the end of the honeymoon period. Eating slowly and taking small bites can help you to feel more satisfied and ward off hunger. In addition, getting 48 to 64 ounces of fluid in between meals really helps.

Typically, my patients report an increasing appetite within 4 to 6 months after the surgery, although I know a few who still seem to be in the honeymoon even 2 years after their surgery. Although it may seem wonderful not to have any appetite after surgery, don't skip meals or forget to eat, because this may wreak havoc on your nutritional status and your weight loss success as well. However, by meals, I'm talking about a small light yogurt or high-protein, low-sugar shake. These meals right after weight-loss surgery may seem like snacks, but most people are not able to ingest much at one time right after surgery. Please don't push yourself to eat too much in one sitting. Listen to your body.

Your New Stomach

Your new stomach, which is about the size of an egg, may take 6 to 8 weeks to heal. To facilitate the healing process, you will progress through five diet stages, which I will talk about in detail later in this chapter. Basically, you will be on a liquid diet for 2 to 3 weeks before advancing to ground (and if necessary, pureed) foods, and finally to soft, moist, whole foods. Your meal plan will be high in protein, which is very important for healing and weight loss. Your diet needs to always be low in fat and concentrated sweets.

It's important that you eat slowly. Your meals should last for 30 minutes to an hour. It is recommended that you take about 10 minutes to eat each ounce of food (for example, one egg is 1 ounce.) Eat slowly and mindfully, taking pencil-eraser-size bites of food. Chew each bite 15 times before you swallow it. Food should be at a liquid consistency in your mouth before you swallow. Mindful eating is always a priority. Don't eat in front of the television or computer, but rather at the dinner table (ideally), and focus solely on your eating. Also, it's a good idea to put your eating utensil down in between bites, if possible for 1 to 2 minutes before taking your next bite. See how your body feels after that last bite before you go for another one. It takes your brain about 20 minutes to figure out you're full, so slow eating is important to help you avoid feeling overly full or uncomfortable.

Sip liquids slowly, between meals only, so you will still have room in your stomach for meals.

If you are experiencing any cramps, gas, or diarrhea in the early stages, you might have developed a problem digesting lactose, or milk sugar, called lactose intolerance. This is fairly common after gastric bypass surgery. I see it in about 20 percent of my patients, and it may occur because the first part of the small intestine, the duodenum, which is bypassed in gastric bypass surgery, is responsible for how your body handles sugars, including milk sugar, or lactose. Changing your diet to one that is lactose-free—avoiding milk and milk products—should alleviate the problem. If you'd rather not omit these foods or beverages, you can purchase the enzyme that digests milk sugar at your local pharmacy. This enzyme is called lactase, and taken with lactose-containing foods and beverages, it should solve the problem. In addition, you may purchase foods that have already been treated with the lactase enzyme (such as low-fat cottage cheese), so you can have your cottage cheese and eat it, too! Alternatively, keep in mind that there are now a number of options on the market you can use in place of milk, such as lactose-free milk and a variety of soy milk products that taste great and have plenty of protein. And remember, probiotics may also help with lactose intolerance. These are the "good bacteria" that help your body digest milk sugar so that you don't have the resultant gas, bloating, or diarrhea. Probiotics can also be found in yogurt, although in much lower amounts. There are typically around 4 strands of active culture in the Greek yogurt called for in some of the recipes in this book.

As you advance through the diet stages, you will always be able to consume any food or beverage you were allowed in the previous stage(s). When advancing, it's important to try only one new food at a time, so that if you don't tolerate it (for example, notice it feels stuck in your chest, even when eating slowly and mindfully), you'll be able to better determine which food was the culprit. Eliminate the offending food from your diet for a few weeks and try again.

Food Diary

Keep an accurate food diary of what you eat, how quickly or slowly you ate, and also how you tolerated the foods. You may find that you might not be able to tolerate foods that were your favorites before surgery. Many people also comment that foods taste different or that their preferences have changed. Some cite issues with the taste of water. If that happens to you, try adding lemon or lime to it.

Keeping a food diary will also help you to plan your meals and keep your nutritional goals on track. It may be helpful to review your food diary with your dietitian.

Stop When You're Full

Stop eating as soon as you feel full so that you better tolerate your food and minimize risks for chest pain or discomfort. And certainly, stop eating the instant you feel chest pressure or discomfort. If necessary, put away the food you didn't finish and eat it later. However, ensure that it isn't dried out, because that may increase the chances it will not be well-tolerated. You can add low-fat salad dressing or lime juice to leftovers to re-moisten them. Also, you could keep a bowl of hot, low-fat gravy or sauce nearby to add to your meat or chicken, for example, if it starts to get cold, tough, or both. Food tastes better hot to a lot of people, too, so you might want to make a habit of doing this for the long run.

Dumping Syndrome

Gastric bypass patients may experience something called dumping syndrome, which occurs when a sugary food, such as syrup or a cookie, is eaten. Because the duodenum, the first part of the small intestine, is bypassed in GBP surgery, and it handles sugars, water will go rushing into the small intestine to try to lessen the concentration. When this happens, a vaso-vagal response may occur, leaving the person feeling dizzy, shaky, sweaty, and overall, very lethargic. Some of my GBP patients report that after an episode of dumping, their energy is zapped and they're too tired to do anything else. It's not a good feeling, so it's best not to see whether you can tolerate chocolate and other sweets. Keep in mind that dumping may also occur with nonsugary foods, such as high-fat or greasy foods, or even protein, especially if you're drinking super-concentrated protein drinks (those that contain more than 50 grams of protein per serving). I've actually had patient reports of dumping, including cramping, sweating, and a low blood sugar–type of reaction when they drank concentrated protein drinks too quickly. This is because the bottom portion of your stomach, the pylorus, which is a "fluid manager" and is also involved in the tolerance of foods and beverages, is no longer "available" to your digestive tract after gastric bypass. The pylorus is, however, still in your body, along with the duodenum and the rest of your stomach, making hormones and juices that meet further down the digestive tract. This is yet another reason why I discourage consuming more than about 30 grams of protein per serving of protein supplement. Sure, it's highly possible your body can absorb it if it's high-quality protein, but it's certainly dehydrating because your kidneys have to process all that protein at once. I don't have my patients count protein supplements as fluid if they drink more than 40 grams of protein at one sitting. Although I have worked with several GBP patients who stated they didn't dump at all, others avoid sweets altogether and convince themselves they'll be ill if they eat sweets. This approach may work well for you if you're a lover of sweets. Even if you don't have dumping when you eat sugary foods or beverages, it's best to avoid them anyway. They're just empty calories and may also increase the appetite by stimulating more insulin in response to the sugar intake.

Hair Loss

Another problem that is not uncommon for gastric bypass surgery patients is hair loss. Hair loss can be caused by many things, including the stress caused by rapid weight loss or by nutritional inadequacies. This is just one more reason why it's important to meet your dietary goals. Eating enough protein, taking your vitamins (zinc and iron deficiency may cause hair loss), and drinking enough fluid may help to minimize your hair loss, if it does occur. But even if you find you are losing quite a bit of hair after surgery, many of my patients find that the cycle reverses itself within 3 to 6 months. It's believed the main cause of this overall shedding of the hair within the first months after bariatric surgery is due to a condition with the fancy term "telogen effluvium," which is hair loss due to a variety of causes, including physical stress. This stress could include both the stress of the surgical procedure itself, as well as the perceived "stress" of significant weight loss. Keep in mind your body doesn't "know" that you had surgery of your own accord, and your body "stresses out" with all of the resultant changes after surgery, including (hopefully) significant weight loss. If your hair doesn't start to grow back, talk to your surgical team, since other factors, such as thyroid issues, stress, or lack of sleep, could be the culprit.

Decrease in Weight Loss

Gastric bypass surgery patients also often experience a slowdown in weight loss. You may find that sometimes your weight loss slows down, even just a few months after your gastric bypass surgery. It may sound counterintuitive, but you want to make sure you're eating enough. Yes, you heard right! Sometimes my patients come to see me and are a little discouraged that they've stopped losing weight a few months after their surgery, despite consuming only 500 calories. I'm not saying this happens to a lot of people, but I've had patients who were afraid to eat and felt tired all the time. When I looked at their diet, I found they were only eating chicken or turkey (and nothing else, sometimes) months after surgery. Often they complained of no energy and didn't understand why they felt this way. While I think it's always a good idea to check with your doctor at the surgery center if you're not feeling great, also check in with your dietitian to ensure you're getting enough protein and the minimum amount of nutrition to have enough energy to work, exercise, and have fun.

Our bodies are magnificent in that they will do everything they can to help us not only survive, but thrive. For example, if we're eating very little for long periods of time (such as 200 to 300 calories a day for several weeks), it's possible that the body's metabolism—the way it burns calories—could slow down, sometimes a great deal, to adjust for the decrease in calories. Ensure that you're consuming an adequate amount of calories and protein to offset the plateau and get the weight loss back on track. Another possibility when you see weight loss stop for a while is that you're losing inches, which you may not see on the scale but might see in your loose clothing or belt. Check in with your dietitian or doctor regarding whether you're eating an adequate diet after your surgery. Take your food diary to the center so that they can better assess your overall dietary intake for adequacy and appropriateness.

Protein Goals

Some people have a hard time meeting their protein goals. Weighing your food on a scale after it has been cooked may better guarantee that you are meeting your protein needs. If you don't have a food scale, a regular deck of playing cards or a computer mouse can serve as size guidelines for approximately 3 ounces of protein (such as chicken and fish), which is often the goal I ask my patients to attain for lunch and dinner, at least within a couple of months of their gastric bypass surgery. But remember that you should be able to get your protein without feeling chest discomfort or vomiting, which can be potentially dangerous. If getting this in solids is hard for you, you might want to use the high-protein liquid supplements from the earlier diet stage to help you meet your protein goal. If you find you have an issue with persistent chest pain and/or vomiting, please check in with your doctor right away. Persistent vomiting is not normal after this surgery.

Exercise

If cleared by your doctor or exercise physiologist, exercise may greatly help to jump-start your metabolism and speed up weight loss. We often suggest walking right away after weight-loss surgery and within 8 weeks adding abdominal exercises and weight-lifting. (Please consult with your doctor before engaging in exercise after your surgery.) It's important to know that exercise helps "tell" your body to be happier at a new lower weight and may really help establish a new "happy weight" or set point. Gastric bypass surgery is a procedure that helps your brain to want to stay at a much lower, much healthier weight, but of course it's still just a tool. Healthy eating (3 meals a day with protein and healthy carbs, no more than 5 hours apart) and exercise really help enhance your chances of staying at that happy weight and/or keeping within about a 5-pound range of that new healthy weight or set point. If you don't like to exercise or find you have obstacles, like inclement weather, talk to your center's professionals about alternatives. You might want to take dance classes or try free programs available from your cable TV provider or a walk-in-place program (I often recommend Leslie Sansone's Walk Away the Pounds program, as another alternative).

Your New Body

Especially in the first few months after your weight-loss surgery, you may start to feel anxious about comments and compliments about your weight loss or your new body. You may feel uncomfortable with an enhanced amount of attention or find that new issues may replace old ones in your life as a result of your weight loss. Please know that this uneasiness is common. The decision to pursue gastric bypass surgery often involves a major change in your lifestyle, which may affect all areas of your life. Remember that you are not alone in this process. It is important to involve yourself in postoperative support groups and to meet regularly with the members of your health care team, including your nutritionist, doctor, and psychologist.

Your Diet Following Gastric Bypass Surgery

Since having your gastric bypass surgery, your stomach has been altered, in both its anatomy and function. You need to make special dietary changes to ensure successful weight loss while lowering the risk of malnutrition. In this section, I describe what may happen at a "typical" center, which I hope will help you understand the various stages of your diet. Once again, you may find that your center has somewhat different guidelines. The diet after gastric bypass surgery may vary quite a bit among surgical centers. These instructions are only suggestions. Please check with your center's dietitian for your personal meal plan and pre- and postoperative nutritional instructions.

STAGE 1: CLEAR LIQUIDS

The first day of you can have liquids, including, broth, protein supplement powder, diet gelatin, and a diet (noncarbonated) beverage. While every center is different, it's fairly common to start with clear liquids as the first diet stage (again, please check your center's recommendations). At my current center, the first day patients receive a tray after gastric bypass surgery, they're given small (1-ounce) medicine cups and are told to *slowly* drink one medicine cup, or 1 ounce, per hour. The following day, they advance to 2 ounces per hour, and, if still in the hospital on the following day, increase to 3 to 4 ounces per hour, as tolerated. When they disconnect the intravenous fluid, I reinforce the importance of aiming for a minimum of 4 to 8 ounces per hour to help meet the 48- to 64-ounce-per-day fluid goal. This may be challenging at first, since during the first week there is often a great deal of postoperative swelling and an 8-ounce protein drink may take up to 2 hours to drink. Slow and easy is key, but not so slowly that dehydration sets in. Patients are told to stop if they feel chest pressure or pain and also are told that vomiting, extreme chest pain, and/or hiccoughs may be a sign they are drinking too quickly and/or not tolerating fluids. In that case, they're then evaluated by the surgical team.

Flattened diet carbonated beverages are okay, but we discourage drinking regular, unflattened carbonated beverages because they may cause a great deal of gas to become trapped in the connection (or anastomoses) where the new stomach pouch meets the middle part of the small intestine. This gas bloat may cause a great deal of discomfort. Also, it's possible that continued increased pressure in the new connection (anastomosis) from chronic use of carbonated beverages after gastric bypass surgery could stretch this outlet and cause a decreased feeling of fullness, which could lessen weight loss and/or cause weight regain after GBP surgery. It's not proven, but why risk stretching out your new connection from your pouch?

We encourage our patients to stop sipping or eating as soon as they feel full or nauseated. They are advised to drink slowly, and not to gulp fluids.

Our patients are also encouraged to walk as much as they can, even while in the hospital. Often our patients will walk down the hospital halls with their nurse and/or a friend. This is really key to get the blood circulating and possibly decrease your risk of getting a blood clot after surgery. (This risk is not unique to weight-loss surgery. If you're not moving or walking after just about any kind of surgery, you could be at risk for a blood clot, according to many doctors with whom I've talked.) If you feel pain, weakness, or dizziness, of course you should stop, but if you feel good, walking could also help get rid of postoperative gas pain and discomfort. Sometimes I see my GBP patients walking at a pretty good clip! (Check with your doctor before starting to exercise, including walking, after your surgery.)

STAGE 2: FULL LIQUIDS

These items, as recommended at my current center, might be what you have at home the first week: skim or 1 percent milk, unsweetened soy milk, whey or soy protein supplement, noncaloric and noncarbonated diet beverages, fat-free (or sometimes low-fat is okay) ricotta or cottage cheese, diet or light yogurt, plain fat-free or low-fat Greek yogurt (my favorite yogurt to recommend since it's higher in protein), broth, fat-free cream soups, decaffeinated tea or coffee, etc. I generally recommend no more than 15 grams of sugars per serving of any item to decrease the risk of dumping syndrome (for gastric bypass patients). Even patients who have had other procedures, such as gastric banding, are encouraged not to consume more sugars than this at a sitting in order to lower their overall intake of simple sugars. Of course, fruit and milk have natural simple sugars, but in general, every 4 grams of sugar on a food label is roughly equivalent to one teaspoon of table sugar.

Note that this is commonly where some centers differ in their postop GBP surgery diet. Some centers have you eat all pureed foods for weeks after your weight-loss surgery to minimize the risks of solid food getting stuck in the new passageway from your new stomach into the middle part of your small intestine. Always follow the advice of your surgery center doctor and/or dietitian regarding when and how to advance your diet.

Our patients are encouraged to eat slowly and mindfully and to sip all liquids slowly. In addition to the meals, they are also advised to try to drink at least 3 high-protein drinks per day. If your urine is dark and concentrated, it may be a good indicator that you need to get more fluid in, but remember not to gulp, but rather sip fluids slowly.

In addition, it is highly recommended that our patients keep food diaries, including protein and fluid records, to better ensure they are meeting their nutritional goals. My patients bring their food diaries with them to visits with me, and it's very helpful to see how they're doing. Your dietitian may also recommend that you bring logs into the center for your nutrition appointments.

Diarrhea and/or stomach cramps during this stage may stem from lactose-intolerance, so lactase pills can come in very handy (or you could switch to lactose-free products). Some of my patients switch to soy products.

STAGE 3: PUREE

An American dietitian survey revealed that there's a wide variety of ways in which centers advance the diet after bariatric surgery. Pureed texture, at least in my practice, involves putting all food, including meat, chicken, and turkey, through a blender. Alternatives include mashed tofu or pureed beans, eggs, and low-fat cheeses. These are advised from weeks 2 to 4 at my current center, but some centers may start earlier or later, or may forego purees and advance to soft and/or minced texture. Keep in mind, there's no "correct" way to do it, but follow your center's advice. I often advise my patients to put their pureed protein in an ice cube holder. Each cube is equivalent to about 1 ounce, which is about 7 grams of protein. Since it's common for only about 1 ounce of pureed protein to be tolerated at one sitting this soon after surgery, 5 to 6 small meals, and the use of high-quality protein supplements (e.g., whey protein isolate or soy protein isolate), is highly recommended.

While it may be difficult to get to 60 to 80 grams of protein—our goal for patients—by 2 to 4 weeks out, try to get close to 50 or 60 grams if you can for the day, with the help of supplements. Keep in mind that getting adequate fluid (48 to 64 ounces per day, minimum) is absolutely imperative to help lower your risk for dehydration, decrease your risk for constipation, and help your body work better overall.

STAGE 4: MECHANICAL SOFT

Usually about 4 to 6 weeks postop, patients begin on soft, "mushy," or minced foods. Since these could be interpreted very differently among patients, it's important to clearly review your choices with your doctor or dietitian prior to advancing to this stage. This diet stage consists of 3 to 6 meals per day of high-protein ground or soft foods, or slow cooker consistency. A serving may be as small as 1 ounce of ground beef or chicken.

Acceptable foods for most of my patients involve lean (93 percent lean or leaner) ground beef (yes, you can have a hamburger!), lean ground chicken, lean ground turkey, or soft, low-fat fish. Some of my patients try pureed meat first, but for my patients, ground meat is just fine. Veggie burgers are a great alternative.

If ground white meat chicken or turkey is too dry for you, try the dark meat instead. Because it's moister than the white meat, it may go down better, but please remove the skin first because the high fat content and texture may not be too well tolerated.

If you prefer fattier fish, such as salmon, to lower-fat fish, such as scrod or haddock, start with a smaller portion, such as 1 to 2 ounces. Although fattier fish is very healthy, the higher fat content may cause it to take a little longer to empty from your new stomach pouch than other foods. Because your stomach is about the size of an egg at this stage postop GBP surgery, you may find that even 2 ounces of salmon (less than a deck of playing cards) causes you to feel a little heavy, and it may even cause diarrhea for some individuals. This is an excellent example of why it's always a good idea to start slowly when you're first adding foods to your diet, especially if they're a little higher in fat.

Steak and chicken are the toughest foods to tolerate on this stage, since the fibers are tough. I discourage my patients from eating dry, tough foods such as barbecued or grilled chicken or steak, particularly right after gastric bypass surgery, because they will make you thirsty, and patients aren't supposed to drink fluids with meals—or even 30 minutes before or 30 minutes after meals. Therefore, tough, dried-out steak or chicken has a much higher chance of causing chest pain or pressure, and it can cause you to vomit, because of its low moisture content and tough fibers. If you have a hankering for a piece of steak or chicken, you may find that canned chicken or a lean, ground hamburger fit the bill just fine.

Low-fat cheeses (less than 5 grams of fat per ounce), whole eggs, beans, low-fat chili, and tofu are all allowed at this stage. (Please be sure to eat only one new food at a time, and consult with your dietitian if you're having any dietary issues, such as food intolerance.)

Whatever you eat at this stage, make sure the food is a liquid consistency in your mouth before you swallow. Take pencil-eraser-size bites, and you may need to chew each bite up to 25 times. Eat very slowly, allowing about 30–45 minutes per meal. If you find that you don't have this time to devote to some of your meals—for example if you returned to work and have a short lunch break—you can always refer back to previous stage meals, such as stage 2 and the high-protein, low-sugar drinks. I tell my patients they could have these shakes at breakfast and lunch, and then allow increased time for a varied meal in the comfort of their home, when they can really take their time and experiment with different foods (one new food only at a time) within their allowed stage.

Around 1 to 2 weeks after your surgery, if not sooner, your center will suggest you start your multivitamins, calcium, and other vitamin/mineral supplements. Due to postoperative swelling and the risk of pills getting stuck, the first 4 weeks after surgery you'll typically be given vitamins that are sublingual (under the tongue), such as vitamin B_{12} (if applicable), or that come in a chewable, liquid, or powder form. There is also a suggestion in the medical community that solid multivitamins and calcium tablets may not be as well absorbed, especially with gastric bypass surgery or duodenal switch procedure, where there is a malabsorptive component. Although more research is needed in this area, I don't recommend solid multivitamin tablets or calcium pills after any weight-loss surgery, including the gastric band.

Also at this time, we recommend our patients begin taking calcium supplements, 600 milligrams 2 or 3 times per day. But because our bodies can only absorb 600 milligrams of calcium at one time, you need to space your calcium tablets at least a few hours apart. Also, don't take calcium at the same time as your multivitamin because the iron in the multivitamin may decrease the absorption of the calcium. There are several types of calcium supplements, including calcium citrate and calcium carbonate. Calcium citrate is far preferable to calcium carbonate because calcium carbonate requires stomach acid for your body to absorb it. Since you don't have much acid left in your pouch after GBP surgery, you may not have very good absorption of the calcium carbonate.

For the first 6 months following gastric bypass surgery, our patients are on antacid therapy. This helps prevent ulcers and other problems. If you still have your gallbladder after your weight-loss surgery, many centers will recommend you take a specific medication (e.g., ursodiol) to help decrease the risk of gallstones. It's important to tell your surgical team if you have any onset of sudden pain, including to your right rib area, since it may be a sign of gallstone problems.

Here's a sample day in the later stages of the postop gastric bypass surgery diet, 6 weeks or more after surgery:

BREAKFAST

1 whole egg, preferably using a cooking spray rather than oil, butter, or margarine to keep the fat in the diet low and help improve tolerance in the early days after your gastric bypass surgery.

LUNCH

1 to 3 ounces of fish. Fish, in general, is nice and soft and high in protein, so it's generally better-tolerated than steak or a tough, grilled piece of chicken. Seafood—such as shrimp, lobster, and scallops—may be well-tolerated if moist (add lemon and lime instead of high-calorie butter) and chewed well. Shellfish, such as clams and mussels, are a bit "slimy" going down and hard to cut into pencil-eraser-sized bites, so they may not be the best choice in the early postop period, but everyone is different. I recommend people stay away from raw fish for the first month or so after surgery, just in case it's tainted. Chopsticks are a great way to help make sure you're eating slowly and mindfully.

SNACK

Low-fat, low-sugar yogurt.

DINNER

Small to medium bowl of low-fat chili or lentil soup. It's a good source of fiber; just check with your surgery center because some centers may have you puree beans, etc., for several weeks after your surgery.

SNACK

8-ounce glass of nonfat or 1% milk or a high-protein, low-sugar, low-fat liquid shake. It's a great source of calcium as well.

Keep in mind that you have what I describe to my patients as "a baby stomach in training." That is, it's tiny in area, and you may not be able to tolerate foods that never caused you problems before, such as spicy foods and lactose-containing foods and beverages. Your tastes may be very different too, so please allow your new palate to adjust to one new food at a time.

STAGE 5: LOW-FAT, LOW-SUGAR SOLID FOODS

About 5 to 8 weeks after surgery, you will begin stage 5. Congratulations! This is the final stage a healthy, balanced diet of low-fat, low-sugar solid foods. Dietary goals include 64 ounces or more of fluids per day and 60 to 80 grams of protein per day. It includes fruits, vegetables, and starches, but we urge our patients to always avoid commonly ill-tolerated foods, such as doughy breads, rolls, pasta, rice, and skins, such as potato skins, apple skins, and cucumber skins.

It's very important to continue to eat slowly and mindfully. Also continue to avoid drinking fluids with meals, as well as 30 minutes before and after meals. Please make sure you add only one new food at a time to better ensure you can tolerate it. When in doubt, try only a small amount. Continue keeping your food diaries.

At stage 5, the foods that many of my patients report as problems include red meat, doughy breads, pasta, rice, tomato sauce, dry or tough chicken or turkey, and raw fruits and vegetables (the skins in particular). Easier foods to digest and tolerate in the beginning of this stage include toast, cereal, crackers, pita bread, and well-cooked vegetables and fruits.

If you're a vegetarian, especially if you're vegan (no eggs, dairy products—only vegetable proteins), check with your dietitian to better ensure you're meeting your protein needs with your vegetable sources, such as tofu, beans, and veggie burgers. But if you have a problem with excessive gas from eating beans and lentils, you can buy pills that contain natural enzymes to help you digest beans and lentils. Also, mashing the beans well may better ensure tolerance. Some commercial bean and chili dishes (especially canned) are high in sugar. Always check labels, including those of beans, to confirm that you're not consuming more than 15 grams of sugar per serving. Other commercial bean and chili dishes are high in fat. Aim for less than about 10 grams of fat per serving, because fats slow down the emptying of your stomach, which is still only the size of an egg.

Incorporating All Food Groups

Here in stage 5, your dietitian can help you incorporate all of the food groups from the food guide pyramid, although the portion sizes will be smaller. The food groups include grains and starches, fruits, vegetables, protein, and dairy. Within these groups, it is important to emphasize high-protein, low-fat, low-sugar foods in order to minimize stomach upset.

Even after advancing to stage 5, the final diet stage, my patients often find it takes a month or two (and in some cases, several months) to expand their diet repertoire to include a wide variety of foods. Over time, you'll be able to tolerate more foods as well as a larger quantity at one time, because it's common for the stomach pouch outlet (new passageway from your new stomach to the middle part of the small intestine) to expand to twice the size it was right after surgery (to the size of two eggs instead of one), even if you're eating slowly and mindfully. That should make it a little easier to get the protein and other nutrients in, including fruits and vegetables, which are often filling because of their higher fiber content. Please don't drink any fluids with meals or within the first 30 minutes or so after eating to help your new pouch hold onto food longer before it empties into the new passageway. If food travels through the new passageway too fast, it could leave you feeling hungry and dissatisfied, which you don't want, because it may cause you to overeat and regain weight. It may take work to remember these tips and remain consistent, but they can help you lose weight and keep it off. I know you can do it!

Gastric Banding Surgery

Congratulations on your gastric banding surgery!

Although the anatomy of your body wasn't changed with this surgery, the silicone band you had placed in your stomach separates your stomach into two chambers, similar to an hourglass. The very small upper chamber is connected by a narrow channel to the much larger lower chamber, which includes most of your stomach's storage capacity. Because of this, food moves through your stomach more slowly.

After your initial surgery, when the surgeon placed the band near the top of your stomach, your body will need time to heal, since it typically swells a little bit during this procedure. This may leave you with little or no appetite at first.

Feeling Hungry

However, after the swelling goes down, you may feel hungry, perhaps much hungrier than you imagined you would even 1 to 2 weeks postop. Don't worry; this is why your surgeon will schedule fills or adjustments, which typically involve injections of a small amount of saline (salt solution) into your abdomen, where your "port" is located. (Your port is the spot where your surgeon or other clinician at your center will inject the salt solution in order to tighten your band and create a more narrow passageway from the top of your stomach, above your band, to the lower larger part of your stomach, below your band. Your port is about the size of a quarter, and it is under your skin, usually in the area above your belly button and just below your rib cage, although centers vary in terms of exactly where they place the port within your abdominal cavity. This is under your skin, so no one will see your port, and many of my patients tell me they can't feel it and/or it doesn't bother them. This should cause more of a bottleneck at the top of your stomach, which should increase your feeling of fullness. After this, the small top part of your stomach will fill up faster and the large bottom part of your stomach will empty slower.

After your surgery, your diet will go through several stages, which I'll discuss in more detail later in this chapter. In order to help your tissues heal after your gastric banding surgery, your postop diet will be high in protein, and primarily liquid. Then, after 2–3 weeks, you should be able to advance to pureed or ground foods. (Check with your center's doctor or nutritionist regarding whether you need pureed texture.)

Changing the Way You Eat

After having gastric banding surgery, you will need to change the way you eat. Although your stomach has not been cut into two parts, the top part of your stomach, above where the band was placed, is going to do the mechanical chewing job that your whole stomach was previously doing. Because your whole stomach is about the size of a football, but the part that's now doing the work is only the size of your thumb, you will need to chew your food much more carefully to decrease the chances that food will get stuck in the narrow hourglass part where your band is sitting. That bottleneck may be as narrow as your little finger. Take pencil-eraser-size bites of food and chew each bite 15 to 25 times, until the food is a liquid consistency.

This will help to prevent food from getting "stuck" in the upper part of your stomach, just above your silicone band. If you feel intense chest pressure, pain, or experience persistent vomiting after eating a large piece of food, call your doctor.

Avoid Drinking Fluids with Meals

After your surgery, it's important not to drink fluids with meals, as well as 30 minutes after meals. Drinking fluids during and right after a meal flushes the food through the band, or backfires, and causes regurgitation. As you graduate from liquids to ground foods to soft solids, it is very important to limit the amount of high-calorie liquids that you drink. For example, juices and soda are discouraged. Your gastric band is designed to limit the solid foods you eat rather than liquids. That means, unfortunately, that some very weight unfriendly items—such as juice, soda, milkshakes, and even ice cream—tend to go down easily, which is not a good thing for weight loss. Specifically, try to avoid soda, even diet, because it tends to cause quite a bit of gas and bloating, and drinking it may prevent you from reaching your fluid and protein goals.

Eat Slowly

Eat very slowly. It's recommended that you allow about 5 to 10 minutes for each ounce of food that you eat. (An ounce of chicken is about one-third the size of a standard deck of playing cards or a computer mouse.) That translates into about 15 to 30 minutes for a 3-ounce portion of fish, for example. It's key that you put down your eating utensil between bites. Eating slowly and mindfully may help you to better tolerate your diet and lower the risk of food getting stuck because you didn't chew thoroughly enough. Don't force yourself to finish your food within a specific time or to ingest a particular amount of food in at one sitting. You're much better off stopping your meal as soon as you feel chest fullness or pressure than continuing to eat and vomiting.

Introducing New Foods

When advancing through the dietary stages, it is important to try only one new food at a time. This way, if you don't tolerate a particular food, you'll be able to ascertain which one didn't sit well with you. Also, I always tell my patients "when in doubt, only try a small amount." That is, if you're trying a food for the first time, go with a tiny amount, like you would give a baby just starting table foods. Also, even though your stomach wasn't cut into with the gastric band, you may find that your tastes have changed and that foods you could always tolerate before are not tolerated or liked now.

Other Important Considerations

To help your body heal, it is vital that you eat a minimum of 3 protein meals per day. You may find that your new pouch may only hold only a small amount, especially after a fill or adjustment by your surgeon. Therefore, you may prefer 4 to 6 small, high-protein meals, such as light yogurt or an 8-ounce glass of nonfat or 1% milk to help you meet your protein goal. However, I typically discourage "grazing," which involves increased snacking, such as with foods like crackers, nuts, and cookies. These foods tend to go down very well, but are not nutrient-dense, nor are they very weight-friendly.

After having banding surgery, avoid chewing gum altogether. It tends to introduce a lot of air, and it may cause gas and discomfort, especially if you select one with sugar alcohols, such as sorbitol.

As you know, the band is a tool for weight loss, but is not magic that will do the work for you. You're still responsible for making healthy food choices, but the portions will be controlled by the band. Regular visits with your doctor after your band is placed can help you to achieve the optimal level of fullness with the band and better allow you to be successful in meeting your long-term weight loss goals.

Your Diet Following Gastric Banding Surgery

The diet after gastric banding surgery may vary quite a bit among surgical centers. These instructions are only suggestions. Please check with your center's dietitian for your personal meal plan and pre- and postoperative nutritional instructions. to avoid gulping. We urge them to stop if they feel full or nauseated. (Note that some surgeons don't allow their patients to even drink until the day after surgery.)

STAGE 1

DIET: Clear liquids

DIETARY GOALS: Progression of the diet after gastric banding is similar to that of gastric bypass surgery at my center, except that the initial fluid goal the first day after the procedure is 2 ounces, or 2 medicine cups, per hour versus 1 ounce per hour for GBP patients. Most patients go home the next day on the minimum goal of 4 to 8 ounces per hour to reach the fluid goal of 48 to 64 ounces of fluid per day (more if urine isn't light or clear).

INSTRUCTIONS: This stage also begins in the hospital on the day of surgery, and it lasts until patients are discharged from the hospital, about a day or two. Patients are given sugar-free clear liquids to drink, such as beef, chicken, or vegetable broth.

Although sugars do not cause dumping among gastric banding patients like they do for gastric bypass patients, diet beverages are recommended to keep simple calories and sugars low. Some centers give their patients gelatin at this stage, but others have their patients avoid it because of its consistency. Some surgeons report patients getting dysphagia (difficulty swallowing) or even vomiting from gelatin. Check with your surgical center regarding whether it allows gelatin at this stage.

STAGE 2

DIET: Full liquids

DIETARY GOALS: Drink at least 64 ounces of fluid per day and eat a minimum of 50 to 60 grams of protein per day.

INSTRUCTIONS: This stage usually begins on the second day after surgery. It lasts for about 1 week. Note that some surgical centers have their gastric banding patients stay on liquids for 2 weeks, and others have them stay on liquids for 4 weeks after their band is placed. Please check with your center regarding your specific dietary recommendations after your banding surgery.

This stage may include high-protein, low-sugar drinks (the low sugar is for keeping empty calories low); low-fat cottage cheese; fat-free cottage cheese; egg whites; whole eggs (if desired); sugar-free, fat-free pudding; low-fat cream soups; and low-fat, low-sugar yogurt.

The most important thing at this stage, even more than getting enough protein, is getting enough fluid into your body, because dehydration is common right after surgery. This may stem from the decreased amount of time in your day for drinking because you are discouraged from drinking with meals, or 30 minutes after meals.

Sip fluids slowly over a 45- to 60-minute period (as if you are drinking hot tea). Don't gulp them. If you're drinking your goal of 64 ounces of fluid per day but find you have a very dry mouth, your urine is dark, and/or you're feeling dizzy when you stand up, you may need to increase your fluid intake further.

In order to meet your fluid goals and also your protein goals, try to drink at least 1 high-protein drink per day. These high-protein drinks are a meal, not a snack, and they could be used up to three times a day to replace a meal.

Foods with protein, such as low-fat cottage cheese or eggs, may help you feel more satisfied than carbohydrate-rich foods, such as crackers, which are not allowed during this stage anyway.

STAGE 3

DIET: Puree

INSTRUCTIONS: Please follow the pureed texture guidelines provided under the gastric bypass surgery section (page 30), if your center utilizes this stage. Some centers forego this stage and advance to soft solids and/or minced foods at this point.

STAGE 4

DIET: Soft and moist diced foods

DIETARY GOALS: Drink at least 64 ounces of fluid per day and get a minimum of 50 to 60 grams of protein per day.

INSTRUCTIONS: Most patients begin stage 4 between 4 to 6 weeks after the gastric band is placed. It usually lasts for 3 to 4 weeks. This stage includes very soft and moist high-protein foods, such as lean ground hamburger, lean ground chicken and turkey, veggie burgers, low-fat cheeses (less than 5 grams per ounce), low-fat chili, fish, and lentils.

Some people may find they still can't tolerate lean ground hamburger, even with low-fat gravy, so they may need pureed meat or chicken. In fact, many band surgeons around the country who do large numbers of gastric banding surgeries keep their patients on liquids for two weeks, then purees for two weeks, and then solids by week five. Check with your surgical center regarding its specific guidelines for advancing your diet after your banding surgery.

However, the vast majority of my patients are able to tolerate ground or very soft foods included in this stage, especially if they add moisture (such as lemon to fish or low-fat gravy to chicken). The big problem foods for many people after banding surgery are steak and chicken, along with doughy breads, rice, and pasta.

My patients typically are started on chewable multivitamins/minerals and chewable calcium with vitamin D by postop week one.

When in stage 4, ensure that you try only one new food at a time. Also, when in doubt, try only a small amount. This will help you to tolerate the diet and decrease your risk for vomiting, which is never a good thing. Persistent vomiting is never normal and should necessitate a visit with your surgeon for assessment.

Continue to eat slowly, take pencil-eraser-size bites, and chew your food thoroughly. Remember to chew all foods to a liquid consistency and stop eating when you feel full. Mindful eating includes not only eating slowly but also removing distractions during a meal, such as the television or computer. It may take quite a bit of getting used to, but you may find a new-found pleasure in really savoring your meals, and your dining companions may learn how to eat mindfully as well, which is certainly a bonus!

Employing moist cooking methods, such as baking, roasting, steaming, or poaching is preferable to grilling or barbecuing foods. Since fluids are not permitted with meals, or 30 minutes after meals, consuming dry, tough foods, such as grilled steak, may increase your risk of the food getting "stuck" in your chest area and/or may greatly increase the chance you will vomit, which is unpleasant and potentially dangerous.

Foods that are not very well-tolerated in stage 4 include red meat, pasta, doughy breads, rice, dry or tough chicken or turkey, skins of certain vegetables and fruits such as potatoes and apples, and the membranes of citrus fruits.

STAGE 5

DIET: A healthy diet of low-fat, low-sugar solid foods

DIETARY GOALS: Drink at least 64 ounces of fluid per day and get approximately 60 to 80 grams of protein daily.

INSTRUCTIONS: Usually about 5 to 6 weeks after gastric banding surgery, you may be advanced to the fifth and final stage of the postop gastric banding diet: a solid, low-fat, low-sugar healthy diet. This is the final stage! It includes fruits, vegetables, and starches, as well as protein foods and dairy, and it is considered an overall healthy diet.

Please remember to add only one new food at a time. Certain foods you ate your whole life may not go down well now, such as grilled beef. Keeping an accurate food diary may help you to better ascertain which foods are well-tolerated, and which foods may just not be right for you. You can try offending foods again later, but there may be some foods that may just not sit right in your body after your gastric banding surgery. That may be true for a few weeks, or perhaps that food may never settle right in your stomach after your surgery. Because there are so many potential foods you may be able to tolerate well, stick to those rather than continually getting ill by trying to force your body to tolerate a food that just doesn't go down or settle well.

Although banding patients don't experience the dumping syndrome from sugars typically seen with gastric bypass patients, it's important to select lower calorie alternatives for weight loss.

As you go through stage 5, always eat and drink mindfully, chewing foods to a liquid consistency. Continue avoiding fluids with meals and 30 minutes after meals.

Chewable multivitamin/mineral and calcium supplements with vitamin D are continued daily.

It's always a good idea to keep in close contact with your surgical center, especially after surgery, in order to make certain that you're meeting your nutritional needs, and that everything is going well overall after your gastric banding surgery. Please ensure that you keep all of your appointments with your clinicians, including those with your surgeon for a potential fill or adjustment. Our gastric banding patients are often asked to see their surgeon or nurse practitioner once a month for the first year postop, to confirm that they are doing well, and to evaluate whether they need a fill or adjustment to increase their restriction (increased level of fullness while eating). Our patients typically receive an adjustment to their band if they are feeling continuously hungry, and/or weight loss has stopped or slowed dramatically (or weight has gone up).

Vertical Sleeve Gastrectomy

Congratulations on your vertical sleeve gastrectomy (VSG)! During this procedure, commonly called "the sleeve," the surgeon cuts and discards the majority of your stomach (primarily the outer part known as the "greater curve", including the upper right part, called the fundus. The fundus is the site of 90 percent of your body's production of ghrelin, the chief hunger hormone. As a result, as well as what's believed to be the release of weight friendly hormones, like PYY and GLP-1 (abbreviated here), this surgery often will alleviate hunger for about 3 to 6 months, called "the honeymoon period."

VSG is a procedure that's really growing in popularity, and the results thus far—in terms of 5-year U.S. data on weight loss and remission of some diseases—are very promising. But some barriers still exist, including the fact that, as I write this revision, some insurance companies do not cover this procedure; more and more companies, however, are covering it.

The sleeve may be done as the first of two procedures. That is, if you have a higher weight or medical complications (or both), your surgeon may suggest you have the sleeve first, and then possibly have, for example, gastric bypass surgery 9 to 12 months later, when, hopefully, you've lost a good amount of weight and your liver is also most likely smaller to help with surgery. (If you have weight challenges, you may have an enlarged or fatty liver, which is the major obstacle for the surgeon getting underneath it to your stomach.) If you have a good deal more weight to lose, the less commonly performed biliopancreatic diversion with a duodenal switch, or "the switch," may be done as the secondary procedure, but there aren't a great number of surgeons who do it. (See the next section for more information on this procedure.)

Advantages to the sleeve include pretty good weight loss. Five-year U.S. data cites 40 to 60 percent excess body weight lost, or about 40 to 60 pounds lost for every extra 100 pounds of weight. I use a body mass index (BMI) of 25 as the point of "no excess weight" to do this calculation. For example, if you're 5'7" and weigh 360 pounds, you're roughly 200 pounds overweight, since a BMI of 25 for this height is 160 pounds. Therefore, average weight loss at the lowest weight after the sleeve would be about 80 to 120 pounds. Of course, there are "intangibles" involved, such as your age (younger often means faster metabolism), sex (men lose more weight, on average, than women do), ability or willingness to exercise, height (taller is better for weight loss), diet (at least 3 meals a day with protein, no more than 5 hours apart), proper sleep (at least 7 hours of uninterrupted sleep per night), and good stress management. I've had some patients, male and female alike, who have lost 60 to 70 percent of their excess weight (which is more along the lines of gastric bypass surgery weight-loss expectations) after the sleeve and didn't need a second procedure. Others have failed to lose the average, perhaps for strong genetic reasons or an inability to exercise.

I've read quite a few research reports that cite the sleeve helping with diabetes and other diseases, despite the fact that the only anatomical change is making the stomach banana size rather than football size. This may be due to suspected complex changes in hormones that help the body want to "settle in" at a lower set point. Although the sleeve is believed to do this to a lesser extent than gastric bypass surgery, it may be an excellent "middle of the road" procedure for some people with moderate weight issues.

Vitamin and Mineral Absorption

Since there is much less stomach area after the sleeve, certain vitamins and minerals may not be absorbed as well, despite the fact that your surgeon has not touched your small intestines, as he or she would with gastric bypass surgery. Iron needs acid to be absorbed well, so we carefully check iron levels after the sleeve and recommend at least 100 percent of the daily value for iron, or 18 milligrams of elemental iron per day (more if women have heavy menstrual periods or if iron deficiency is present before surgery). Vitamin B12 requires a certain amount of acid to tear itself apart from the protein in the food its bound to, so we also recommend additional vitamin B_{12} supplements after the sleeve (e.g., 500 micrograms sublingual [under the tongue] daily, or a 1000-microgram shot once a month, perhaps from your primary care doctor). There's still much research that needs to be done with this surgery, but those who've had the sleeve should be taking a high-quality multivitamin (ideally, chewable, liquid, or powder) with iron, along with vitamin B_{12} and 500 to 600 milligrams (3 times daily) of calcium (as calcium citrate only, since calcium carbonate requires acid for absorption). As with all other procedures, iron and calcium should never be taken at the same time, since they compete for the same receptor sites, so at least 2 hours in between each is strongly recommended.

Diet Advancement after the Sleeve

The advancement of the diet, once again, may vary among surgical centers. At my current hospital, we advance the diet essentially the same as we would for someone who had gastric banding (see page 35), although VSG patients are typically in the hospital an extra day, so they would have one more day of clear liquids than banding patients do.

Biliopancreatic Diversion, with or without a Duodenal Switch

Congratulations on your biliopancreatic diversion (BPD), with or without a duodenal switch surgery!

The BPD surgery has two components. The first part of this procedure is a limited gastrectomy—partial removal of up to two-thirds the stomach. This makes people eat less, so they lose weight, especially in the first year after the surgery. The second part of this procedure involves construction of a long limb Roux-en-Y anastamosis. This is a connection that in some cases is similar to that seen in gastric bypass surgery, where the new stomach is connected to the small intestine at a lower level, but has a short common alimentary channel (the part where food travels through) of 50 centimeters in length.

This part of the procedure causes food to pass straight through the body, and not be absorbed by the body, which is key to maintaining long-term weight loss.

Sometimes the BDP surgery is done with a duodenal switch (D/S). In this procedure, the pylorus, the common alimentary channel, is 75 to 100 centimeters. This is probably more information than you need to know, but the BPD with the duodenal switch may help improve tolerance to the diet after your surgery, compared to the classic BPD surgery.

Vitamin and Mineral Absorption

The most serious nutritional risk of BPD surgery is malabsorption of protein, vitamins, and minerals. To combat this, people who have undergone BPD surgery need to take extra calcium and vitamins—especially fat-soluble vitamins A, D, E, and K—for the rest of their lives. Vitamin A deficiency causes night blindness. Vitamin D deficiency causes hyperparathyroidism, which leads to premature osteoporosis. Iron deficiency is sometimes seen, which leads to anemia. Other malabsorption problems are linked to low protein (hypoalbuminemia), edema (fluid build-up), and alopecia (hair loss). In light of possibly serious nutritional complications, individuals who have undergone this procedure need to ensure they follow up with their surgical centers for the rest of their lives.

One of the benefits of this surgery is that 75 percent of the fat you eat is discharged through bowel movements as waste. However, about 50 percent of protein is also discharged, which supports the need for at least 80 grams of protein per day. High-protein foods, such as fish, eggs, soft chicken or turkey, and tofu are possible sources in the diet to help meet your higher protein needs. (Please see the sample menu for "later stages" under the gastric bypass diet guideline in this book for a visual of a potential daily menu suggestion for you to follow after this surgery.)

Mealtime Considerations

It is important not to drink liquids with your meals, or approximately 30 minutes after your meals, because it may not only decrease nutrient absorption, but may also keep you from meeting your protein needs, which are higher than those for gastric banding and gastric bypass surgery. Because your stomach may only hold a maximum of 4 to 6 ounces after your BPD surgery, you may feel full after eating only a few tablespoons of food. Even if you're eating slowly and mindfully (pencil-eraser-size bites, chewing 15 times before swallowing, etc.), your stomach typically stretches over time. However, it may take several months, even up to one year, for your new stomach to stabilize and for you to figure out how much food your body can handle at one sitting.

As with the other weight-loss surgeries, it's important to eat slowly and mindfully. Mindful eating is extremely important, not only for long-term weight loss, but to help decrease the risk of stretching your new stomach, as well as worsening potential issues related to loose stools and gas. Keeping the picture (or actual model!) of a pencil eraser while you're eating your meals should help remind you of the ideal bite size. Also, you should chew each bite at least 15 times, until the food is a liquid consistency.

Because there is more intestinal bypassing in this surgery (more than gastric bypass surgery, for example), you may want to limit high-fat foods, such as fried foods and fatty meats, because they may greatly increase your risk for diarrhea, gas, and a "blah" feeling because fats really delay the emptying of your stomach. Also, the BPD surgery already increases your chances of having frequent loose stools and gas, and high-fat foods will just magnify these issues.

However, some people who have had BPD surgery lose more weight when eating certain higher fat foods (preferably healthy foods, like salmon and other fatty fish) because it fills them up quickly, but only about 25 percent gets absorbed. Conversely, if they eat foods low in fat, and high in carbs, they may gain weight. This weight gain may happen because the overall transit time is much faster with fats among people who have had this surgery.

BPD surgery affects absorption of not only vitamins, but also medications. Many people may not realize the possible issues seen with malabsorption in this surgery, such as excessive loose stools, which may cause issues with low potassium, for example, and can be potentially dangerous because your heart needs a normal potassium level to beat properly. Also, malabsorption after BPD surgery may result in hair loss, skin dryness, and dry and brittle nails. It's important to take all of the vitamins and other supplements, such as calcium with vitamin D, exactly as your surgical center recommends to help lower your risks for nutritional deficiencies.

The Importance of Protein

After your surgery, you will have a goal of how much protein to eat each day. Protein is essential for preserving lean or muscle mass, and it is vital for wound healing, so it's imperative right after surgery that you try to get in at least 60 to 70 grams of protein within the first few weeks of your surgery. Ideally, you'll be able to reach the 100-gram protein mark (about 15 ounces total of chicken, fish, etc.) within a few months of your procedure.

To help guarantee that you meet your protein needs, you should try to include protein in every meal and snack. The latter should not include things like crackers, chips, and other high-carbohydrate foods that may be very well-tolerated but could fill you up, possibly keeping you from getting enough protein, and potentially resulting in weight gain down the road (if you "graze" or eat these snack foods continuously throughout the day). Snacks that I recommend, within the proper diet stage, include low-fat cheeses (less than 3 grams of fat per ounce, ideally); low-fat, low-sugar yogurts; low-fat cottage cheese; fat-free ricotta cheese; and egg whites. People who have undergone the BPD procedure may need as much as 120 grams (about 16 ounces) of protein a day, which is the equivalent of six decks of cards worth of chicken! That's a lot of chicken (or equivalent) in one day, especially if you're not feeling at all hungry after your surgery. Therefore, I often encourage my BPD patients to consume up to six small, high-protein meals per day (such as 2 ounces chicken at lunch, ½ cup low-fat cottage cheese in between lunch and dinner, 2 ounces of fish at dinner, ½ cup fat-free ricotta cheese at night, etc.).

If adequate protein intake is still a struggle several weeks after surgery, I often recommend a very high-protein, no-carbohydrate, fat-free drink, found in most health food stores. These drinks contain about 40 grams of protein (soy or whey are good quality protein sources to look for) per 20 ounces of liquid supplement, so I recommend splitting it into 8- or 10-ounce glasses, up to 4 times per day (total of 80 grams of protein for 40 ounces) as needed to help meet protein needs while solid high-protein food intake is suboptimal. I don't advise drinking more than 30 grams of protein at one time because protein requires water to flush out the breakdown products, and therefore can be dehydrating, as well as potentially taxing to your kidneys.

Decreased Appetite

A decreased appetite is quite common after BPD, and it is thought to be related to minimization of hunger hormones after this surgery. It's sometimes called the "honeymoon period," and it can last more than a year postoperatively. Believe it or not, you may need to constantly remind yourself to eat for some time after your surgery. This may sound ideal before surgery, but in reality can sometimes feel like a part-time job, at least per some of my BPD patients' comments.

As with the other weight-loss surgeries, it is really important to introduce only one new food at a time. This way, if you feel sick or vomit after you eat it, you'll have a better idea of what the offending food or beverage was.

Avoid Concentrated Sugars

Concentrated sugars, like table sugar (sucrose), should be avoided after BPD without the duodenal switch. Done more frequently outside the United States, especially in Europe, in this procedure the surgeon removes the lower part of the stomach, including the lower part going into the small intestine, called the pylorus. Since the pylorus is removed, patients who have this procedure have the potential for dumping syndrome, as with gastric bypass surgery. In contrast, BPD with D/S involves the removal of the outer right part of the stomach, including the fundus, where 90 percent of ghrelin, the body's chief hunger hormone, is made. It is rather involved, but think "banana stomach," like that of the sleeve procedure, so dumping syndrome is not an issue for D/S patients. Carbohydrates are, however, the Achilles heel of this procedure, since fat is vastly malabsorbed, as is protein, to a lesser extent; yet carbohydrates are well absorbed. Thus, some patients who are "carbohydrate addicts" may find it more difficult to lose the estimated excess body weight of 80 to 90 percent with this procedure (or about 80 to 90 pounds lost for every 100 pounds of excess weight, using a body mass index of 25 as the cutoff for no extra weight).

Regardless of whether you had the BPD or new D/S procedure, simple carbohydrates are discouraged overall. It's best to just say no to sweets to not only feel better overall, but to also aid in long-term weight loss success.

Lactose Intolerance

Milk and milk products can also be a problem. If you find you have more gas, abdominal bloating, or diarrhea after eating or drinking milk products, lactose intolerance may be an issue. You can purchase pills, and in some cases drops, which contain the enzyme lactase, which breaks down the milk sugar, lactose, avoiding the symptoms of lactose intolerance. Please keep in mind that even if you purchase low-fat or nonfat milk that has been treated with this lactase enzyme, if you add a protein powder with lactose in it, you will probably feel the symptoms of lactose intolerance, because the enzyme-treated milk will not break down the lactose in the protein powder. However, taking the lactase enzyme pill, or adding the lactase drops, will resolve the problem.

Additional Considerations

A potential problem after BPD surgery is bacterial overgrowth. So if you have had BPD surgery and you have a terrible cramping pain and bloating after eating, you may need to see your surgeon for antibiotics. Probiotics may also be helpful with bacterial overgrowth, so ask your surgical team about this. With this kind of malabsorptive surgery, the bacteria in your large intestine can really change to incorporate more "bad bacteria," which may be a culprit in gas, bloating, and diarrhea. Probiotics may help with constipation issues, as well as loose stools. Anecdotally, I have at least a few D/S patients who have gone from loose stools to formed stools within days of starting probiotics. But be sure to ask your doctor or surgical team if this is appropriate in your particular situation.

Avoid carbonated beverages. They tend to cause a great deal of gas and abdominal distention or discomfort, which could already be an issue after BPD surgery. In addition, carbonated beverages, such as diet soda, could cause you to feel very full and decrease your chances of getting in enough protein during the day.

Your Diet after BPD Surgery

As with the gastric bypass sleeve, and gastric banding surgeries, the diet immediately after BPD surgery may vary quite a bit among surgical centers throughout the world.

Although people who have had this procedure have a larger workable stomach for digestion than gastric bypass (GBP) patients, I often find that my D/S patients do very well following the dietary guidelines we suggest for GBP, with the exception that I recommend at least 30 more grams protein per day (compared with gastric bypass patients) and additional fat-soluble (A, D, E, K) vitamins and calcium because of the significant malabsorptive nature of this surgery.

Some centers have designed postoperative D/S diets that allow patients to immediately try such foods as unsweetened applesauce, meat loaf, ripe bananas, oatmeal, crackers, and well-cooked vegetables. Crackers are typically very popular and well-tolerated at any diet stage, but please be careful not to eat them on a regular basis, because even just a few may fill you up in the beginning, and could potentially prevent you from meeting your protein needs. You may find these foods are well-tolerated, even during your first weeks after your BPD procedure.

Everyone is different, but I tend to suggest a postoperative D/S diet inline with the GBP diet. (Please see those postop nutrition guidelines and stages beginning on page 22.)

Congratulations, once again, on your weight-loss surgery and your new life! We're absolutely thrilled you've included us in your journey toward nourishing the new you.

In the next section, we'll answer common questions that patients have about cooking with artificial sweeteners and protein powders. After that, we'll describe some useful time-saving and stress-reducing tips for stocking your kitchen, and then finally we'll dive right in to our nutrious and tasty recipes.

Artificial Sweeteners: How Sweet They Are

Artificial sweeteners, also known as sugar substitutes, are designed to replace table sugar (or sucrose) in order to sweeten foods and beverages. You need to use less sugar substitute than sugar because artificial sweeteners are many times sweeter than table sugar. These sweeteners are regulated by the U.S. Food and Drug Administration (FDA).

Here are the most common artificial sweeteners found on the market and some general information regarding their uses:

SPLENDA (SUCRALOSE)

This artificial sweetener was approved by the FDA as a tabletop sweetener in 1998, and then as a general-purpose sweetener in 1999. Splenda is often regarded as "natural" because it's made from real sugar, although it's chemically combined with chlorine, a process most would consider unnatural. Splenda is 600 times sweeter than table sugar. It may be of benefit for people with diabetes, because it has been deemed to have no effect on carbohydrate metabolism, short- or long-term blood sugar control, or insulin secretion.

Splenda is considered to be very stable, so it's a popular ingredient in almost every type of food and beverage, including diet sodas, juice drinks, and teas. However, the biggest selling point is the ability to bake with Splenda, which isn't possible with most of the other artificial sweeteners.

EQUAL AND NUTRASWEET (ASPARTAME)

Aspartame, distributed under the trade names Equal and Nutrasweet, was approved in 1981 by the FDA, and it became the artificial sweetener of choice when saccharin decreased in popularity many years ago. It's derived from the amino acids (building blocks of protein) aspartic acid and phenylalanine. People who have a rare genetic disorder called PKU (phenylketonuria) can't break down phenylalanine, so they must totally avoid aspartame. However, it has been deemed safe for people with diabetes, as it seems to produce a very small rise in blood sugar.

This sweetener is 200 times sweeter than table sugar, and it is often used in beverages, ice cream, and puddings. Aspartame's sweetness is enhanced by other flavors and sweeteners, but it loses its sweetness when heated. Therefore, it is not ideal for baking. However, Sugar Lite, a new product that is a combination of table sugar and aspartame, can be used in baking. One teaspoon of this product contains 8 calories, which is half the calories of a teaspoon of pure table sugar.

SWEET'N LOW AND SUGAR TWIN (SACCHARIN)

Saccharin, which is sold as Sweet'N Low and Sugar Twin, is the oldest of the approved artificial sweeteners. In 1977, the FDA tried to ban saccharin based on research indicating it caused cancer in animals. However, it remained on the shelves, but with a warning regarding this finding. In 2000, the National Institutes of Health (NIH) removed saccharin from its list of cancer-causing agents (carcinogens), and the necessity of including the warning label regarding the animal studies was waived. Although saccharin has been cleared by the FDA, it continues to be a bit controversial.

Like other artificial sweeteners, saccharine produces no sugar (or glycemic) response. It is 300 times sweeter than table sugar, and it is used in many products. Sugar Twin, which is a combination of malto-dextrin and sodium saccharin, contains 0 calories per teaspoon, but it measures the same as sugar, cup for cup. However, the label on the box states that Sugar Twin is not appropriate for recipes calling for more than $1/2$ cup of sugar. Therefore, this product is not ideal for baking overall. It may be ideal though, for sweetening coffee or tea.

STEVIA (SWEET LEAF)

This sweetener is considered the ultimate "natural" sweetener, and it has been quite popular lately in the United States. It is extracted from a shrub that grows in South America. Because our bodies can't metabolize sweet leaf or break it down, it does not provide calories.

SUNETTE (ACESULFAME POTASSIUM)

This artificial sweetener was approved by the FDA in 1988. It is 200 times sweeter than table sugar, and it produces no blood sugar response. It is often found in diet sodas, juice drinks, gums, and ice cream. However, it's not available for use in baking or cooking.

SUGAR ALCOHOLS (SORBITOL, MANNITOL)

For many years, people with diabetes have used products with sugar alcohols—such as sorbitol, mannitol, xylitol, and malitol—to sweeten foods without the sugar or glycemic response seen with table sugar. These are natural sweeteners that do not trigger an insulin reaction. Sugar alcohols contain half the calories of sugar, and they are not digested by the small intestine.

It is important to realize that sorbitol, one of the sugar alcohols commonly found on the market, is a natural laxative, and it may cause diarrhea, bloating, and flatulence. I often tell my patients not to try sugar alcohols for the first time while you're on a camping trip, since the potential laxative effect could be quite embarrassing and uncomfortable. However, for people having constipation issues, sugar-alcohol-sweetened products, in moderation, may help alleviate this problem. It is often found in sugar-free candies, as well as some high-protein bars.

Try these Web sites for more information regarding artificial sweeteners:

Splenda: www.splenda.com

Stevia: www.stevia.com

Sweet'N Low: www.sweetnlow.com

Equal: www.equal.com

Sugar Twin: www.sugartwin.com

Saccharin: www.saccharin.org

The following cookbooks feature artificial sweeteners:

Cooking Healthy with Splenda, by JoAnna M. Lund and Barbara Alpert, Perigee Trade Books, 2004.

Graham Kerr's Simply Splenda Cookbook, by Graham Kerr, American Diabetes Association, 2004.

Unbelievable Desserts with Splenda: Sweet Treats Low in Sugar, Fat and Calories, by Marlene Koch, M. Evans & Company, Inc., 2001.

500 Low-Carb Recipes, by Dana Carpender, Fair Winds Press, 2002.

Protein Powders: What's the Scoop?

In this section, we discuss commonly found, high-quality protein powders, starting with the most commonly found and recommended variety, whey protein powder. It's important to check with your medical center's dietitian regarding the protein quality score (Protein Digestibility-Corrected Amino Score, or PDCAAS), which relates to the quality and absorption of the protein powders. I always discourage poor-quality protein, such as collagen (often marketed as "test tubes," "bullets," or "shots"); it's not highly absorbed, even if it's fortified, due to missing amino acids, or building blocks of protein, that our bodies cannot make. Some studies suggest absorption to be anywhere from 15 to 40 percent of the protein those collagen-based and/or "predigested" protein supplements claim you're getting. There are also a number of newer vegetarian protein powder options, including hemp, but their protein absorption may be suboptimal. In general, it's better to stick with whey or soy protein isolate, since they're lactose free and well digested and absorbed. Many of my weight-loss surgery patients ask me about protein powders, and it seems there are new ones cropping up almost daily. How do you know which ones are best? Also, are there any possible things to watch out for with some of the protein powders, such as intolerance issues?

Protein powders can vary greatly in terms of quality, and they may be a mixture of two or more different kinds of proteins. In terms of pure sources of protein, there are four general types: whey, soy, egg, and rice. Let's talk about each in turn.

WHEY PROTEIN

This is taken from milk, and is the most popular type of protein supplement on the market. Because it is a derivative of milk, it contains some lactose, or milk sugar. People who are lactose intolerant shouldn't take whey protein. Also, because gastric bypass and biliopancreatic diversion patients may have lactose intolerance issues after surgery, whey protein can cause a problem. If you have gas, abdominal bloating, cramping, and/or diarrhea every time you take whey protein, you may be lactose intolerant. Try taking the whey protein along with the enzyme lactase, which you can purchase over the counter at any pharmacy and many supermarkets. When taken with whey protein powder, this enzyme should eliminate the problem by breaking down the milk sugar (lactose) to lactic acid, thereby doing away with the symptoms.

Whey protein powders contain both essential amino acids (building blocks of protein the body cannot make) and nonessential amino acids (building blocks of protein that can be made in the body). Whey is easily taken up and used by the muscles in the body, and it is considered very safe to use.

There are two types of whey protein powders: concentrate and isolate. The concentrate form is more common, easier to find, and less expensive. It contains between 30 and 85 percent protein. Whey isolate is a higher quality protein, so it's more expensive than the concentrate. Because whey isolate contains more than 90 percent protein, it's more easily absorbed by the body, and it also contains less fat and lactose (milk sugar).

Benefits of whey protein: Whey protein may help boost immunity. It is an ideal source of amino acids. It also may help prevent muscle breakdown and speed up muscle recovery after exercise.

SOY PROTEIN

Soy protein comes from soy flour, so it is a good protein source for vegans. Soy is the most complete vegetable protein available. Like whey protein powders, soy protein also has two varieties: concentrate and isolate. The isolate is the more expensive form, because it is more pure and has a higher percentage of protein, compared to the concentrate. Soy protein is typically very easy to digest, and it can be considered as high a quality protein as milk and meat. I often recommend soy protein powders to my weight-loss surgery patients who have a milk allergy or lactose intolerance issues.

Benefits of soy protein: Soy protein is ideal for vegans, and it's perfect for people with milk intolerance or allergies. There are studies suggesting moderate soy consumption may help lower cholesterol and possibly reduce the risk of heart disease, although some recent studies seem to be challenging this claim.

EGG PROTEIN

Egg protein powders are made from egg whites, so they are very high in protein and essentially fat-free. Egg protein is considered a perfect protein, with a grade of 100 in terms of biological value. Egg protein is complete in essential amino acids, and it also has other amino acids, such as branched chain amino acids (leucine, isoleucine, and valine) and glutamic acid. The branched chain amino acids and glutamic acid may be especially useful after weight-loss surgery, because they tend to help muscles recover more quickly. However, egg protein powders should not be used by anyone with an egg allergy.

Benefits of egg protein: Egg protein is fat-free, fairly inexpensive, and not an issue for people with milk or lactose intolerance or soy intolerance or sensitivity.

RICE PROTEIN

Rice protein is made by carefully extracting the protein from brown rice. Although rice is often overlooked because of its incomplete amino acids, or building blocks of protein, rice powders are typically supplemented with L-amino acids to make them complete.

Benefits of rice protein: Rice protein is hypoallergenic, so it's ideal for people with soy, milk, or egg allergies or sensitivities. It is also perfect for vegans or strict vegetarians.

Lynette's Tips for Stocking an Efficient Kitchen

I can't count the number of times I've heard people say, "If only I could just make a few things turn out right in the kitchen!" Maybe you've uttered the same words. We are so pleased to present this cookbook to you that will guide you step-by-step through producing these user-friendly and delicious recipes and also help you become aware of some basic and essential culinary rules to live by. From cooking for your family to entertaining, there is something here for everyone. Let's begin with your kitchen. Here are a few good tips to follow to make your culinary adventures easy, fun, and educational.

It's essential to have a few standard pieces of equipment in your kitchen, which will make preparing any meal faster. **A set of good sharp knives** is an absolute must, along with a block to store them in to keep them from becoming dull quickly. A chef's blade (8- to 10-inch, or 20 to 25 cm), a fillet or boning knife, a serrated knife, and a small paring knife will get you through just about any recipe you'll ever prepare.

A pair of ordinary kitchen shears is also a good idea. Shears are wonderful for removing skin and fat from meat and poultry, for trimming vegetables of their stems and other unwanted parts, and for opening stubborn packages.

A set of nonstick pots and pans is a good item to have. Choose one that has thicker-gauged bottoms, which will promote even heat distribution and help to avoid constant scorching. Find the set that looks right for you in your local department store. A 7- or 9-piece set is sufficient to begin with, and then as you become more adventurous, you'll soon learn what additional pieces you wish to add to your collection.

Next, **a set of stainless-steel mixing bowls** can make your kitchen endeavors easier and more efficient. I prefer stainless steel over glass or plastic because it is light-weight but sturdy enough to handle an electric mixer or being dropped without breaking. In addition to being sturdy, stainless steel holds temperatures more efficiently than plastic or glass, neither of which conducts heat or cold. In other words, the item you are mixing in stainless steel will hold its temperature longer rather than rise or fall to room temperature like it will in glass or plastic. Choose a set of mixing bowls ranging in size from 1 to 5 quarts (1 to 5 liters) to meet all of your mixing needs. When mixing anything in your mixing bowls, be sure to leave plenty of room for the product to be sufficiently manipulated. Always use a bowl that is twice the size of the product you are mixing.

A food processor is essential for preparing purees and certain types of sauces. A blender can be used in place of a food processor. However, a blender may not be sufficient for certain applications, such as finely chopping onions and peppers or grinding meat and other products. Since blenders are essentially designed for liquids, gravity plays an important role in their design. A food processor, however, is designed to expose more surface area of the product being processed by the working blade and so that gravity is not such a factor. There are a variety of processors on the market today, and you can buy a decent one at a department store.

It is a good idea to keep **one colander** and **one fine mesh strainer or sieve** in your kitchen. It is important to wash vegetables before preparing them, and these are the tools to use. You will find many other uses for these simple and inexpensive items as well.

Eventually you will learn what works best for your kitchen and your own style as it develops. That's true for kitchen equipment, but also for food. Here are a few of my own essentials items I recommend having on hand at all times.

Ordinary table salt may be easily accessible, although it may not be the best choice for cooking. A **good sea salt** can be found at the grocer, as well as **kosher salt.** A little bit of either of these salts goes a long way.

Fresh cracked or fresh ground pepper can have a great deal more flavor compared to prepackaged ground pepper. Oil in the peppercorn dehydrates at a much faster rate after it is ground, and so the flavor dissipates as well. Truly fresh black pepper will have a fruity aroma and a hearty bite. In addition, I find that it's worth researching where your spices come from. Dried spices and seasonings will lose the intensity of flavor as they age. Quality ingredients, including spices and seasonings, can contribute a world of difference to your recipes.

Lemons are also essential in your kitchen. You will find many recipes in this book that require fresh lemon juice and lemon zest. Zest is the outer portion of the rind that is grated off with a zester or a fine grating surface. The flavor is very intense, and not at all bitter like the inner white portion of the rind. You will also find recipes using fresh lime and orange zest.

There are many **substitutes available for butter,** such as light butters, margarines, and butter alternatives. I recommend reduced-fat and reduced-calorie butter in place of margarine, because of the usually high sodium content in margarine. Some spreads contain olive oil and offer a rich flavor and good heat conduction when using for a sauté. When using a butter alternative or oil to sauté foods, always be sure to thoroughly heat it before adding the ingredients to be sautéed, unless the recipe states otherwise.

Quite a few recipes in the book call for **wine.** If you prefer not to cook using alcohol, any of our recipes calling for the use of wine can be made without compromising flavor or consistency simply by substituting chicken or vegetable broth or water with a bit of lemon juice for the wine.

You'll find that the recipes often offer ranges of time for cooking, such as bake for 20 to 30 minutes, instead of exact numbers. That's because each oven, stovetop, refrigerator, and freezer varies in temperature. Likewise, different pots, pans, and baking dishes will all conduct temperatures to varying degrees, and so it is necessary to make adjustments to cooking time and temperatures as you progress through any recipe.

As you're cooking, to save time and also to stay organized in your kitchen, it's always best to have all of the measured, cut, and prepared ingredients ready to use before you begin the recipe.

Here's an important food safety note. **It's important to keep the work surfaces, such as counter tops and cutting boards, clean and sanitized.** An ordinary kitchen sponge will transfer concentrated amounts of bacteria from every surface it has touched since it was placed into use. One of the best solutions for sanitizing is simply bleach and tap water, in the proportion of one capful of bleach to one gallon of water. If too much bleach is used, the solution will evaporate before it has sufficient time to sanitize. Also, bleach in the solution will evaporate if the temperature of the water is too hot.

Now that you have the basic recommendations for setting up your kitchen, we hope all of your culinary endeavors are delicious, nutritious, exciting, and fun!

CHAPTER 2

Breakfasts and Brunches

All-American Scramble

To save time, prepare the turkey bacon ahead of time per the package instructions. Serve this, or any of the scrambles in this book, with a slice of whole grain toast or English muffin for a complete breakfast. You can leave out the cheese from any of these scrambles.

TEXTURE: Soft

INGREDIENTS

- 1 teaspoon light butter
- 1 slice turkey bacon, crumbled
- $^1/_4$ cup (60 ml) liquid egg substitute
- 1 tablespoon (7 g) reduced-fat shredded Cheddar cheese

In an omelet pan, melt the butter over medium heat, swirling the pan to coat evenly.

Add the turkey bacon and sauté 4 to 5 minutes, until it becomes soft and just begins to brown. Add the egg substitute, stirring gently but constantly with a heat-resistant rubber spatula, scraping the bottom of the pan to keep the eggs moving to avoid browning. When the eggs are almost finished, add the cheese and turn off the heat. Gently fold the cheese into the eggs, turning over with the spatula. When the cheese becomes soft, but not dissolved, turn the scramble onto a plate.

YIELD: Makes 1 serving.

NUTRITIONAL ANALYSIS
Each with: **Calories:** 118.13 **Protein:** 11.03 g **Carbs:** 0.59 g **Total Fat:** 7.89 g **Sat Fat:** 2.09 g **Cholesterol:** 14.38 mg **Sodium:** 379.82 mg **Sugars:** 0.40 g **Fiber:** 0.00 g

Denver Scramble

TEXTURE: Soft

INGREDIENTS

- 1 teaspoon light butter
- 1$\frac{1}{2}$ teaspoons chopped green bell pepper
- 1$\frac{1}{2}$ teaspoons chopped yellow onion
- 1$\frac{1}{2}$ teaspoons chopped tomato
- 1 slice (1 ounce, or 28 g) reduced-sodium, reduced-fat ham, chopped
- $\frac{1}{4}$ cup (60 ml) liquid egg substitute
- 1 tablespoon (7 g) reduced-fat shredded Cheddar cheese

In an omelet pan over medium heat, melt the butter, swirling the pan to coat evenly.

Add the pepper, onion, and tomato and cook 4 to 5 minutes, until they become soft. Add the ham and continue cooking, until heated through. Add the egg substitute, stirring gently but constantly with a heat-resistant rubber spatula, scraping the bottom of the pan to keep the eggs moving to avoid browning. When the eggs are almost finished, add the cheese and turn off the heat. Gently fold the cheese into the eggs, turning over with the spatula. When the cheese becomes soft but not dissolved, turn the scramble onto a plate.

YIELD: Makes 1 serving.

NUTRITIONAL ANALYSIS

Each with: **Calories:** 126.55 **Protein:** 13.96 g **Carbs:** 3.48 g **Total Fat:** 6.34 g **Sat Fat:** 1.60 g
Cholesterol: 17.38 mg **Sodium:** 381.03 mg **Sugars:** 1.15 g **Fiber:** 0.39 g

Ground Beef and Spinach Scramble

TEXTURE: Soft

INGREDIENTS

- 1 teaspoon light butter
- 6 teaspoons lean, browned ground beef
- 1/3 cup (10 g) chopped fresh spinach leaves, stems removed
- 1/4 cup (60 ml) liquid egg substitute
- 1 tablespoon (5 g) shredded Parmesan cheese

In an omelet pan over medium heat, melt the butter, swirling the pan to coat evenly. Add the ground beef and sauté 4 to 5 minutes, until warmed through. Add the spinach and continue cooking, until the spinach is completely wilted. Add the egg substitute, stirring gently but constantly with a heat-resistant rubber spatula, scraping the bottom of the pan to keep the eggs moving to avoid browning. When the eggs are almost finished, add the cheese and turn off the heat. Gently fold the cheese into the eggs, turning over with the rubber spatula. When the cheese becomes soft but not dissolved, turn the scramble onto a plate.

YIELD: Makes 1 serving.

NUTRITIONAL ANALYSIS
Each with: **Calories:** 141.75 g **Protein:** 17.45 g **Carbs:** 0.93 g **Total Fat:** 7.29 g **Sat Fat:** 2.47 g **Cholesterol:** 24.92 mg **Sodium:** 250.21 mg **Sugars:** 0.61 g **Fiber:** 0.22 g

Mushroom and Swiss Cheese Scramble

TEXTURE: Soft

INGREDIENTS

- 1 teaspoon light butter
- $1/4$ cup (15 g) sliced mushrooms
- $1/4$ cup (60 ml) liquid egg substitute
- 1 slice (1 ounce, or 28 g) low-fat Swiss cheese, cut into strips

In an omelet pan over medium heat, melt the butter, swirling the pan to coat evenly.

Add the mushrooms and sauté about 4 to 5 minutes, until they become soft and just begin to brown. Add the egg substitute, stirring gently but constantly with a heat-resistant rubber spatula, scraping the bottom of the pan to keep the eggs moving to avoid browning. When the eggs are almost finished, add the cheese and turn off the heat. Gently fold the cheese into the eggs, turning over with the rubber spatula. When the cheese becomes soft but not dissolved, turn the scramble onto a plate.

YIELD: Makes 1 serving.

NUTRITIONAL ANALYSIS

Each with: **Calories:** 171.85 **Protein:** 19.29 g **Carbs:** 2.24 g **Total Fat:** 9.27 g **Sat Fat:** 3.57 g **Cholesterol:** 17.63 mg **Sodium:** 223.34 mg **Sugars:** 1.46 g **Fiber:** 0.68 g

Greek Scramble

TEXTURE: Soft

INGREDIENTS

- 1 teaspoon light butter
- $1/2$ teaspoon chopped fresh thyme leaves
- $1/4$ cup (60 ml) liquid egg substitute
- 2 large pitted black olives, sliced
- 2 teaspoons finely diced green bell pepper
- 2 teaspoons feta cheese crumbles

In an omelet pan over medium heat, melt the butter, swirling the pan to coat evenly. Add the thyme and sauté about 1 to 2 minutes, until it begins to bubble and sweat. Add the egg substitute, stirring gently but constantly with a heat-resistant rubber spatula, scraping the bottom of the pan to keep the eggs moving to avoid browning. When the eggs are almost finished, add the olives, pepper, and cheese and turn off the heat. Gently fold the ingredients into the eggs, turning over with the rubber spatula. When the cheese becomes soft but not dissolved, turn the scramble onto a plate.

YIELD: Makes 1 serving.

NUTRITIONAL ANALYSIS

Each with: **Calories:** 96.95 **Protein:** 8.61 g **Carbs:** 1.78 g **Total Fat:** 5.97 g **Sat Fat:** 1.68 g **Cholesterol:** 6.19 mg **Sodium:** 247.13 mg **Sugars:** 1.42 g **Fiber:** 0.38 g

Tomato and Fresh Basil Scramble

TEXTURE: Soft

INGREDIENTS

- 1 teaspoon light butter
- 2 tablespoons (20 g) chopped tomato
- 1½ teaspoons chopped fresh basil leaves
- ¼ cup (60 ml) liquid egg substitute
- 1 tablespoon (5 g) shredded Parmesan cheese

In an omelet pan over medium heat, melt the butter, swirling the pan to coat evenly. Add the tomato and continue cooking 4 to 5 minutes, until soft. Add the basil and egg substitute, stirring gently but constantly with a heat-resistant rubber spatula, scraping the bottom of the pan to keep the eggs moving to avoid browning. When the eggs are almost finished, add the cheese and turn off the heat. Gently fold the cheese into the eggs, turning over with the spatula. When the cheese becomes soft but not dissolved, turn the scramble onto a plate.

YIELD: Makes 1 serving.

NUTRITIONAL ANALYSIS
Each with: **Calories:** 98.72 **Protein:** 9.82 g **Carbs:** 2.53 g
Total Fat: 5.58 g **Sat Fat:** 1.63 g **Cholesterol:** 4.23 mg
Sodium: 228.78 mg **Sugars:** 1.38 g **Fiber:** 0.74 g

Zucchini, Bacon, and Swiss Cheese Scramble

To save time, prepare the turkey bacon ahead of time per the package instructions.

TEXTURE: Soft

INGREDIENTS

- 1 teaspoon light butter
- 1 tablespoon (5 g) turkey bacon crumbles
- ¼ cup (30 g) chopped spring zucchini
- ¼ cup (60 ml) liquid egg substitute
- 1 slice (1 ounce, or 28 g) low-fat Swiss cheese, cut into strips

In an omelet pan over medium heat, melt the butter, swirling the pan to coat evenly. Add the bacon and continue cooking 4 to 5 minutes, until heated through. Add the zucchini and cook, until soft. Add the egg substitute, stirring gently but constantly with a heat-resistant rubber spatula, scraping the bottom of the pan to keep the eggs moving to avoid browning. When the eggs are almost finished, add the cheese and turn off the heat. Gently fold the cheese into the eggs, turning over with the spatula. When the cheese becomes soft but not dissolved, turn the scramble onto a plate.

YIELD: Makes 1 serving.

NUTRITIONAL ANALYSIS
Each with: **Calories:** 179.08 **Protein:** 18.88 g **Carbs:** 1.35 g
Total Fat: 10.39 g **Sat Fat:** 3.81 g **Cholesterol:** 22.69 mg
Sodium: 320.08 mg **Sugars:** 0.89 g **Fiber:** 0.31 g

Fresh Herb and Goat Cheese Scramble

TEXTURE: Soft

INGREDIENTS

- 1 teaspoon light butter
- 1 teaspoon chopped fresh parsley
- 1 teaspoon chopped fresh chives
- 1 teaspoon chopped fresh tarragon
- $1/4$ cup (60 ml) liquid egg substitute
- 2 teaspoons goat cheese crumbles

In an omelet pan over medium heat, melt the butter, swirling the pan to coat evenly.

Add the parsley, chives, and tarragon and sauté 1 to 2 minutes, until they begin to bubble and sweat. Add the egg substitute, stirring gently but constantly with a heat-resistant rubber spatula, scraping the bottom of the pan to keep the eggs moving to avoid browning. When the eggs are almost finished, add the cheese and turn off the heat. Gently fold the cheese into the eggs, turning over with the spatula. When the cheese becomes soft but not dissolved, turn the scramble onto a plate.

YIELD: Makes 1 serving.

NUTRITIONAL ANALYSIS
Each with: **Calories:** 103.94 **Protein:** 9.90 g **Carbs:** 0.98 g
Total Fat: 6.66 g **Sat Fat:** 2.51 g **Cholesterol:** 8.07 mg
Sodium: 166.70 mg **Sugars:** 0.58 g **Fiber:** 0.11 g

Italian Scramble

TEXTURE: Soft

INGREDIENTS

- 1 teaspoon light butter
- $1/8$ teaspoon dried oregano
- 2 teaspoons finely chopped yellow onion
- 1 tablespoon (10 g) chopped tomato
- $1/4$ cup (60 ml) liquid egg substitute
- 1 slice (1 ounce, or 28 g) part skim mozzarella, cut into strips

In an omelet pan over medium heat, melt the butter, swirling the pan to coat evenly. Add the oregano and sauté 4 to 5 minutes, until it begins to sweat. Add the onions and continue cooking, until they become soft. Add the tomato and stir just enough to evenly distribute. Add the egg substitute, stirring gently but constantly with a heat-resistant rubber spatula, scraping the bottom of the pan to keep the eggs moving to avoid browning. When the eggs are almost finished, add the cheese and turn off the heat. Gently fold the cheese into the eggs, turning over with the spatula. When the cheese becomes soft but not dissolved, turn the scramble onto a plate.

YIELD: Makes 1 serving.

NUTRITIONAL ANALYSIS
Each with: **Calories:** 158.21 **Protein:** 15.05 g **Carbs:** 1.86 g
Total Fat: 9.63 g **Sat Fat:** 4.41 g **Cholesterol:** 18.92 mg
Sodium: 343.86 mg **Sugars:** 1.08 g **Fiber:** 0.27 g

Spanish Omelet

This is a delicious (and nutritious) way to start your day!

TEXTURE: Soft

INGREDIENTS

- 3 teaspoons drained and chopped roasted red pepper
- 2 tablespoons (20 g) chopped tomato
- 1/2 teaspoon fresh minced garlic
- 3 or four 1-inch (2.5-cm) button mushrooms, cleaned and sliced
- 2 tablespoons (20 g) 95% fat-free ham, diced
- 1/4 cup (60 ml) liquid egg substitute
- 1 slice soy cheese, cut into strips
- 1 1/2 teaspoons fresh cilantro, chopped
- 2 tablespoons (35 g) Fresh Salsa Caliente (page 162)
- Fresh strawberries

Coat a 6-inch (15-cm) nonstick omelet pan with cooking spray and heat to medium high.

Add the roasted pepper, tomato, garlic, mushrooms, and ham and sauté for about 4 minutes, or until the mushrooms are soft. Transfer the mixture to a bowl, drain off excess liquid, and set aside.

Wipe clean the pan with paper towels and coat again with nonstick spray. Heat over medium heat and add the egg substitute. Using a rubber spatula, carefully lift the sides of the omelet up to let the egg substitute spill underneath the cooked, solid bottom. Repeat this process until the egg mixture is almost done, then turn off the heat. Immediately add the cheese and cilantro to the bottom half of the omelet, followed by the sauté mixture. Gently fold the top half of the omelet over the bottom half and carefully slide it onto a serving plate. Top the omelet with the salsa and garnish the plate with the strawberries.

YIELD: Makes 2 (about 1/2-cup) servings.

NUTRITIONAL ANALYSIS

Each with: **Calories:** 83.85 g **Protein:** 10.21 g **Carbs:** 5.15 g **Total Fat:** 3.77 g **Sat Fat:** 0.52 g **Cholesterol:** 7.12 mg **Sodium:** 303.63 mg **Sugars:** 3.13 g **Fiber:** 0.84 g

Cheese and Pepper Omelet

TEXTURE: Soft

INGREDIENTS

- $1/4$ cup (35 g) finely diced red bell pepper
- $1/4$ cup (35 g) finely diced yellow bell pepper
- $1/4$ teaspoon minced fresh garlic (about one small clove)
- $1/4$ cup (25 g) thinly sliced green onions
- $1^1/4$ cups (295 ml) liquid egg substitute
- $1/8$ teaspoon salt
- $1/8$ teaspoon ground black pepper
- 2 tablespoons (15 g) nonfat shredded Cheddar cheese
- 2 tablespoons (15 g) nonfat shredded Swiss cheese

Coat a 9- or 10-inch (22.5- or 25-cm) nonstick skillet with cooking spray and heat to medium-high. Add the red pepper, yellow pepper, garlic, and green onions. Cook for about 3 minutes, until the peppers just begin to soften, stirring occasionally. Pour the egg substitute into the pan and sprinkle in the salt and black pepper. Add the Cheddar and Swiss and cook without stirring for about 3 to 4 minutes, until the underside begins to brown. (Check the underside by using a rubber spatula to loosen and lift up the edges.) Loosen the omelet with a rubber spatula, and fold it in half. (A firmer spatula may be required to fold the omelet.) Cook for about 2 additional minutes, until the egg mixture is set and the cheese begins to melt. Cut the omelet in half and slide the halves onto serving plates.

YIELD: Makes 2 (3–4 ounce) servings.

NUTRITIONAL ANALYSIS

Each with: **Calories:** 146.76 **Protein:** 19.79 g **Carbs:** 5.04 g **Total Fat:** 5.03 g **Sat Fat:** 1.35 g
Cholesterol: 2.51 mg **Sodium:** 477.30 mg **Sugars:** 2.55 g **Fiber:** 1.35 g

Mark's Fruity French Toast

Mark is a gastric bypass surgery patient in the Boston area who makes this recipe for himself almost every morning and loves it.

TEXTURE: Regular

INGREDIENTS

- $1/4$ cup (60 ml) liquid egg substitute
- 1 tablespoon (14 ml) nonfat milk
- $1/2$ teaspoon allspice
- 2 slices reduced-calorie whole-wheat bread
- $1/4$ cup (40 g) sliced fresh strawberries
- $1/3$ cup (50 g) fresh blueberries
- $1/8$ cup (30 ml) sugar-free maple syrup

Coat a medium (big enough to hold two slices of bread) nonstick pan with cooking spray.

In a small mixing bowl combine the egg substitute, milk, and allspice. Dip the bread into the egg batter to coat both sides.

Heat the pan over medium heat. Place the bread into the pan and cook on both sides, until golden brown. Transfer the French toast to a serving plate and top with the strawberries, blueberries, and maple syrup.

YIELD: Makes 1 (2-slice) serving.

NUTRITIONAL ANALYSIS

Each with: **Calories:** 221.36 **Protein:** 12.91 g **Carbs:** 39.31 g **Total Fat:** 3.52 g **Sat Fat:** 0.63 g **Cholesterol:** 0.93 mg **Sodium:** 408.18 mg **Sugars:** 9.14 g **Fiber:** 7.65 g

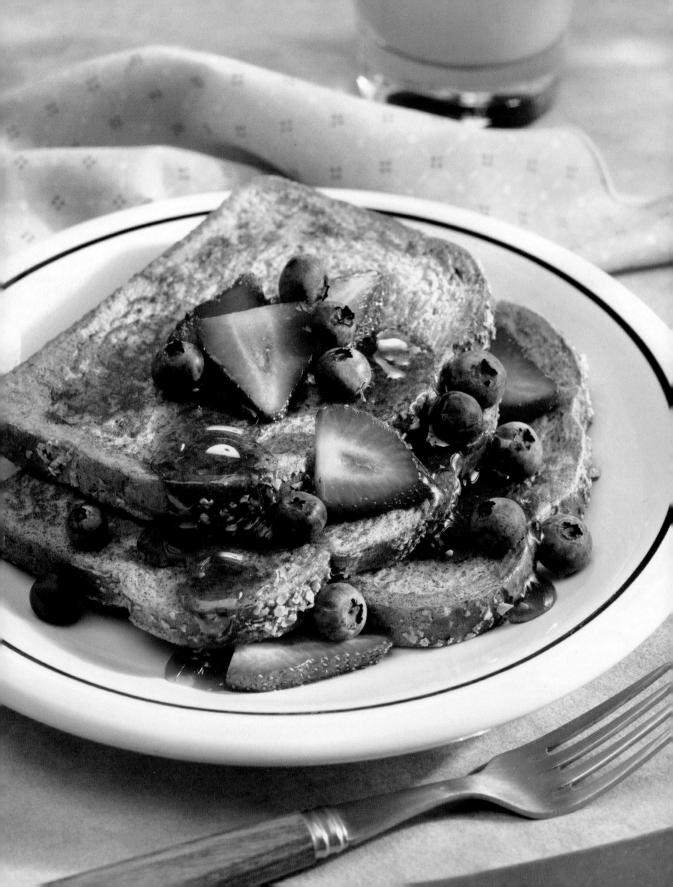

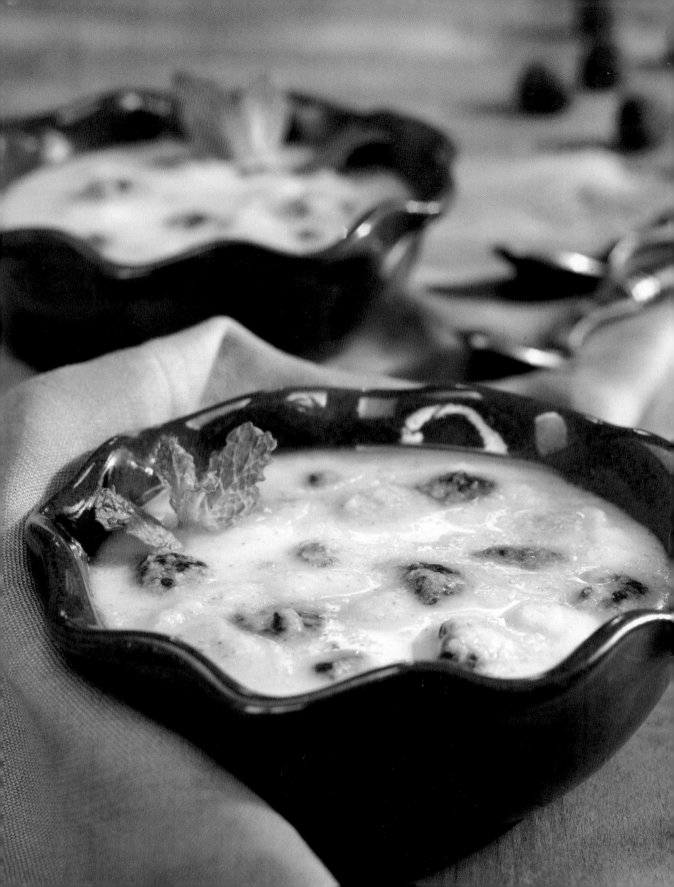

Berry Delicious Cream of Wheat

TEXTURE: Soft

INGREDIENTS

- ³/₄ cup (135 g) instant Cream of Wheat, no salt added
- ¹/₂ teaspoon vanilla extract
- ¹/₂ cup (60 g) fresh raspberries
- 2 tablespoons (15 g) protein powder supplement (see note)
- 2 tablespoons (28 ml) nonfat milk or low-fat, low-sugar soy milk
- 2 sprigs spearmint

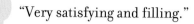

"Very satisfying and filling."

—Julie,
a gastric bypass surgery patient in the Boston area

Prepare Cream of Wheat per the package instruction for 2 servings, adding the vanilla to the water before boiling. Just before removing the Cream of Wheat from the pan, stir in the raspberries. Add the protein powder just prior to serving. Serve in warmed bowls, topped with the milk and garnished with fresh spearmint sprigs.

YIELD: Makes 2 servings.

NUTRITIONAL ANALYSIS

Each with: **Calories:** 219.29 **Protein:** 24.88 g **Carbs:** 23.10 g **Total Fat:** 3.21 g **Sat Fat:** 0.07 g **Cholesterol:** 0.28 mg **Sodium:** 83.74 mg **Sugars:** 4.04 **Fiber:** 4.36 g

MARGARET'S NOTES

Although raspberries contain the highest fiber of all berries, you may substitute blueberries, blackberries, strawberries, or huckleberries.

It is essential to select a protein powder that is appropriate for hot foods and beverages for this recipe to optimize the quality of the protein (avoid protein breakdown) when exposed to heat, a process known as denaturing. This is also why you add the protein powder after heating the Cream of Wheat, just prior to serving it.

Cumin Mushroom Omelet

This is simple and delicious! For a complete breakfast, serve this delicious omelet with a whole-wheat English muffin half and fresh fruit. Serve it with Fresh Salsa Caliente (page 162).

TEXTURE: Soft

INGREDIENTS

- ½ pound (225 g) mushrooms
- 1 tablespoon (14 g) low-fat butter alternative
- 1 teaspoon olive oil
- 1 small clove garlic, minced
- 2 teaspoons ground cumin
- ⅛ teaspoon cayenne pepper (optional)
- ¼ teaspoon paprika
- ¼ teaspoon kosher salt or sea salt
- 2 tablespoons (25 g) nonfat sour cream
- 1 cup (235 ml) liquid egg substitute
- ¾ cup (85 g) reduced-fat shredded Cheddar cheese
- ¼ cup (4 g) chopped fresh cilantro
- Fresh cilantro sprigs

Clean the mushrooms with a mushroom brush or paper towels. Cut the end of the stems away and discard. Slice the mushrooms into thin slices.

In a medium nonstick skillet, heat the butter alternative and oil over medium heat. Add the mushrooms, garlic, cumin, pepper, paprika, and salt. Sauté, stirring often, for about 8 minutes, until the mushrooms become soft. Stir in the sour cream and continue cooking for 2 minutes, stirring once or twice. Remove the pan from the heat.

Coat a 7-inch (17.5 cm) nonstick skillet with cooking spray and heat to medium. Add the egg substitute and cook until the bottom becomes solid, but not browned. Using a rubber spatula, carefully lift the sides of the omelet up to let the egg substitute spill underneath the cooked, solid bottom. Repeat this process until the egg mixture is entirely cooked, then turn off the heat. Add the cheese and cilantro to the bottom half of the omelet. Fold the top half over the bottom half and gently press down with the rubber spatula. Cut the omelet in half and slide the halves onto serving plates. Garnish with the cilantro sprigs and salsa.

YIELD: Makes 4 (about ½-cup) servings.

NUTRITIONAL ANALYSIS
Each with: **Calories:** 160.93 **Protein:** 14.59 g **Carbs:** 5.09 g **Total Fat:** 9.11 g **Sat Fat:** 3.39 g **Cholesterol:** 13.13 mg **Sodium:** 408.90 mg **Sugars:** 1.99 g **Fiber:** 1.19 g

Berry-Mango Breakfast Shake

This is a great shake to share with friends before a Saturday morning walk. Add a scoop of whey or soy protein powder to this shake for more protein. It's yummy and helps meet your protein needs.

TEXTURE: Pureed. May be allowed on some full liquid meals

INGREDIENTS

- 1½ cups (385 g) frozen berries (see note)
- 1 cup (165 g) fresh or canned mango slices, chilled
- 1 cup (240 g) soft, silken, low-fat tofu
- 1 cup (235 ml) diet cranberry juice cocktail
- ½ teaspoon vanilla extract
- 6 teaspoons sugar substitute
- 4 sprigs mint

In a blender, process the berries, mango, tofu, juice, vanilla, and sugar substitute, until consistency is smooth. Pour into glasses and top with the mint.

YIELD: Makes 4 (1-cup) servings.

NUTRITIONAL ANALYSIS
Each with: **Calories:** 103.60 **Protein:** 3.52 g **Carbs:** 19.27 g **Total Fat:** 2.13 g **Sat Fat:** 0.05 g
Cholesterol: 0.00 mg **Sodium:** 6.75 mg **Sugars:** 13.44 g **Fiber:** 4.69 g

NOTE

If you should avoid seeds, choose blueberries.

Greek High-Protein Berry-Licious Milkshake

Delicious Greek yogurt makes this creamy and super nutritious. If you've recently had your weight-loss surgery and can't seem to get solid food in, you could make this shake and have 1 serving (about 1 cup) three times a day for your 3 meals. (Just place the rest in your refrigerator for later use). It will provide more than 60 grams of protein for the 3 servings, which should meet your basic protein needs. The fiber in the berries may help with any constipation problems, which are quite common, especially within the first month or two of weight loss surgery.

TEXTURE: Pureed. May be allowed on some full liquid meals

INGREDIENTS

- 1 cup (235 ml) nonfat milk or low-fat, low-sugar soy milk (see note)
- 1 cup (150 g) fresh or frozen blueberries, raspberries, strawberries, or blackberries
- 2 ounces (55 g) protein powder supplement
- 7 ounces (200 g) Greek yogurt (2% fat)
- 1 tablespoon (14 ml) sugar-free vanilla syrup
- 1 cup (150 g) crushed ice (optional) (see Lynette's note)

LYNETTE'S NOTE

Add ice cubes to make the shake thicker. But if you add ice cubes, the shake will not hold in the refrigerator.

"Yummy and creamy ... I used frozen blueberries instead of ice, and it worked great. I used Stevia to sweeten it even more."

—Julie,
a gastric bypass surgery patient in the Boston area

In a blender, combine the milk, blueberries, protein powder, yogurt, syrup, and ice (if using). Blend until the ingredients are emulsified. (The milkshake will be a creamy consistency and blue color throughout.)

YIELD: Makes 3 (about 1-cup) servings.

NUTRITIONAL ANALYSIS
Each with: **Calories:** 179.65 **Protein:** 23.13 g **Carbs:** 15.55 g **Total Fat:** 3.36 g **Sat Fat:** 1.11 g **Cholesterol:** 4.97 mg **Sodium:** 107.57 mg **Sugars:** 11.53 g **Fiber:** 1.16 g

MARGARET'S NOTE

Make sure the soy milk contains no more than 14 grams of sugar per cup.

Lisi's "Berry Kool" Smoothie

This is a great smoothie to run out the door with in the morning; the sweet and tart taste of delicious fresh berries with the addition of extra vitamins and minerals found in the greens will really amp up your day. It was created by Lisi Deswart, dietetic intern at the University of Maryland Eastern Shore, class of 2011.

TEXTURE: Pureed. May be allowed on some full liquid meals.

INGREDIENTS

- $1/2$ cup (65 g) fresh raspberries
- $1/2$ cup (75 g) fresh blackberries
- $1/2$ cup (115 g) 2% Greek yogurt
- $1/2$ cup (120 ml) skim milk
- 2 stalks kale, leaves removed and finely chopped

Add the raspberries, blackberries, yogurt, milk, and kale leaves to blender. Blend until smooth.

YIELD: Makes 2 (8-ounce) smoothies.

NUTRITIONAL ANALYSIS
Each with: **Calories:** 94.65 **Protein:** 8.11 g **Carbs:** 14.67 g **Total Fat:** 1.47 g **Sat Fat:** 0.80 g **Cholesterol:** 4.97 mg **Sodium:** 52.02 mg **Sugars:** 6.94 g **Fiber:** 2.14 g

JOE'S TIP

To cut cost, it's perfectly fine to use frozen berries instead of fresh. Frozen berries are always good to have on hand for many recipes. Try them in different combinations to spice up your favorite protein powder.

Frozen Fruit Smoothie

MARGARET'S NOTE

You may substitute raspberries, strawberries, or blackberries for the blueberries, because the calories and carbohydrates are equivalent. Raspberries are the highest in fiber among these fruits, but all contain healthy antioxidants, which are wonderful cancer-fighting agents.

NOTES

Make sure the soy milk contains no more than 14 grams of sugars per cup.

Generic (low-sugar) protein powders are fine, but please ensure they're appropriate for cold beverages.

Frozen fruit smoothies can become a high-protein, easy-to-digest meal when you're on the go, or in the earlier stages of your postoperative diet. You can incorporate them into your diet up to twice a day if you're very busy or if you find your weight is inching upward and you'd like to reverse the trend. If you freeze the bananas for a few hours before making this shake, it will be even thicker and more delicious.

TEXTURE: Pureed. May be allowed on some full liquid meals

INGREDIENTS

- 4 ounces (115 g) banana, sliced (approximately 8- to 8⁷/₈-inches long)
- 1 cup (150 g) fresh or frozen blueberries (see note)
- 1 cup (235 ml) soy milk, unsweetened (see note), or 1 to 1¹/₂ cups (235 ml) nonfat milk
- 2 ounces (55 g) protein powder supplement (see note)
- 2 sprigs mint

In a blender, combine the bananas, blueberries, soy milk, and protein powder. Blend for 10 to 15 seconds, until a smooth consistency is reached. Garnish with the mint.

YIELD: Makes 2 servings.

NUTRITIONAL ANALYSIS
Each with: **Calories:** 250.73 **Protein:** 27.09 g **Carbs:** 26.33 g **Total Fat:** 5.01 g **Sat Fat:** 0.06 g **Cholesterol:** 0.00 mg **Sodium:** 85.00 mg **Sugars:** 13.93 g **Fiber:** 5.47 g

"I love this smoothie. I never liked the protein shakes, and I found that I could tolerate the protein in this recipe. In fact, my 3-year-old son loves it too, and we call it "fruit milk." Definitely freeze the bananas. It makes a tasty treat that has some nice chunks in it. I have tried this with blueberries and strawberries in it together, and it is delicious. This is great if you have no time and really want something yummy."

—Julie, *a gastric bypass patient in the New Bedford, Massachusetts, area*

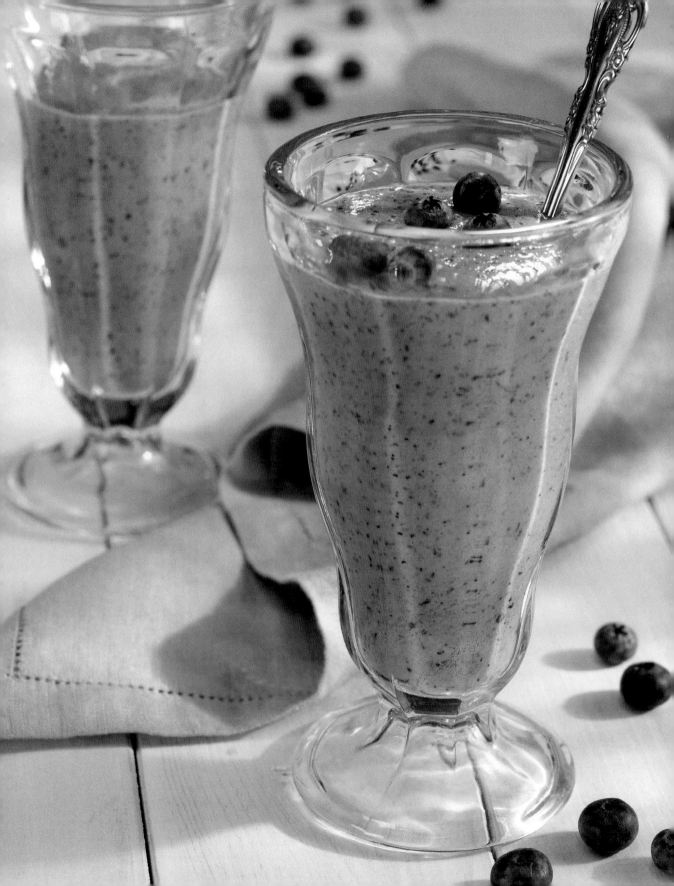

Zucchini Frittata with Capers and Olives

This is great served with the Chive-Yogurt Sauce to the right.

TEXTURE: Regular

INGREDIENTS

- 2 teaspoons extra-virgin olive oil
- 2 cloves garlic, minced
- 1/2 cup (70 g) finely diced red bell pepper
- 1 cup (160 g) finely diced yellow onion
- 2 cups (250 g) grated zucchini
- 2 tablespoons (20 g) capers, drained
- 1/4 cup (35 g) finely diced, pitted black or Greek olives
- 1/2 cup (75 g) feta cheese crumbles
- 2 tablespoons (8 g) chopped fresh parsley
- 2 1/2 cups (590 ml) liquid egg substitute

Preheat the oven to 375°F (190°C, or gas mark 5). Spray cooking spray around the inside edges of an 8-inch (20-cm) cast iron skillet. In the skillet, heat the oil over medium-high, stirring occasionally. Sauté the garlic, bell pepper, and onion for about 5 minutes, until soft but not brown. Remove the skillet from heat and add the zucchini, capers, and olives. Arrange the cheese and parsley evenly over the sauté mixture. Slowly pour the egg substitute over the top of the mixture in the skillet.

Place the skillet in the oven and bake for 40 minutes, until the center of the frittata rises to match the outer edges. (The frittata should be just beginning to brown when it's finished cooking. If it begins to brown too quickly, reduce the oven temperature to 350°F, 180°C, or gas mark 4.) Serve on warmed plates with Chive-Yogurt Sauce drizzled over the top of each slice.

YIELD: Makes 6 (1 1/2-cup) servings.

NUTRITIONAL ANALYSIS
Each with: **Calories:** 172.69 **Protein:** 15.32 g **Carbs:** 7.03 g **Total Fat:** 8.86 g **Sat Fat:** 2.80 g **Cholesterol:** 12.17 mg **Sodium:** 506.49 mg **Sugars:** 4.01 g **Fiber:** 1.25 g

Chive-Yogurt Sauce

This is a light, clean-tasting sauce that would be great with lamb, chicken, beef, and even as a dip for pita bread or vegetables.

TEXTURE: Pureed. May be allowed on some full liquid meals.

INGREDIENTS

- ¼ cup (50 g) nonfat sour cream
- ¼ cup (60 g) nonfat plain yogurt
- ½ teaspoon salt
- ⅛ teaspoon ground white pepper
- 1 tablespoon finely chopped chives

In a small mixing bowl, combine the sour cream, yogurt, salt, pepper, and chives. Vigorously mix with a fork or wire whip.

YIELD: Makes 6 (1-tablespoon) servings

NUTRITIONAL ANALYSIS
Each with: **Calories:** 16.13 **Protein:** 1.06 g **Carbs:** 2.68 g **Total Fat:** 0 g **Sat Fat:** 0 g **Cholesterol:** 1.88 mg **Sodium:** 110.43 mg **Sugars:** 1.30 g **Fiber:** 0.03 g

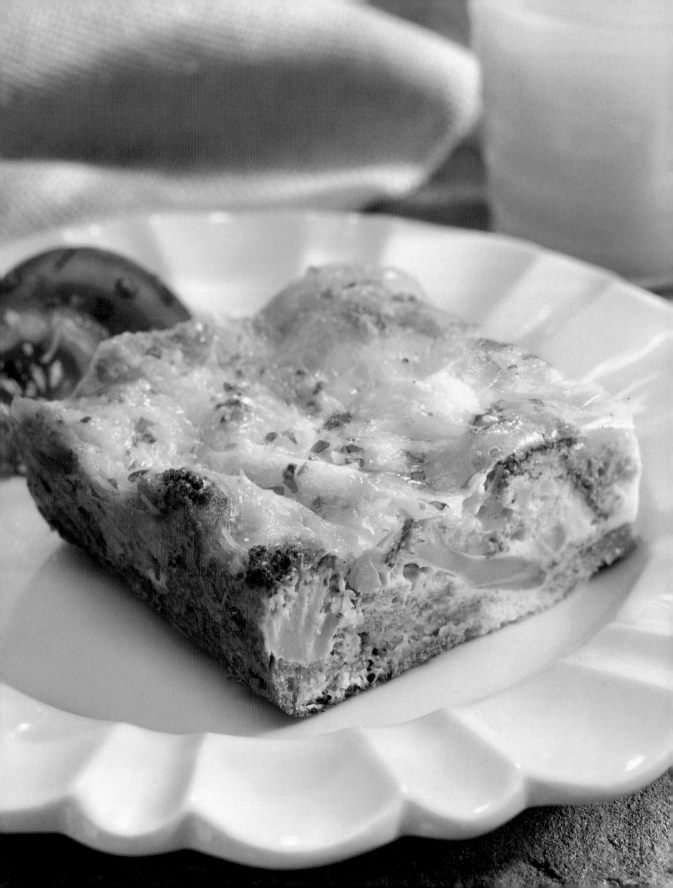

Savory Broccoli and Cheese Bread Pudding

This is an elegant breakfast, lunch, or dinner.

TEXTURE: Regular

INGREDIENTS

- 2 teaspoons olive oil
- 1 medium sweet onion, diced (about 1¹/₂ cups, or 240 g)
- ¹/₂ teaspoon dried oregano
- ¹/₂ teaspoon dried basil
- ¹/₄ teaspoon granulated garlic
- 5–6 whole-wheat English muffins, toasted and cut into ¹/₂-inch (1.25-cm) croutons
- 1 package (14 ounces, or 400 g) chopped frozen broccoli, thawed and drained
- 1¹/₂ cups (170 g) reduced-fat shredded Cheddar cheese
- 2 tablespoons (10 g) shredded Parmesan cheese
- 3 large eggs, beaten
- 2 tablespoons (8 g) chopped fresh parsley
- ¹/₂ cup (120 ml) nonfat half-and-half

Preheat the oven to 350°F (180°C, or gas mark 4).

In a medium skillet, heat the oil over medium-high heat. Add the onion and sauté until it begins to soften. Add the oregano, basil, and garlic and continue cooking for an additional 2 minutes, stirring once or twice. Remove the mixture from heat and set aside.

Coat a 7- x 9-inch (17.5- x 22.5-cm) baking dish with cooking spray. Place the croutons and broccoli in the baking dish. Evenly distribute the sauté mixture over the bread and broccoli. Sprinkle the Cheddar and Parmesan over the croutons and broccoli.

In a small (1 quart, or 1 L) mixing bowl, combine the eggs, parsley, and half-and-half, then pour the egg mixture evenly over the cheese. Bake for 35 minutes, until the center of the dish has risen to meet the level at the edges and the top is golden brown.

YIELD: Makes 12 (²/₃-cup) servings.

NUTRITIONAL ANALYSIS
Each with: **Calories:** 196.14 **Protein:** 11.01 g **Carbs:** 25.80 g **Total Fat:** 6.36 g **Sat Fat:** 2.70 g **Cholesterol:** 68.50 mg **Sodium:** 480.27 mg **Sugars:** 6.13 g **Fiber:** 4.49 g

Breakfast Turkey Sausage Patties

Serve these breakfast sausages with any of our egg dishes, frittatas, or egg scrambles and whole-wheat English muffins for a satisfying breakfast or brunch.

TEXTURE: Regular

INGREDIENTS

- 1 pound (455 g) lean ground turkey (93% fat-free or leaner)
- ¼ cup (25 g) fine, plain bread crumbs
- 2 teaspoons ground sage
- 1 teaspoon ground coriander
- 1 teaspoon ground oregano
- ½ teaspoon ground thyme
- ½ teaspoon black pepper
- ¼ teaspoon sea salt or kosher salt
- ¼ teaspoon cayenne pepper (optional)
- ½ teaspoon paprika
- ½ teaspoon garlic powder
- ½ cup (120 ml) low-sodium chicken broth

In a large (4 quart, or 4 L) mixing bowl, combine the turkey, bread crumbs, sage, coriander, oregano, thyme, black pepper, salt, cayenne pepper (if using), paprika, and garlic powder. Stir to incorporate completely. Add the broth, stir again, and let stand in the refrigerator for about 20 minutes. Form the mixture into 8 patties, about ½-inch (1.25 cm) thick.

Coat a nonstick skillet with cooking spray and heat over medium-high. Cook the patties for about 7 minutes on each side, until browned and done in the center.

YIELD: Makes 8 (about 2-ounce) patties.

NUTRITIONAL ANALYSIS
Each with: **Calories:** 78.73 **Protein:** 14.25 g **Carbs:** 3.32 g **Total Fat:** 1.06 g **Sat Fat:** 0.32 g **Cholesterol:** 27.54 mg **Sodium:** 166.32 mg **Sugars:** 0.27 g **Fiber:** 0.49 g

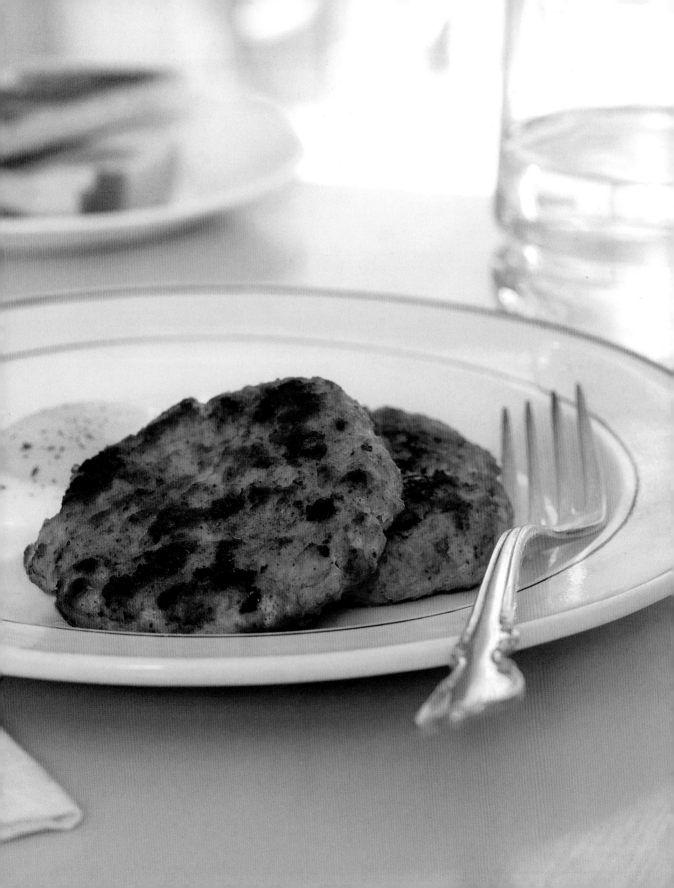

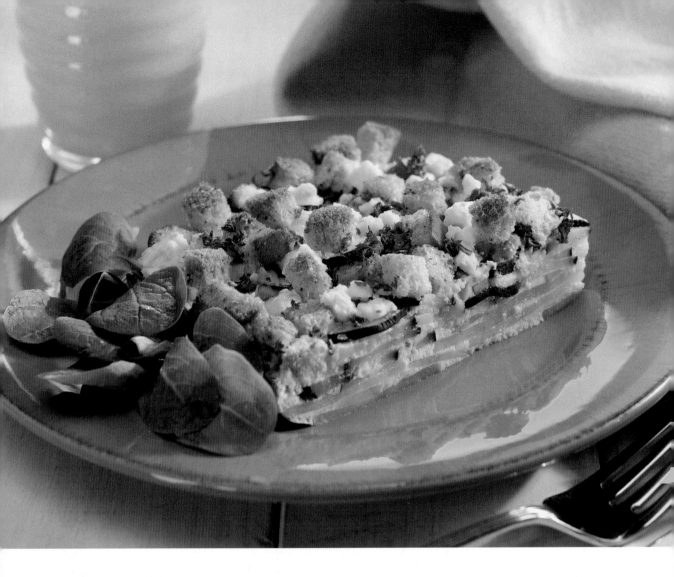

MARGARET'S NOTE

If you'd like to pack even more protein into this dish, sprinkle part-skim shredded mozzarella cheese or shredded vegetarian (soy) cheese over your frittata, then melt under the broiler until bubbly and golden brown.

Zucchini and Potato Strata

If you like omelets, you'll love this dish. This is a fantastic brunch-style main course that can be prepared the night before and refrigerated. Be sure to bring it just to room temperature before placing it in the oven to avoid cracking the dish.

TEXTURE: Regular

INGREDIENTS

- $3/4$ pounds (340 g) Yukon gold potatoes
- $1^1/2$ cups (355 ml) liquid egg substitute
- $2/3$ cup (150 ml) nonfat half-and-half
- $1/4$ cup (15 g) chopped fresh parsley
- $1/8$ teaspoon granulated garlic
- $1/4$ teaspoon salt
- $1/8$ teaspoon black pepper
- 2 cups (240 g) zucchini slices (cut into thin circles)
- 1 cup (40 g) seasoned croutons
- $1/2$ cup (75 g) feta cheese crumbles
- Sprigs fresh parsley

LYNETTE'S NOTE

A lovely topping of warm Pomodoro Sauce (page 286) makes this wonderful dish unforgettable! (3 tablespoons each)

Wash, drain, and peel the potatoes. Using a mandolin slicer or a large chef's knife, slice the potatoes approximately $1/8$-inch (3-mm) thick. Place the potatoes into a medium saucepan and cover them with cold water to 1 inch (2.5 cm) above the level of the potatoes. Bring the potatoes just to a boil, then immediately drain them in a colander. Rinse the potatoes in cold water to stop the cooking process and let stand to continue draining.

In a medium mixing bowl, combine the egg substitute, half-and-half, chopped parsley, garlic, salt, and pepper, then whisk together with a wire whip or hand-held blender.

Coat a 9- x 13-inch (22.5- x 32.5-cm) baking dish with cooking spray. Arrange the potatoes in a single layer. Arrange the zucchini on top of the potatoes. Evenly distribute the croutons over the zucchini. Evenly distribute the cheese over the croutons. Pour the egg mixture evenly over top and let stand in the refrigerator for 20 minutes, until the croutons have softened by absorbing the egg mixture.

Preheat the oven to 375°F (190°C, or gas mark 5). Bake the strata for 40 minutes, until the egg mixture is done in the center of the dish and the top is golden brown. Garnish with the parsley sprigs and serve warm.

YIELD: Makes 10 (1-cup) servings.

NUTRITIONAL ANALYSIS
Each with: **Calories:** 192.79 **Protein:** 19.46 g **Carbs:** 11.51 g **Total Fat:** 7.23 g **Sat Fat:** 2.40 g **Cholesterol:** 9.14 mg **Sodium:** 440.91 mg **Sugars:** 3.36 g **Fiber:** 1.08 g

Spring Herb and Zucchini Muffins

Muffins are not your typical post-weight-loss surgery food, but many of my gastric bypass and band patients tell me they can tolerate them if they're not doughy. I usually don't encourage muffins from a calorie and nutrition perspective, but Lynette concocted some healthy, non-doughy muffins that are as tasty as they are nutritious. Serve these muffins for an elegant accompaniment to a festive and special brunch.

TEXTURE: Regular

INGREDIENTS

- 1 cup (110 g) all-purpose flour
- ¹/₂ cup (55 g) oat bran flour
- 1 teaspoon baking powder
- 1 teaspoon baking soda
- ¹/₂ teaspoon salt
- 1 egg
- 1 tablespoon (14 ml) vegetable oil
- 1 cup (240 g) nonfat plain or vanilla yogurt
- ³/₄ cup (95 g) grated zucchini (press out the moisture by squeezing it in paper towels)
- ¹/₄ cup (60 g) unsweetened applesauce
- 1 tablespoon (3 g) chopped chives
- 1 tablespoon (4 g) chopped fresh parsley
- 1¹/₂ teaspoons chopped fresh tarragon

Preheat the oven to 375°F (190°C, or gas mark 5). Spray a muffin tin with cooking spray. In a large mixing bowl, combine the all-purpose flour, oat bran flour, baking powder, baking soda, and salt. Stir to combine.

In medium mixing bowl, whisk together the egg, oil, yogurt, zucchini, applesauce, chives, parsley, and tarragon, just enough to combine. (The batter should be slightly lumpy.)

Fill the muffin cups two-thirds full with batter. Bake for 20 to 25 minutes, until a toothpick inserted into the middle of a muffin comes out clean. Let the muffins cool for 15 minutes before turning the tin over to release the muffins. (If the muffins stick to the pan, a slight tap on the back should help to release them.)

YIELD: Makes 12 (2-ounce) muffins.

NUTRITIONAL ANALYSIS

Each with: **Calories:** 85.22 **Protein:** 3.03 g **Carbs:** 14.21 g **Total Fat:** 1.87 g **Sat Fat:** 0.23 g **Cholesterol:** 20.42 mg **Sodium:** 206.11 mg **Sugars:** 2.05 g **Fiber:** 0.92 g

Lavender-Blueberry Muffins

Enjoy the delicious and delightful combination of lavender and blueberries.

TEXTURE: Regular

INGREDIENTS

- ¹⁄₃ cup (65 g) sugar or ¹⁄₃ cup (9 g) baking sugar substitute (see page 50) (see Margaret's Note)
- 1 cup (110 g) oat bran flour
- ¹⁄₂ cup (55 g) all-purpose flour
- 1 teaspoon baking powder
- 1 teaspoon baking soda
- ¹⁄₂ teaspoon salt
- ¹⁄₄ cup (60 g) dried lavender (no stems)
- 1 egg
- 1 tablespoon (14 ml) vegetable oil
- 1¹⁄₂ teaspoons vanilla extract
- 1 cup (240 g) nonfat plain or vanilla yogurt
- ³⁄₄ cup (110 g) fresh or frozen blueberries
- ¹⁄₄ cup (60 g) unsweetened applesauce

Preheat the oven to 375°F (190°C, or gas mark 5). Spray a muffin tin with nonstick spray.

In a large mixing bowl, combine the sugar or baking sugar substitute, oat bran flour, all-purpose flour, baking powder, baking soda, salt, and lavender. Stir to combine.

In a medium mixing bowl, whisk together the egg, oil, vanilla, yogurt, blueberries, and applesauce, just enough to combine. (The batter should be slightly lumpy.)

Fill the muffin cups two-thirds full with batter. Bake for 20 to 25 minutes, until a toothpick inserted into the middle of a muffin comes out clean. Let the muffins cool for 15 minutes before turning the tin over to release the muffins. (If the muffins stick to the pan, a slight tap on the back should help to release them.)

YIELD: Makes 12 (2-ounce) muffins.

NUTRITIONAL ANALYSIS

Each with: **Calories:** 113.45 **Protein:** 2.94 g **Carbs:** 21.64 g **Total Fat:** 2 g **Sat Fat:** 0.22 g **Cholesterol:** 20.42 mg **Sodium:** 205.71 mg **Sugars:** 9.20 g **Fiber:** 1.39 g

MARGARET'S NOTE

The nutritional analysis is based on the recipe made with table sugar. If you use a sugar substitute instead, the nutritional analysis will be: Calories: 90 Protein: 3 g Carbs: 15 g Total Fat: 2 g Sugars: 2.87 g. (The sugar substitute won't change the fat, cholesterol, sodium, or fiber content.)

Carrot Muffins with Fresh Dill

Serve these savory muffins with soup or salad for a special luncheon.

TEXTURE: Regular

INGREDIENTS

- ¹/₄ cup (40 g) light brown sugar or brown sugar substitute (see note)
- 1 cup (110 g) oat bran flour
- ¹/₂ cup (55 g) all-purpose flour
- 1 teaspoon baking powder
- 1 teaspoon baking soda
- 1 teaspoon onion powder
- ¹/₂ teaspoon salt
- 1 egg
- 1 tablespoon (14 ml) vegetable oil
- ¹/₃ cup (65 g) sugar
- 1 teaspoon lemon juice
- 1 cup (240 g) nonfat plain or vanilla yogurt
- ³/₄ cup (85 g) finely grated carrots
- 2 tablespoons (4 g) chopped fresh dill
- ¹/₄ cup (60 g) unsweetened applesauce

Preheat the oven to 375°F (190°C, or gas mark 5). Spray a muffin tin with nonstick spray.

In a large mixing bowl, combine the light brown sugar, oat bran flour, all-purpose flour, baking powder, baking soda, onion powder, and salt. Stir to combine.

In a medium mixing bowl, whisk together the egg, oil, sugar, juice, yogurt, carrots, dill, and applesauce, just enough to combine. (The batter should be slightly lumpy.)

Fill the muffin cups two-thirds full with batter. Bake for 20 to 25 minutes, until a toothpick inserted into the middle of a muffin comes out clean. Let the muffins cool for 15 minutes before turning the tin over to release the muffins. (If the muffins stick to the pan, a slight tap on the back should help to release them.)

YIELD: Makes 12 (about 2-ounce) muffins.

NUTRITIONAL ANALYSIS
Each with: **Calories:** 104.71 **Protein:** 3.03 g **Carbs:** 19.5 g **Total Fat:** 2 g **Sat Fat:** 0.22 g **Cholesterol:** 20.42 mg **Sodium:** 215.52 mg **Sugars:** 6.63 g **Fiber:** 1.59 g

MARGARET'S NOTE

If you leave out the brown sugar, each serving will provide: Calories: 90 Protein: 3 g Carbs: 15 g Total Fat: 2 g Sugars: 3 g. (The sugar substitute won't affect the saturated fat, cholesterol, sodium, or fiber.)

Fresh Strawberry Muffins

When strawberries are in season, these muffins are as good for dessert as they are for breakfast.

TEXTURE: Regular

INGREDIENTS

- $^1/_3$ cup (65 g) sugar or $^1/_3$ cup (9 g) baking sugar substitute (see page 50) (see note)
- 1 cup (110 g) oat bran flour
- $^1/_2$ cup (55 g) all-purpose flour
- 1 teaspoon baking powder
- 1 teaspoon baking soda
- $^1/_2$ teaspoon salt
- 1 egg
- 1 tablespoon (14 ml) vegetable oil
- $1^1/_2$ teaspoons vanilla extract
- 1 cup (240 g) nonfat vanilla yogurt
- $^1/_4$ cup (60 g) unsweetened applesauce
- $^3/_4$ cup (120 g) sliced fresh strawberries

LYNETTE'S NOTE

For dessert: Slice a muffin in half horizontally and fill the middle with 2 tablespoons (35 g) nonfat, sugar-free vanilla pudding. Replace the top and add a dollop of nonfat whipped cream topping and a few fresh strawberry slices.

Preheat the oven to 375°F (190°C, or gas mark 5). Spray a muffin tin with nonstick spray.

In a large mixing bowl, combine the sugar or sugar substitute, oat bran flour, all-purpose flour, baking powder, baking soda, and salt. Stir to combine.

In a medium mixing bowl, whisk together the egg, oil, vanilla, yogurt, and applesauce, just enough to combine. (The batter should be slightly lumpy.) Gently fold in the strawberries.

Fill the muffin cups two-thirds full with batter. Bake for 20 to 25 minutes, until a toothpick inserted into the middle of a muffin comes out clean. Let the muffins cool for 15 minutes before turning the tin over to release the muffins. (If the muffins stick to the pan, a slight tap on the back should help to release them.)

YIELD: Makes 12 (about 2-ounce) muffins.

NUTRITIONAL ANALYSIS
Each with: **Calories:** 111.53 **Protein:** 2.94 g **Carbs:** 21.11 g **Total Fat:** 2 g **Sat Fat:** 0.22 g **Cholesterol:** 20.42 mg **Sodium:** 205.71 mg **Sugars:** 8.79 g **Fiber:** 1.37 g

MARGARET'S NOTE

If you omit the sugar, each serving will provide: Calories: 88 Protein: 3 g Carbs: 15 g Total Fat: 2 g Sugars: 2 g. (The saturated fat, cholesterol, sodium, and fiber won't change.)

Green Chili and Cheese Cornbread Muffins

These muffins are perfect with soup or chili.

TEXTURE: Regular

INGREDIENTS

- ¹/₂ cup (55 g) all-purpose flour
- ¹/₂ cup (70 g) coarse yellow cornmeal
- 1 teaspoon baking powder
- ¹/₂ teaspoon baking soda
- ¹/₄ teaspoon salt
- 1¹/₂ teaspoon onion powder
- ¹/₂ cup (120 ml) low-fat buttermilk
- 1 egg
- 2 tablespoons (12 g) diced mild green chilies, drained
- ¹/₂ cup (55 g) reduced-fat shredded Cheddar cheese

Preheat the oven to 400°F (200°C, or gas mark 6). Spray a muffin tin with cooking spray.

In a large mixing bowl, combine the flour, cornmeal, baking powder, baking soda, salt, and onion powder. Stir to combine.

In a medium mixing bowl, whisk together the buttermilk, egg, chiles, and cheese, just enough to combine. (The batter should be slightly lumpy.)

Fill 8 of the muffin cups two-thirds full with batter. Bake for 20 to 25 minutes, until a toothpick inserted into the middle of a muffin comes out clean. Let the muffins cool for 15 minutes before turning the tin over to release the muffins. (If the muffins stick to the pan, a slight tap on the back should help to release them.)

YIELD: Makes 8 (2-ounce) muffins.

NUTRITIONAL ANALYSIS

Each with: **Calories:** 93.10 **Protein:** 4.35 g **Carbs:** 13.36 g **Total Fat:** 2.43 g **Sat Fat:** 1.17 g **Cholesterol:** 34.36 mg **Sodium:** 254.99 mg **Sugars:** 1.09 g **Fiber:** 0.92 g

Zucchini-Bran Muffins

These muffins are great for breakfast or a mid-day snack. They hold well in the freezer for several weeks.

TEXTURE: Regular

INGREDIENTS

- ¹/₃ cup (50 g) unpacked light brown sugar or brown sugar substitute (see note)
- ³/₄ cup (30 g) bran cereal
- 1 cup (110 g) oat bran flour
- ¹/₂ cup (55 g) whole wheat flour
- 2 teaspoons baking powder
- ¹/₂ teaspoon salt
- 1 teaspoon cinnamon
- ¹/₄ teaspoon nutmeg
- 1 egg
- 1 tablespoon (14 ml) vegetable oil
- ¹/₄ teaspoon vanilla extract
- ¹/₄ teaspoon almond extract
- 1 cup (240 g) nonfat plain or vanilla yogurt
- ³/₄ cup (95 g) grated zucchini (press out the moisture by squeezing it in paper towels)
- ¹/₄ cup (60 g) unsweetened applesauce

Preheat the oven to 375°F (190°C, or gas mark 5). Spray a muffin tin with cooking spray.

In a large mixing bowl, place the brown sugar or sugar substitute, bran cereal, oat bran flour, whole wheat flour, baking powder, salt, cinnamon, and nutmeg. Stir to combine.

In a medium mixing bowl, whisk together the egg, oil, vanilla, almond extract, yogurt, zucchini, and applesauce, just enough to combine. (The batter should be slightly lumpy.)

Fill the muffin cups two-thirds full with batter. Bake for 20 to 25 minutes, until a toothpick inserted into the middle of a muffin comes out clean. Let the muffins cool for 15 minutes before turning the tin over to release the muffins. (If the muffins stick to the pan, a slight tap on the back should help to release them.)

YIELD: Makes 12 (about 2-ounce) muffins.

NUTRITIONAL ANALYSIS

Each with: **Calories:** 121 **Protein:** 3.8 g **Carbs:** 23.6 g **Total Fat:** 2.18 g **Sat Fat:** 0.26 g **Cholesterol:** 20.42 mg **Sodium:** 157.62 mg **Sugars:** 8.72 g **Fiber:** 3.39 g

MARGARET'S NOTE

If you leave out the brown sugar, each serving of this recipe will provide: Calories: 101 Protein: 4 g Carbs: 18 g Total Fat: 2 g Sugars: 3 g.

Bacon-Cheddar Muffins

You can't go wrong with the flavors of bacon and cheese. To save time, prepare the bacon strips per the package instructions, then chop or break them into crumbles.

TEXTURE: Regular

INGREDIENTS

- ¹/₂ cup (55 g) all-purpose flour
- ¹/₂ cup (70 g) coarse yellow cornmeal
- 1 teaspoon baking powder
- ¹/₂ teaspoon baking soda
- ¹/₈ teaspoon salt
- ¹/₂ cup (120 ml) low-fat buttermilk
- 1 egg
- 2 tablespoons (15 g) chopped green onion
- ¹/₂ cup (55 g) reduced-fat shredded Cheddar cheese
- ¹/₄ cup (20 g) turkey bacon crumbles, prepared as per package instructions (about 4 strips)

Preheat the oven to 375°F (190°C, or gas mark 5). Spray a muffin tin with cooking spray.

In a large mixing bowl, combine the flour, cornmeal, baking powder, baking soda, and salt. Stir to combine.

In a medium mixing bowl, whisk together the buttermilk, egg, green onion, cheese, and bacon, just enough to combine. (The batter should be slightly lumpy.)

Fill 8 of the muffin cups two-thirds full with batter. Bake for 20 to 25 minutes, until a toothpick inserted into the middle of a muffin comes out clean. Let the muffins cool for 15 minutes before turning the tin over to release the muffins. (If the muffins stick to the pan, a slight tap on the back should help to release them.)

YIELD: Makes 8 (2-ounce) muffins.

NUTRITIONAL ANALYSIS
Each with: **Calories:** 101.19 **Protein:** 5.47 g **Carbs:** 12.34 g **Total Fat:** 3.65 g **Sat Fat:** 1.38 g **Cholesterol:** 39.36 mg **Sodium:** 380.42 mg **Sugars:** 0.91 g **Fiber:** 1.01 g

CHAPTER 3

Lunches

Cumin Mushroom Quesadillas

Quesadillas are a great appetizer, or double the amount of mushrooms for a quick and easy entrée. Serve them with Fresh Salsa Caliente (page 162).

TEXTURE: Regular

INGREDIENTS

- $1/2$ pound (225 g) white or crimini mushrooms
- 1 tablespoon (14 g) low-fat butter alternative
- 1 tablespoon (14 ml) olive oil
- 1 small clove garlic, minced
- 2 teaspoons ground cumin
- $1/8$ teaspoon cayenne pepper (optional)
- $1/4$ teaspoon paprika
- $1/2$ teaspoon kosher salt or sea salt
- 2 tablespoons (25 g) nonfat sour cream
- 4 low-carb whole-wheat tortillas
- $3/4$ cup (85 g) reduced-fat shredded Cheddar cheese
- $1/4$ cup (4 g) chopped fresh cilantro

Clean the mushrooms with a mushroom brush or paper towels. Cut the end of the stems away and discard. Slice the mushrooms into thin pieces.

In a medium nonstick skillet, heat the butter alternative and oil over medium heat. Add the mushrooms, garlic, cumin, pepper (if using), paprika, and salt. Sauté, stirring often, for 8 minutes, until the mushrooms become soft. Stir in the sour cream and continue cooking for 2 minutes, stirring once or twice. Remove the pan from the heat.

Preheat the oven to 375°F (190°C, or gas mark 5). Place the tortillas on a baking sheet. Equally divide the mushrooms on half of each tortilla. Equally divide the cheese and distribute over the mushrooms.

Fold the empty half of each tortilla over the mushroom half. Bake the quesadillas for about 12 minutes, until the cheese has melted.

YIELD: Makes 4 quesadillas.

NUTRITIONAL ANALYSIS
Each with: **Calories:** 168.22 **Protein:** 12.06 g **Carbs:** 16.69 g **Total Fat:** 9.03 g **Sat Fat:** 2.98 g **Cholesterol:** 12.50 mg **Sodium:** 635.33 mg **Sugars:** 1.59 g **Fiber:** 10.19 g

Classic Turkey and Swiss Wrap

Many people have a hard time with breads after any kind of weight-loss surgery, but many of my patients tell me they can tolerate pita bread, wrap or lavash bread, and thin and/or toasted breads. As always when trying a new food for the first time after your weight loss surgery, try only a small amount at a time and listen to your body.

Here's a wrapped version of the classic turkey and Swiss cheese sandwich, only with less carbs, calories, and fat.

TEXTURE: Regular

INGREDIENTS

- 2 tablespoons (30 g) nonfat mayonnaise
- 2 teaspoons prepared sweet mustard
- 1/8 teaspoon black pepper
- 4 (9-inch, or 22.5-cm) low-carb tortillas
- 4 whole green or red leaf lettuce leaves
- 12 ounces (340 g) thin sliced roasted turkey, skin and fat removed
- 4 slices (4 ounces, or 115 g) low-fat, low-sodium Swiss cheese
- 2 Italian plum tomatoes, cored and cut lengthwise into 8 slices
- 8 thin red onion ring slices

In a small bowl, combine the mayonnaise, mustard, and pepper. Spread the mixture equally onto 4 tortillas. Next, layer the lettuce, then the turkey, Swiss cheese, tomato, and onion.

Wrap the tortillas tightly around the filing, wrap the roll in plastic wrap, and refrigerate for at least one hour before serving. To serve, cut each wrap in half.

YIELD: Makes 8 (1/2-wrap) servings

NUTRITIONAL ANALYSIS
Each with: **Calories:** 151.44 **Protein:** 17.23 g **Carbs:** 11.63 g **Total Fat:** 6.54 g **Sat Fat:** 2.01 g **Cholesterol:** 32.50 mg **Sodium:** 438.73 mg **Sugars:** 2.02 g **Fiber:** 7.31 g

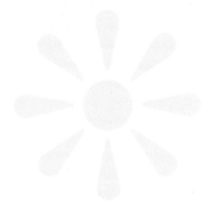

Spinach-Turkey Wraps

These wraps are an easy and nutritious lunch and a great way to use up leftover turkey!

TEXTURE: Regular

INGREDIENTS

- 4 ounces (115 g) nonfat cream cheese
- 2 tablespoons (15 g) sliced green onions
- 1 teaspoon Dijon mustard
- 4 (9-inch, or 22.5-cm) low-carb tortillas
- 1⅓ cups (40 g) fresh spinach, shredded
- 6 ounces (170 g) thinly sliced roasted turkey breast, skin and fat removed
- ¼ cup (25 g) reduced-fat shredded Cheddar or Jack cheese
- 2 tablespoons (20 g) minced red bell pepper

In a small bowl, combine the cream cheese, green onions, and Dijon mustard. Spread the mixture equally onto the tortillas. Next, add in equal portions the spinach, turkey, cheese, and bell pepper. Wrap the tortillas tightly around the filling, wrap the rolls in plastic wrap, and refrigerate for at least one hour before serving.

YIELD: Makes 4 wraps.

NUTRITIONAL ANALYSIS
Each with: **Calories:** 184.53 **Protein:** 23.07 g **Carbs:** 21.83 g **Total Fat:** 6.35 g **Sat Fat:** 1.11 g **Cholesterol:** 28.54 mg **Sodium:** 758.59 mg **Sugars:** 1.39 g **Fiber:** 14.47 g

LYNETTE'S NOTE

Wraps are also great for snacks or appetizers. Simply cut each one into fourths for smaller portions.

We've all undoubtedly heard the quote, "Everything in moderation." It's good advice for so many applications, especially when it comes to foods we love to eat.

This and the sandwiches that follow are worthy of your finest luncheons or special occasions.

When making a sandwich, choose a type of bread that is appropriate for your diet. Breads made with the least processed flours are most beneficial, thus whole grains are non-negotiable. In addition, there are a variety of reduced-fat and reduced-carbohydrate breads. Surgical weight-loss patients generally tolerate toasted breads best, and they don't do well with thicker or doughy breads. Pita and roll-up breads tend to be well-tolerated, but everyone is different, so try a little and see how you feel.

Avocado, Cream Cheese, and Bacon Sandwich

My favorite way to make this sandwich is on toasted honey wheat berry bread.

TEXTURE: Regular

INGREDIENTS

- 1 ounce (28 g) nonfat cream cheese
- 2 slices toasted diet wheat bread
- 2 slices low-sodium turkey bacon, or veggie bacon strips, precooked
- $1/8$ ripe avocado, cut into thin slices

Spread the cream cheese equally on each slice of bread. Break or cut the bacon strips in half, then distribute them on one slice. Next, layer the avocado slices on top of the bacon and top with the other slice of bread. Cut diagonally and serve.

YIELD: Makes 1 serving.

NUTRITIONAL ANALYSIS

Each with: **Calories:** 223.9 **Protein:** 13.12 g **Carbs:** 24.67 g **Total Fat:** 10.27 g **Sat Fat:** 2.16 g **Cholesterol:** 22.27 mg **Sodium:** 770.32 mg **Sugars:** 2.45 g **Fiber:** 7.65 g

Mediterranean Chicken Salad Sandwich

Here's a new twist on an old favorite.

TEXTURE: Regular

INGREDIENTS

- 4 ounces (115 g) cooked boneless, skinless chicken breast, diced small
- 2 large pitted black olives, sliced
- 1 teaspoon minced onion
- 2 teaspoons finely chopped tomato
- 1 teaspoon fresh finely chopped parsley
- Fresh cracked black pepper to taste (optional)
- $^1/_2$ teaspoon capers, chopped or crushed
- 2 teaspoons nonfat mayonnaise
- $^1/_2$ teaspoon lemon juice
- 2 toasted whole grain English muffin halves
- 2 sprigs fresh parsley

In a small bowl, combine the chicken, olives, onion, tomato, chopped parsley, pepper (if using), capers, mayonnaise, and lemon juice. Mix well. Top each toasted English muffin half with half of the chicken salad and garnish with a parsley sprig.

YIELD: Makes 2 ($^1/_2$-sandwich) servings.

NUTRITIONAL ANALYSIS

Each with: **Calories:** 136.93 **Protein:** 15.87 g **Carbs:** 13.93 g **Total Fat:** 1.9 g **Sat Fat:** 0.29 g
Cholesterol: 32.89 mg **Sodium:** 335.21 mg **Sugars:** 3.06 g **Fiber:** 2.15 g

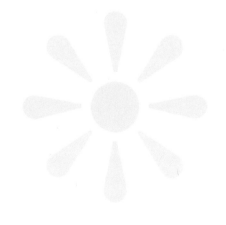

Classic Turkey, Cranberry, and Cream Cheese Sandwich

This is a refreshing, light sandwich you'll want to give thanks for.

TEXTURE: Regular

INGREDIENTS

- 2 slices diet whole grain bread, toasted
- 1 teaspoon nonfat mayonnaise
- 2 teaspoons reduced-fat cream cheese
- 2 tablespoons (25 g) cranberry sauce
- 2 ounces (55 g) sliced turkey meat, no skin or fat
- 1 leaf green or red leaf lettuce

On one slice of the bread, spread the mayonnaise, and spread the cream cheese on the other. On top of the cream cheese, spread the cranberry sauce. Place the turkey on top of the cranberry sauce and the lettuce on top of the turkey. Top with the remaining slice of toast and cut in half.

YIELD: Makes 1 (sandwich) serving.

NUTRITIONAL ANALYSIS
Each with: **Calories:** 214.83 **Protein:** 17.28 g **Carbs:** 27.64 g **Total Fat:** 5.08 g **Sat Fat:** 1.49 g **Cholesterol:** 36.67 mg **Sodium:** 640.71 mg **Sugars:** 8.43 g **Fiber:** 5.76 g

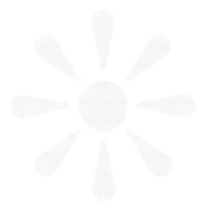

Ultimate Veggie Sandwich

A true-blue vegetarian sandwich should contain a few standard ingredients such as avocado, cucumber, and alfalfa sprouts. After that, it's really up to your personal taste. Here's the recipe for my favorite veggie sandwich.

TEXTURE: Regular

INGREDIENTS

- 2 slices diet whole grain bread, toasted
- $1/4$ ripe avocado (should be slightly soft to the touch on the outside)
- 1 teaspoon nonfat cream cheese
- Small pinch salt
- Small pinch pepper
- 3 thinly sliced red onion rings
- 3 thinly sliced green bell pepper rings
- 2 $5/8$-inch (6.25-cm) thick slices tomato
- 6 thinly sliced cucumber coins, peeled
- 1-inch (2.5-cm) layer alfalfa sprouts

On one slice of bread, spread the avocado, and spread the cream cheese on the other. On top of the avocado, layer the salt, pepper, onion, bell pepper, tomato, cucumber, and sprouts. Top with the remaining slice of bread, spear with toothpicks, cut in half, and serve.

YIELD: Makes 1 (sandwich) serving.

NUTRITIONAL ANALYSIS
Each with: **Calories:** 209.10 **Protein:** 8.05 g **Carbs:** 30.22 g **Total Fat:** 9.02 g **Sat Fat:** 1.76 g **Cholesterol:** 0.76 mg **Sodium:** 291.33 mg **Sugars:** 5.57 g **Fiber:** 10.83 g

Fresh Mozzarella Tomato and Tapenade Sandwich

Tapenade is a delicious (usually pureed) olive spread that can be found in most grocery stores. It's very salty nature is a wonderful complement to the rich creaminess of fresh mozzarella when used in moderation.

TEXTURE: Regular

INGREDIENTS

- 2 slices diet whole grain bread, toasted
- 2 teaspoons nonfat mayonnaise
- 1 teaspoon olive tapenade
- 2 slices (2 ounces, or 55 g) fresh mozzarella cheese (Press the moisture out a bit with paper towels.)
- $2^5/_8$-inch (6.25-cm) thick slices tomato
- Fresh cracked black pepper (optional)

On both slices of bread, spread the mayonnaise evenly. On one slice, spread the tapenade, and then layer the mozzarella, then the tomato. Sprinkle a few turns of pepper on top of the tomatoes (if using). Top with the remaining slice of bread. Spear each corner of the bread with a toothpick about 1 inch (2.5 cm) from the edge of the corner, cut into fourths diagonally, and serve.

YIELD: Makes 1 (sandwich) serving.

NUTRITIONAL ANALYSIS

Each with: **Calories:** 263.70 **Protein:** 14.43 g **Carbs:** 24.70 g **Total Fat:** 13.15 g **Sat Fat:** 0.17 g **Cholesterol:** 40.00 mg **Sodium:** 370.11 mg **Sugars:** 4.87 g **Fiber:** 5.83 g

Baked Ham and Cheese Sandwich

TEXTURE: Regular

INGREDIENTS

- 2 slices fresh diet whole-grain bread
- 2 teaspoons nonfat mayonnaise
- $^1/_2$ teaspoon Dijon mustard
- 2 ounces (55 g) reduced-sodium, reduced-fat sliced ham
- $2^5/_8$-inch (6.25-cm) thick slices tomato
- 1 slice (1 ounce, or 28 g) reduced-fat Swiss cheese

Preheat the oven to 350°F (180°C, or gas mark 4).

On one slice of bread, spread the mayonnaise and spread the mustard on the other. Place the ham on one slice, then the tomato slices, then the cheese. Top with the remaining slice of bread and place on a sheet pan. Bake the sandwich for about 12 minutes, until the bread is nicely toasted and the cheese is melted. Cut in half and serve warm.

YIELD: Makes 1 (sandwich) serving.

NUTRITIONAL ANALYSIS

Each with: **Calories:** 266.32 **Protein:** 24.23 g **Carbs:** 26.99 g **Total Fat:** 8.21 g **Sat Fat:** 2.98 g **Cholesterol:** 43.00 mg **Sodium:** 812.66 mg **Sugars:** 3.83 g **Fiber:** 6.14 g

MARGARET'S NOTE

This recipe is high in sodium because of the ham. If sodium is a problem for you, substitute 2 ounces (55 g) of low-sodium turkey or roast beef for the ham in this sandwich.

Leftover Salmon Sandwich

Delicious and satisfying flavor doesn't get any easier than this! However you prepared your salmon dinner, this easy recipe will make it just as delicious for lunch.

TEXTURE: Regular

INGREDIENTS

- 6 ounces (170 g) leftover salmon, skin and bones removed
- 1 tablespoon (15 g) nonfat mayonnaise
- 2 whole-grain English muffin halves, toasted
- 2 5/8-inch (6.25-cm) thick tomato slices

In a small bowl, mix the salmon with the mayonnaise. Top each muffin half with a tomato slice, then the salmon mixture, and serve.

YIELD: Makes 2 (1/2-sandwich) servings.

NUTRITIONAL ANALYSIS

Each with: **Calories:** 228.31 **Protein:** 24.59 g **Carbs:** 14.82 g **Total Fat:** 7.66 g **Sat Fat:** 1.18 g **Cholesterol:** 60.35 mg **Sodium:** 306.33 mg **Sugars:** 3.79 g **Fiber:** 2.38 g

Turkey Sandwich with Cucumbers and Herbed Cream Cheese

This sandwich is light and refreshing.

TEXTURE: Regular

INGREDIENTS

- 2 ounces (55 g) nonfat cream cheese
- 1/4 teaspoon chopped fresh chives
- 1/4 teaspoon chopped fresh tarragon
- 1/4 teaspoon chopped fresh parsley
- 2 slices diet whole-grain bread, toasted
- 6 thinly sliced cucumber coins, peeled
- 2 ounces (55 g) sliced turkey breast, no skin or fat

In a small bowl, mix together the cream cheese, chives, tarragon, and parsley. Spread half of the mixture on each slice of the bread.

Place the cucumber evenly atop the cream cheese mixture, then place the turkey on top of the cucumber. Top with the remaining slice of bread and serve.

YIELD: Makes 1 (sandwich) serving.

NUTRITIONAL ANALYSIS

Each with: **Calories:** 221.74 **Protein:** 24.68 g **Carbs:** 24.46 g **Total Fat:** 3.92 g **Sat Fat:** 0.68 g **Cholesterol:** 34.54 mg **Sodium:** 865.28 mg **Sugars:** 2.29 g **Fiber:** 5.87 g

Awesome Egg Salad Sandwich

Here's an "egg-citing" sandwich indeed!

TEXTURE: Regular

INGREDIENTS

- 2 whole hard-boiled eggs
- 2 hard-boiled eggs, whites only
- 2 teaspoons nonfat mayonnaise
- 1/4 teaspoon Dijon mustard
- 1 teaspoon finely chopped chives
- 1/8 teaspoon celery seed
- 2 whole-grain English muffin halves, toasted

In a small bowl, crush the hard-boiled eggs and egg whites with a fork. Add the mayonnaise, mustard, chives, and celery seed and mix to combine. Top each muffin half with half of the egg salad and serve.

YIELD: Makes 2 (1/2 sandwich) servings.

NUTRITIONAL ANALYSIS

Each with: **Calories:** 164.78 **Protein:** 13.40 g **Carbs:** 14.57 g **Total Fat:** 5.79 g **Sat Fat:** 1.61 g **Cholesterol:** 240.01 mg **Sodium:** 364.78 mg **Sugars:** 4.07 g **Fiber:** 2.11 g

Bacon, Tomato, Lettuce, and Cream Cheese Sandwich

Add cream cheese to this standard for a delightful combination of flavors.

TEXTURE: Regular

INGREDIENTS

- 2 slices diet whole grain bread, toasted
- 1 ounce (28 g) nonfat cream cheese
- 2 strips reduced-sodium, reduced-fat turkey bacon or veggie bacon
- 2 5/8-inch (6.25-cm) thick slices tomato
- 2 red or green leaf lettuce leaves, stems removed
- Fresh cracked black pepper (optional)

On each slice of bread, evenly spread the cream cheese. Place the bacon strips in a cross from corner to corner on one slice. Layer the tomato, the pepper (if using), then the lettuce leaves, and top with the remaining slice of bread. Spear each half of the sandwich with a toothpick, cut in half, and serve.

YIELD: Makes 1 (sandwich) serving.

NUTRITIONAL ANALYSIS

Each with: **Calories:** 186.63 **Protein:** 12.66 g **Carbs:** 23.50 g **Total Fat:** 6.55 g **Sat Fat:** 1.43 g **Cholesterol:** 22.27 mg **Sodium:** 773.58 mg **Sugars:** 2.64 g **Fiber:** 5.98 g

Best Ever Tofu Burger

Serve with whole wheat and/or low-carb whole-grain pita bread.

TEXTURE: Soft

INGREDIENTS

- 2 pounds (910 g) firm tofu (but not silken tofu), frozen at least 48 hours
- $1/2$ cup (120 ml) water
- 2 tablespoons (28 ml) soy sauce or mushroom soy sauce
- 2 tablespoons (30 g) ketchup
- 2 teaspoons Marmite, Vegemite, or other yeast extract (gives a "beefy" flavor) or 4 teaspoons red miso
- $1/4$ teaspoon fresh minced garlic (one small clove)
- $1/4$ teaspoon dried oregano
- $1/4$ teaspoon dried basil
- 2 tablespoons (20 g) minced fresh onion
- 6 $1/8$-inch- (3 mm-) thick slices tomato
- 6 leaves red leaf lettuce
- 12 slices whole-wheat bread or 6 low-carb, whole grain pitas

Thaw out the tofu. Slice each pound block into 3 thick slices. Place the slices on a cookie sheet covered with a couple of clean, folded tea towels. Cover the slices with more tea towels and another cookie sheet. Weigh this arrangement down with something heavy for about 30 minutes. Place the tofu in a single layer in a shallow container.

In a medium bowl, combine the water, soy sauce, ketchup, yeast extract, garlic, oregano, basil, and onion and pour over the prepared tofu slices. Cover and let marinate for at least 2 hours. (The tofu can marinate for up to 24 hours.)

Spray a heavy skillet or nonstick skillet with cooking spray. Heat it over medium-high heat. Pan-fry the tofu until browned on both sides. Top with the tomato and lettuce. Serve with the bread or pitas.

YIELD: Makes 6 (about 3-ounce) burgers.

NUTRITIONAL ANALYSIS

Each with: **Calories:** 150.68 **Protein:** 16.14 g **Carbs:** 6.98 g **Total Fat:** 6.54 g **Sat Fat:** 0.98 g **Cholesterol:** 0.00 mg **Sodium:** 221.77 mg **Sugars:** 3.43 g **Fiber:** 1.35 g

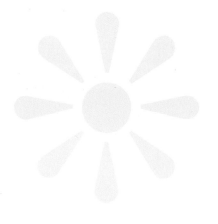

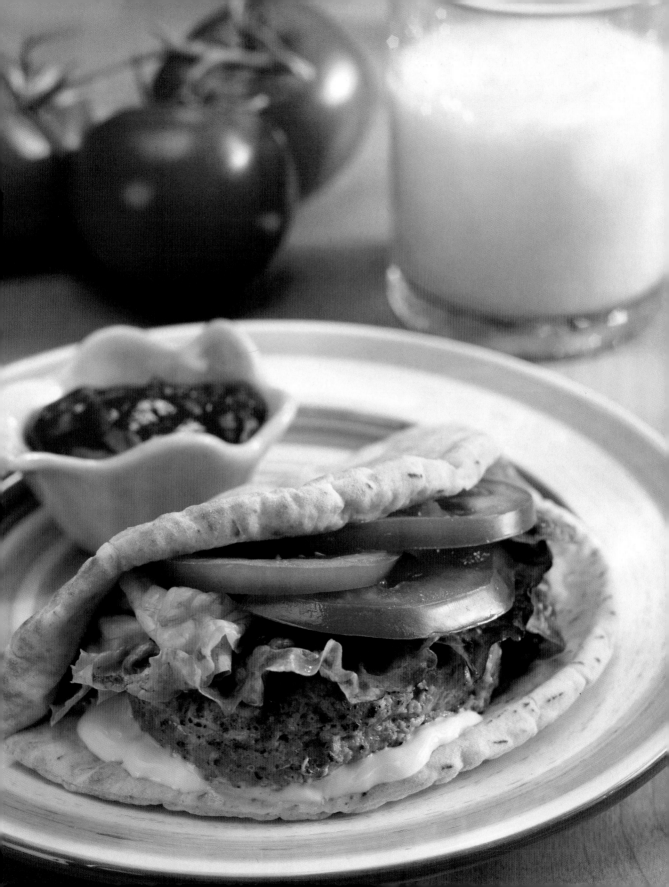

Zesty Turkey Burger Pita Pocket

TEXTURE: Regular

INGREDIENTS

- $^1/_2$ cup (80 g) diced onion
- $^1/_3$ cup (80 g) low-sodium, low-carb ketchup
- 1 teaspoon lemon-pepper seasoning
- 1 teaspoon cumin seed
- $^1/_4$ teaspoon cinnamon
- $^1/_8$ teaspoon black pepper
- 1 tablespoon chopped fresh cilantro
- 1 pound (455 g) extra lean ground turkey (97% fat-free, contains no skin)
- 4 (4-inch, or 10-cm) whole wheat pita pockets
- 4 teaspoons nonfat mayonnaise
- 4 $^1/_8$-inch (3-mm) thick tomato slices
- 4 red leaf lettuce leaves

Preheat the oven to 300°F (150°C, or gas mark 2).

In a medium mixing bowl, combine the onion, ketchup, lemon-pepper seasoning, cumin, cinnamon, pepper, cilantro, and turkey and mix thoroughly. Divide the turkey mixture into 4 equal portions, shaping each into a 1-inch- (2.5-cm-) thick patty.

Place a medium nonstick skillet over medium-heat until hot. Add the patties and cook for about 6 minutes on each side, until no longer pink. Remove burgers from the pan and let rest for 5 minutes.

Wrap the pita pockets in aluminum foil and bake for 10 minutes. Spread 1 teaspoon of mayonnaise inside each pita pocket. Place one burger patty in each pita pocket and top each patty with a slice of tomato and lettuce. Serve immediately.

YIELD: Makes 4 sandwiches.

NUTRITIONAL ANALYSIS
Each with: **Calories:** 239.88 **Protein:** 30.77 g **Carbs:** 25.71 g **Total Fat:** 2.70 g **Sat Fat:** 0.65 g **Cholesterol:** 55.00 mg **Sodium:** 273.07 mg **Sugars:** 6.91 g **Fiber:** 3.15 g

Asian Chicken Wrap

This is a delicious treat worthy of your favorite Asian restaurant. Eaten from the hands, theses wraps are a hit with kids.

TEXTURE: Regular

INGREDIENTS

- 1 tablespoon (14 ml) peanut oil
- 1 tablespoon (14 ml) toasted sesame oil
- 1 tablespoon (14 ml) rice vinegar
- 1 tablespoon (14 ml) low-sodium soy sauce
- 1 teaspoon garlic-chili sauce
- 1 teaspoon fresh grated ginger
- 1/2 teaspoon orange zest (grated orange peel)
- 1 clove fresh garlic, minced
- 4 (4 ounce, or 115 g) boneless, skinless chicken breast halves
- 1 cup (25 g) fresh mint leaves, coarsely chopped
- 1 cup (30 g) fresh baby spinach leaves, stems removed
- 1/2 cup (8 g) cilantro sprigs
- 1/2 cup (50 g) mung bean sprouts
- 8 whole Boston lettuce leaves (about 1 head)
- 1 lime, cut into 8 wedges
- 1 tablespoon (10 g) chopped peanuts (optional)

In a small bowl, combine the peanut oil, sesame oil, vinegar, soy sauce, garlic-chili sauce, ginger, orange zest, and garlic and stir vigorously with a wire whisk. Reserve 2 tablespoons (28 ml) of the mixture and place the rest in a zipper-type plastic bag along with the chicken and marinate in the refrigerator for 1 hour, turning once or twice. Remove the chicken from the bag and discard the marinade.

Coat a medium skillet with nonstick spray and heat it over medium-high heat. Add the chicken to the pan and cook for 6 minutes on each side. Remove the chicken from the pan and let stand while preparing the filling.

In a medium mixing bowl, combine the mint, spinach, cilantro, and bean sprouts. Add the reserved oil mixture and gently toss, just enough to expose all the surface area to the dressing, being careful not to break down the leafy structure.

Slice the chicken into thin strips. Place one sliced chicken breast atop one (or two stacked) lettuce leaves, then top the chicken with the spinach mixture. Garnish equally with chopped peanuts (if using).

YIELD: Makes 4 servings (about 3 ounces chicken and 1/4 cup vegetables each).

NUTRITIONAL ANALYSIS
Each with: **Calories:** 196.76 **Protein:** 29.01 g **Carbs:** 5.79 g **Total Fat:** 6.30 g **Sat Fat:** 0.84 g **Cholesterol:** 65.77 mg **Sodium:** 194.29 mg **Sugars:** 2.19 g **Fiber:** 2.65 g

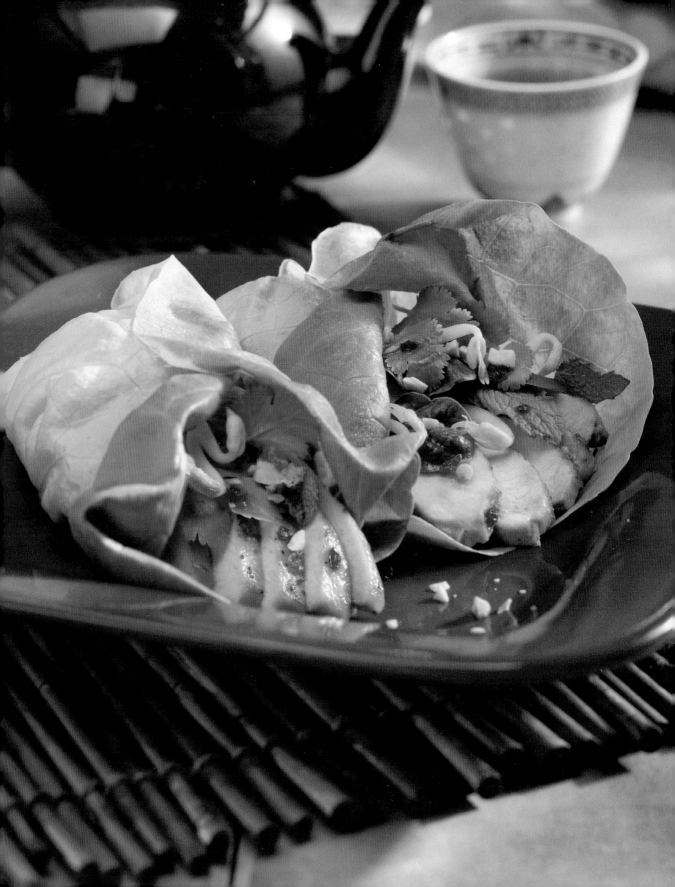

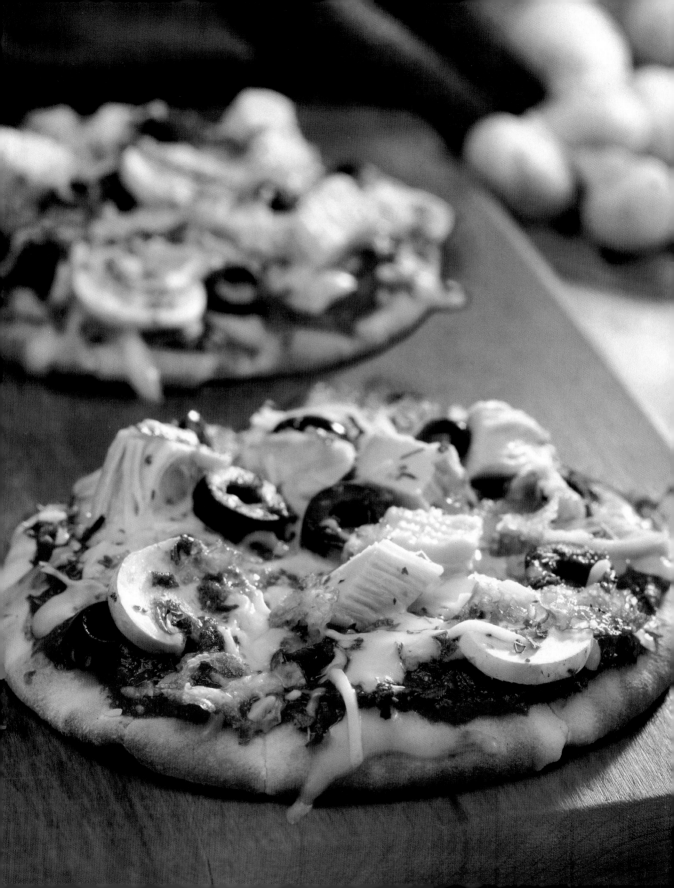

Pita Pizza

Pizza is always a crowd pleaser. Follow these instructions or vary the ingredients to satisfy your pickiest palate.

TEXTURE: Regular

INGREDIENTS

- 4 small (4-inch, or 10 cm) pita breads (whole wheat, preferably)
- 1 can (6 ounces, or 170 g) low-sodium tomato paste
- 1 teaspoon dried oregano
- 1 teaspoon dried basil
- 1 teaspoon dried thyme
- 4 tablespoons (20 g) grated Parmesan cheese
- 1 cup (140 g) cooked, boneless, skinless chicken breast, cut into $1/2$-inch (1.25-cm) cubes
- $1/2$ cup (30 g) sliced fresh mushrooms
- 1 can ($2^1/2$ ounces, or 70 g) sliced olives, drained
- $3/4$ cup (85 g) shredded part-skim mozzarella cheese

Preheat the oven to 375°F (190°C, or gas mark 5). Lightly spray a sheet pan with cooking spray.

Place the pita breads on the sheet pan. Spread about 2 tablespoons (30 g) tomato paste evenly onto each pita bread. Distribute the oregano, basil, thyme, Parmesan, chicken, mushrooms, olives, and mozzarella evenly onto the pizzas. Bake the pizzas for about 15 minutes, until the cheese is bubbly and begins to brown.

YIELD: Makes 4 (4-inch) pizzas.

NUTRITIONAL ANALYSIS
Each with: **Calories:** 284.45 **Protein:** 25.61 g **Carbs:** 24.80 g **Total Fat:** 9.39 g **Sat Fat:** 4.07 g **Cholesterol:** 47.14 mg **Sodium:** 538.32 mg **Sugars:** 5.50 g **Fiber:** 5.09 g

Variations

- In place of the chicken, try a pepperoni alternative (such as soy or vegetable), chicken Italian sausage (skins removed and pre-cooked), leanest ground turkey or beef (precooked and drained of excess grease and liquid).

- In place of the mushrooms and olives, try steamed asparagus tips, drained and sliced artichoke hearts, fresh Roma tomato slices, or fresh spinach leaves.

Vegetarian Sloppy Joe

Serve with vegetables and low-carb pita or lavash bread.

TEXTURE: Soft

INGREDIENTS

- 1 cup (160 g) chopped onion
- ¹/₃ cup (45) diced red bell pepper
- 1 clove fresh garlic, chopped
- ¹/₂ teaspoon ground oregano
- ¹/₂ teaspoon ground basil
- ¹/₂ teaspoon paprika
- ¹/₂ teaspoon cayenne pepper (optional)
- ³/₄ cup (180 g) soy crumbles
- 1 cup (240 g) low-carb ketchup
- 1 cup (244 g) tomato sauce, no added salt

Coat a large skillet with cooking spray and heat over medium-high heat. Add the onion, red pepper, garlic, oregano, basil, paprika, and cayenne pepper (if using). Continue cooking for about 5 minutes, until the onion and pepper begin to soften. Add the soy crumbles and continue cooking for an additional 5 minutes, stirring often. Add the ketchup and tomato sauce and continue cooking for an additional 8 to 10 minutes, stirring occasionally.

YIELD: Makes 4 (about 1-cup) servings.

NUTRITIONAL ANALYSIS
Each with: **Calories:** 208.07 **Protein:** 20.42 g **Carbs:** 18.65 g **Total Fat:** 3.55 g **Sat Fat:** 0.03 g **Cholesterol:** 0.00 mg **Sodium:** 429.05 mg **Sugars:** 9.17 g **Fiber:** 11.44 g

Tuna Salad Wrap To Go

This wrap is great for a healthy lunch or a picnic.

TEXTURE: Soft

INGREDIENTS

- $^3/_4$ cup (115 g) low-sodium tuna, packed in water, drained (see note)
- $^1/_4$ teaspoon salt
- 1 ounce (28 g) low-fat plain yogurt
- 2 teaspoons dill
- 1 teaspoon capers, drained
- $^1/_4$ teaspoon black pepper
- 2 (8-inch, or 20 cm) whole-wheat low-carb tortillas
- $^1/_2$ cup (15 g) alfalfa sprouts, washed, drained, and patted dry
- $^1/_4$ cup (7 g) fresh spinach, washed, drained, and patted dry

In a medium bowl, place the tuna, salt, yogurt, dill, capers, and pepper. Mix thoroughly and squeeze out or drain excess liquid. Place half of the tuna salad mixture in a horizontal line in the middle of each tortilla, leaving a good border for folding at the sides (at least 1½ inches, or 3.75 cm). Top each tortilla with half of the sprouts and half of the spinach. Fold each tortilla over the center from the bottom up. Fold in the sides toward the center. Ensure that you fold the top down snuggly but not so much that you break the tortilla. Wrap the tortillas individually in plastic wrap.

YIELD: Makes 2 sandwiches.

NUTRITIONAL ANALYSIS
Each with: **Calories:** 168.85 **Protein:** 26.33 g **Carbs:** 14.49 g **Total Fat:** 3.09 g **Sat Fat:** 0.27 g **Cholesterol:** 38.35 mg **Sodium:** 568.58 mg **Sugars:** 0.55 g **Fiber:** 9.91 g

LYNETTE'S NOTE

If made the night before and stored in the fridge, these wraps will hold for an easy, on-the-go lunch or dinner.

MARGARET'S NOTE

If you don't have blood pressure issues, are not salt-sensitive, or if you have low blood pressure, you may opt for tuna packed in water that is not low in salt. This will increase the sodium content of this recipe by approximately 750 milligrams. So if you do this, you may wish to omit the salt in the recipe.

CHAPTER 4

Soups

Curried Carrot Soup

TEXTURE: Pureed. May be considered full liquid by some meal programs

INGREDIENTS

- 3 pounds (1.5 kg) carrots, peeled and cut into 2-inch (5-cm) pieces
- 1 large russet potato, diced into $^1/_2$-inch (1.25-cm) pieces
- 4 quarts (4 L) water
- 1 large yellow onion, diced into $^1/_4$-inch (6-mm) pieces
- 4 quarts (4 L) low-sodium vegetable broth
- 3 tablespoons (20 g) curry powder
- 2 teaspoon cayenne pepper (optional)
- 1 teaspoon cinnamon
- 1 teaspoon ground coriander seed
- $^1/_4$ cup (60 ml) lemon juice
- Paprika

In a 6-quart (6-L) soup pot, place the carrots, potato, and water. Bring to a boil, and then add the onion. Continue cooking for 12 to 15 minutes, until the carrots and potatoes are soft throughout. Drain in a colander, reserving half the liquid in a separate container, and set aside. Place the carrot mixture in a food processor fitted with a metal S blade and puree. (You may need to do this in batches.)

Return the pureed mixture to the soup pot. Add the broth, curry powder, cayenne pepper (if using), cinnamon, coriander, and lemon juice. Stir the mixture until an even consistency is reached. Cover and simmer over low heat for about 30 minutes. If a thinner consistency is desired, slowly add the reserved liquid from the carrots and potatoes until the desired consistency is reached. (The more liquid you add, the weaker the flavor becomes.) Serve in warmed bowls with a pinch of paprika sprinkled over the top for garnish.

YIELD: Makes 5 (1-cup) servings.

NUTRITIONAL ANALYSIS
Each with: **Calories:** 233.64 **Protein:** 8.18 g **Carbs:** 49.37 g **Total Fat:** 1.45 g **Sat Fat:** 0.23 g **Cholesterol:** 0.00 mg **Sodium:** 387.76 mg **Sugars:** 14.63 g **Fiber:** 11.51 g

"The carrot soup was absolutely delicious!"

—Mary Kate,
a gastric bypass patient in the Boston area

Green Tomato Soup with Fresh Tarragon

Here's a great way to use the green tomatoes left on the summer gardener's vines.

TEXTURE: Pureed. May be considered full liquid by some meal programs

INGREDIENTS

- 1 tablespoon (14 ml) extra-virgin olive oil
- Olive-oil-flavored cooking spray
- 3 cups (480 g) diced yellow onion
- 8 medium green tomatoes, cored and chopped into 1-inch (2.5-cm) pieces
- 2 teaspoons coriander seed
- 2½ teaspoons fresh tarragon leaves
- 2 cups (475 ml) natural low-sodium chicken broth
- Salt (optional)
- ½ teaspoon fresh cracked black pepper
- ¼ cup (50 g) nonfat sour cream or nonfat plain yogurt (optional)
- 4 sprigs fresh tarragon

In a 6-quart (6-L) stockpot or Dutch oven, heat the oil and cooking spray over medium-high heat. Add the onion, tomatoes, coriander, tarragon leaves, salt (if using), and pepper. Sauté the mixture, stirring just enough to expose all ingredients to the heat surface. Continue to sauté until soft, but do not brown. Remove the pot from the heat and let the mixture cool for 10 minutes.

Place the mixture into a food processor fitted with metal S blade or blender and pulse until almost pureed consistency. Return the mixture to the pot and add the broth. Bring to a simmer, cover, and continue simmering for 20 minutes. Check the seasoning and adjust with salt if necessary. Serve in warmed soup bowls with a dollop of sour cream or yogurt (if using) and the tarragon sprigs.

YIELD: Makes 5 (1-cup) servings.

NUTRITIONAL ANALYSIS
Each with: **Calories:** 123.29 **Protein:** 4.64 g **Carbs:** 20.81 g **Total Fat:** 3.42 g **Sat Fat:** 0.49 g **Cholesterol:** 0.00 mg **Sodium:** 220.90 mg **Sugars:** 11.98 g **Fiber:** 3.87 g

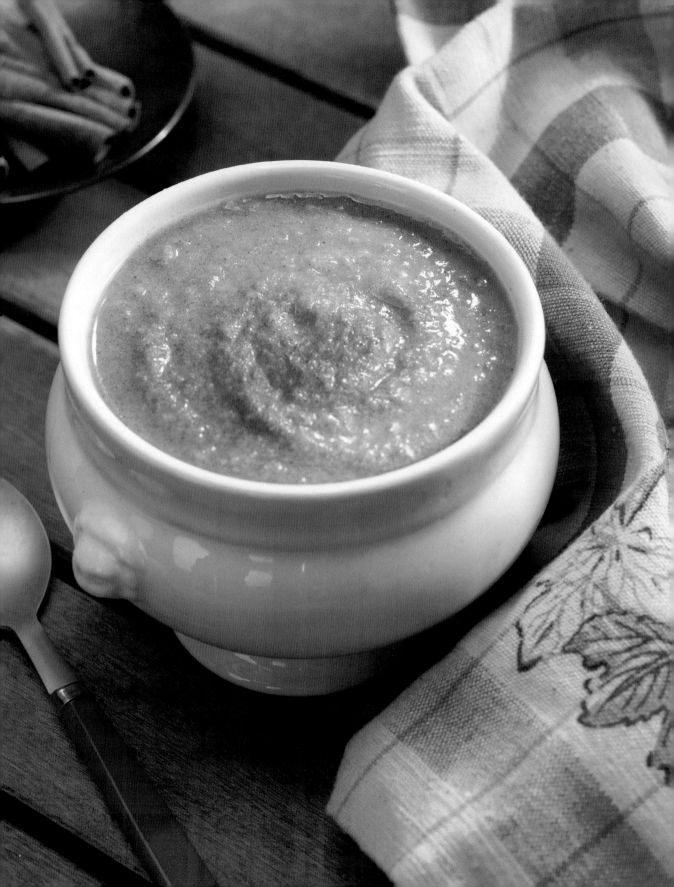

Fall Harvest Pumpkin Soup

This soup is delicious, fun, and a great source of vitamin A. Include the curry powder and cayenne pepper if you like a lot of heat.

TEXTURE: Pureed

INGREDIENTS

- 3 cups (735 g) pureed canned pumpkin (no salt) or 1 (5-pound, or 2.5 kg) sugar pumpkin
- 1 large yellow onion, diced
- 2 large celery ribs cut into $1/2$-inch (1.25-cm) pieces
- 1 quart (1 L) low-sodium chicken stock
- $1/2$ cup (120 ml) white wine, cooking sherry, chicken broth, or vegetable broth
- 2 teaspoons cinnamon, plus more for garnish (optional)
- 2 teaspoons allspice
- 2 teaspoons curry powder (optional)
- 2 teaspoons paprika
- $1/2$ teaspoon cumin
- 1 teaspoon cayenne pepper (optional)
- $1/2$ teaspoon ground white pepper
- $3/4$ cup (175 ml) nonfat half-and-half (see note)

If using fresh pumpkin, preheat the oven to 375°F (190°C, or gas mark 5).

Cut the pumpkin in half and scrape out the seed and strings. Cut the halves into quarters. Place the pumpkin, skin-side down, in a $9^1/_2$- x $13^1/_2$-inch (22.5- x 32.5-cm) or 3-quart (3-L) baking dish, with about $1/2$ inch (1.25 cm) of water in it. Bake the pumpkin for about 60 minutes, until the flesh is tender throughout. Let it cool and scrape out the flesh.

Puree the pumpkin using a hand mixer, blender, or food processor. (You'll have about 3 cups puree.)

In a 4-quart (4-L) soup pot, place the chicken stock, onion, and celery. Cover and bring it to a simmer. Continue cooking for about 15 minutes, until the vegetables are soft and translucent. With a slotted spoon or small mesh strainer, remove the vegetables and puree, using the same method as the pumpkin. Return the vegetables to the chicken stock and add the pumpkin puree. Add the wine (or sherry or broth), cinnamon, allspice, curry powder (if using), paprika, cumin, cayenne pepper (if using), and white pepper. Slowly stir in the half-and-half. Bring it back to a simmer and continue cooking for about 20 minutes, stirring occasionally. Serve in warmed soup bowls, and garnish with a light sprinkle of cinnamon (if using).

YIELD: Makes 6 (1-cup) servings.

NUTRITIONAL ANALYSIS

Each with: **Calories:** 151.17 **Protein:** 5.82 g **Carbs:** 21.99 g **Total Fat:** 3.58 g **Sat Fat:** 0.72 g **Cholesterol:** 4.54 mg **Sodium:** 252.18 mg **Sugars:** 7.44 g **Fiber:** 5.13 g

MARGARET'S NOTE

If you use light half-and-half instead of nonfat, the sugar content will increase to 9 grams per serving, which is still within the 14 grams or less per serving as my general recommendation for weight-loss surgery patients. However, if you use low-sugar, the sugar content will decrease to 3 grams per serving. The taste difference may or may not be noticeable, depending on your individual preferences. Either one is nutritionally acceptable.

Chilled Honeydew Soup with Spearmint

This cold soup is a summertime crowd-pleaser! It can be served as an appetizer, between courses to cleanse the palate, or as a light dessert.

TEXTURE: Pureed

INGREDIENTS

- 1 honeydew melon
- $1/4$ cup (60 ml) lemon juice
- $1/2$ cup (120 ml) cooking sherry or alcohol-free white wine
- 2 tablespoons (11 g) chopped spearmint leaves
- 8 sprigs fresh spearmint (optional)

Cut the melon in half and scrape out and discard the seeds. Using a tablespoon, scrape all of the flesh into a food processor fitted with a metal S blade. Add the lemon juice, sherry or wine, and chopped spearmint. Puree the mixture just until it has a liquid consistency. Place it into a 3-quart (3-L) container with an airtight lid and chill it in the refrigerator for at least 1 hour. Stir and serve in chilled dessert bowls or martini glasses. Garnish with the spearmint sprigs (if using).

YIELD: Makes 8 (about $1/2$-cup) servings.

NUTRITIONAL ANALYSIS:
Each with: **Calories:** 73.60 **Protein:** 0.94 g **Carbs:** 15.39 g **Total Fat:** 0.23 g **Sat Fat:** 0.06 g **Cholesterol:** 0.00 mg **Sodium:** 114.35 mg **Sugars:** 13.25 g **Fiber:** 1.41 g

MARGARET'S NOTE

The serving size above is half the usual serving of soups in this book because the content of sugars is too high using the 1-cup serving (because of the fruit). The $1/2$-cup serving provides 13 grams of sugars, which is within the 14 grams or less per serving needed to avoid dumping syndrome. Gastric banding patients, or those who are not sensitive to sugars, can enjoy a larger portion (such as 1 cup), because this is a low-fat, healthy soup.

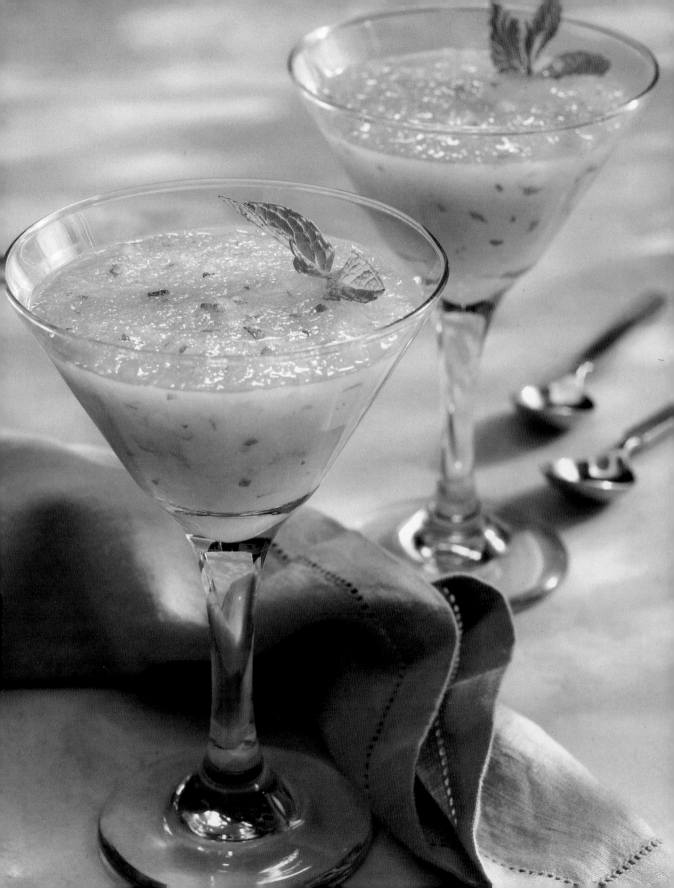

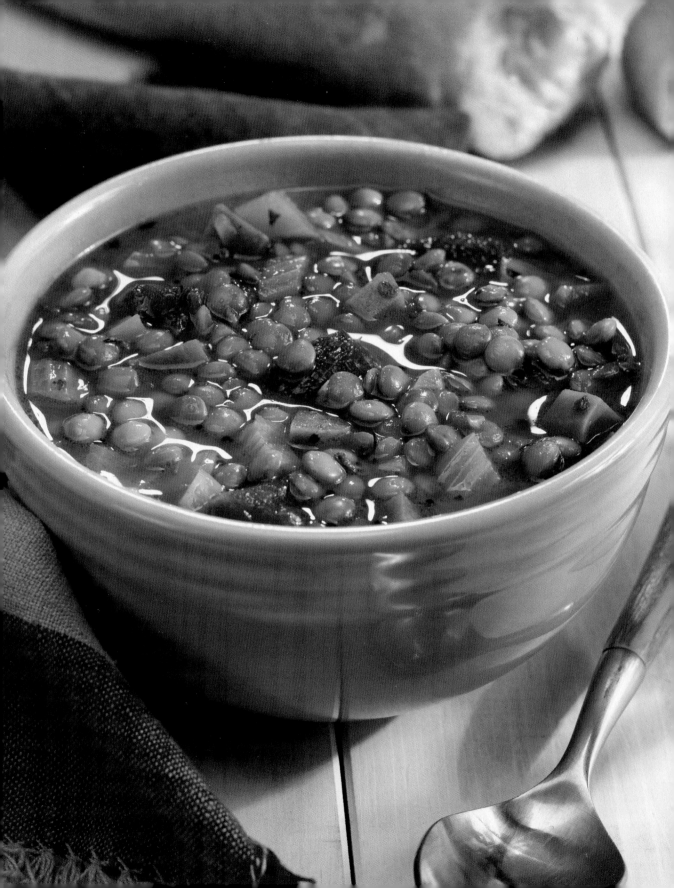

Lentil Soup

Rich in fiber, protein, and iron, this soup is tasty, too.

TEXTURE: Soft

INGREDIENTS

- 1 tablespoon (14 ml) extra-virgin olive oil
- 1 cup (130 g) diced carrot (about 1 large)
- ³/₄ cup (120 g) diced yellow onion (about 1 medium)
- 1 cup (100 g) diced celery (about 1 large rib)
- 2 cloves fresh garlic, chopped
- 2 bay leaves
- 1 tablespoon (14 ml) low-sodium tamari soy sauce
- ¹/₂ teaspoon black pepper
- 1 teaspoon dried oregano
- 1 teaspoon dried thyme
- 1 can (14.5 ounces, or 415 g) plum tomatoes, drained
- 2 cups (385 g) green lentils, soaked for 30 minutes (see note)
- 4¹/₂ cups (1 L) water
- Water or low-sodium vegetable broth (optional)
- 6 sprigs fresh thyme

In a 3-quart (3-L) stockpot or soup pot over medium-high heat, heat the oil. Add the carrot, onion, celery, garlic, bay leaves, tamari soy sauce, pepper, oregano, and dried thyme, and cook until the carrots begin to soften. Break apart the tomatoes by crushing them with your hands, then add them to the pot. Drain the lentils and then add them to the pot. Add the water and bring to a boil. Reduce the heat to a soft boil, cover partially, and cook for 20 minutes, until the lentils become soft throughout. If a thinner consistency is desired, add additional water or low-sodium vegetable broth in small amounts at a time. (Adding too much water to the soup will decrease the strength in flavor.) Remove the bay leaves prior to serving. Garnish with the thyme sprigs and serve in warmed soup bowls.

YIELD: Makes about 6 (1-cup) servings.

NUTRITIONAL ANALYSIS

Each with: **Calories:** 312.58 **Protein:** 20.20 g **Carbs:** 48.78 g **Total Fat:** 4.91 g **Sat Fat:** 1.04 g **Cholesterol:** 0.00 mg **Sodium:** 393.70 mg **Sugars:** 10.79 g **Fiber:** 23.14 g

MARGARET'S NOTE

Although lentils are high in protein, they need to be soaked for at least 30 minutes to help remove the phytates (natural mineral binders) that might impede the absorption of iron.

Creamy Tomato Parmesan Soup

TEXTURE: Pureed

INGREDIENTS

- 1 cup (150 g) peeled and diced Yukon Gold potatoes (about 1 large potato)
- $^1/_2$ cup (80 g) diced yellow onion (about $^1/_2$ large onion)
- 2 cloves garlic, chopped
- $^1/_2$ teaspoon basil
- $^1/_2$ teaspoon oregano
- $^1/_4$ teaspoon black pepper
- $^1/_4$ teaspoon salt
- 2 cans (14.5 ounces, or 415 g each) diced tomatoes in juice (no salt added)
- $^1/_2$ cups (120 ml) 2% milk
- $^1/_4$ cup (60 ml) plain low-fat yogurt
- 2 tablespoons (10 g) grated Parmesan cheese
- 1 tablespoon (4 g) chopped fresh parsley

In a 2-quart (2-L) saucepan, place the potatoes, onion, garlic, basil, oregano, pepper, and salt with enough water to cover 1 inch (2.5 cm) above the level of the vegetables. Bring to a boil, then reduce the heat and simmer uncovered for about 15 minutes, until the potatoes are tender throughout.

Drain the tomatoes, reserving the juice. Place the tomatoes in a food processor or blender and puree. Add the tomatoes and juice to the saucepan.

In a separate 4-cup (1-L) mixing bowl, mix the milk, yogurt, and cheese, stirring until a smooth consistency is reached.

Bring the soup to a simmer and slowly add the yogurt-milk mixture, stirring vigorously with a wire whip until all ingredients are evenly incorporated. Serve in warmed soup bowls and garnish with the parsley.

YIELD: Makes 4 (1- cup) servings.

NUTRITIONAL ANALYSIS
Each with: **Calories:** 92.39 **Protein:** 6.82 g **Carbs:** 15.21 g **Total Fat:** 1.36 g **Sat Fat:** 0.80 g
Cholesterol: 4.75 mg **Sodium:** 363.65 mg **Sugars:** 8.24 g **Fiber:** 2.63 g

Black Bean Soup

High in fiber, this is super tasty, too!

TEXTURE: Pureed

INGREDIENTS

- ½ cup (90 g) long-grain brown rice, raw, rinsed, and drained
- 1 cup (235 ml) water
- 2 cans (16 ounces, or 455 g each) black beans, drained
- 1 tablespoon (14 ml) olive oil
- 1 medium onion, diced
- 1 tablespoon (6 g) finely chopped jalapeño pepper
- 2 cloves garlic, minced
- 1½ teaspoons ground cumin
- ½ teaspoon cayenne pepper (optional)
- 1 teaspoon oregano
- 1 teaspoon paprika
- 1 teaspoon chili powder
- 1 can (11 ounces, or 310 g) diced tomatoes, drained
- 1½ quarts (1.5 L) low-sodium chicken broth
- Juice of ½ fresh lime
- 2 tablespoons (2 g) chopped fresh cilantro
- 1 cup (115 g) reduced-fat shredded Cheddar cheese

In a 1-quart (1-L) saucepan, place the rice and water and bring to a boil.

Immediately reduce the heat to a simmer, then loosely cover and simmer for about 15 minutes, until all the liquid is absorbed. Remove from the heat.

In a food processor, puree the beans and set aside.

In a 3-quart (3-L) saucepan, heat the oil over medium-high heat. Add the onion, jalapeno, garlic, cumin, cayenne pepper (if using), oregano, paprika, and chili powder and sauté until the onion begins to soften. Add the tomatoes and stir. Add the pureed beans, rice, broth, and lime juice and stir with a wire whip. Bring to a soft simmer and continue cooking for 20 minutes, stirring once every 5 minutes. Serve in warmed soup bowls and garnish with the cilantro and cheese.

YIELD: Makes 8 (about 1-cup) servings.

NUTRITIONAL ANALYSIS

Each with: **Calories:** 206.02 **Protein:** 11.28 g **Carbs:** 29.66 g **Total Fat:** 4.38 g **Sat Fat:** 2.21 g **Cholesterol:** 10.00 mg **Sodium:** 535.08 mg **Sugars:** 2.51 g **Fiber:** 5.76 g

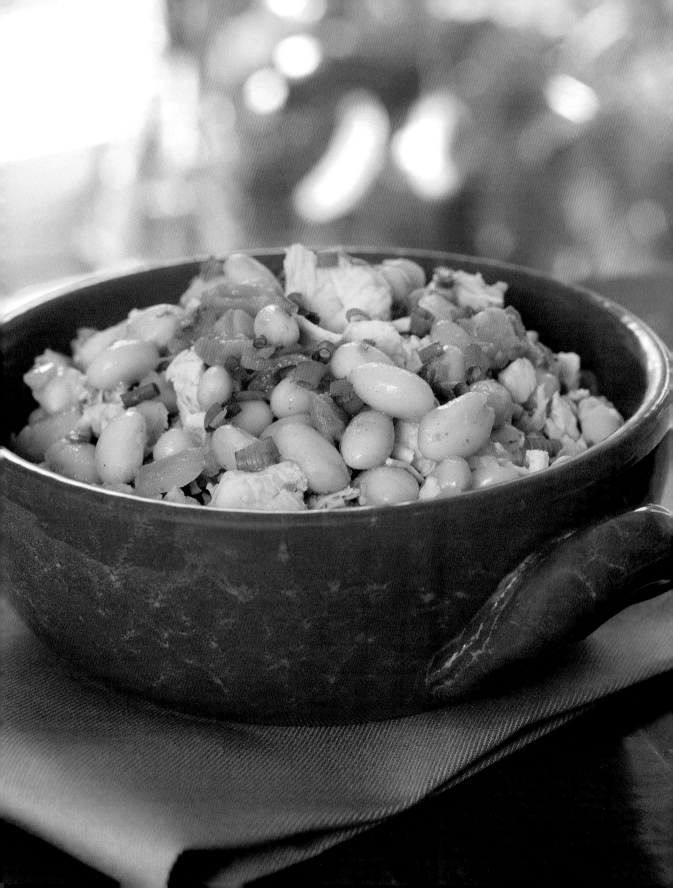

White Chicken Chili

This is a wonderful recipe contributed by a Baltimore woman named Teresa who is having an amazingly successful journey after gastric bypass surgery. This is so quick and easy, you won't believe it!

TEXTURE: Mechanical Soft

INGREDIENTS

- 1 tablespoon (15 ml) canola oil
- 1 1/2 cups (240 g) chopped white onion
- 2 cans (4 ounces, or 113 g each) chopped green chile peppers
- 1 teaspoon dried oregano
- 1 teaspoon ground cumin
- 1 teaspoon ground cumin
- 1/4 teaspoon cayenne pepper
- 2 cans (15 ounces, or 425 g each) great northern beans, rinsed and drained
- 4 cups (946 ml) reduced-sodium chicken broth
- 4 cups (560 g) diced cooked chicken breast
- 2 tablespoons (30 ml) apple cider vinegar

Heat the canola oil in a large pot or Dutch oven over medium-high heat. Add the onion and cook, stirring occasionally, until softened, about 5 minutes.

Stir in the chiles, oregano, cumin, and cayenne. Cook, stirring occasionally, for 5 minutes.

Stir in the beans and broth, and bring to a simmer. Cook, stirring occasionally, for 20 minutes.

Add the chicken and vinegar; cook for 5 minutes more.

YIELD: Makes 14 (1-cup) servings.

NUTRITIONAL ANALYSIS

Each with: **Calories:** 153.62 **Protein:** 23.36 g **Carbs:** 11.72 g **Total Fat:** 25.23 g **Sat Fat:** 3.75 g **Cholesterol:** 54.79 mg **Sodium:** 783.72 mg **Sugars:** 2.72 g **Fiber:** 4.01 g

Potato Leek Soup with Fresh Tarragon

TEXTURE: Pureed

INGREDIENTS

- 1 1/2 to 2 cups (225 to 300 g) peeled and diced russet potatoes
- 1 3/4 pounds (795 g) leeks (2 large or 3 medium)
- 2 tablespoons (28 g) margarine or light butter (see note)
- 2 cloves garlic, minced
- 1 teaspoon black pepper
- 5 cups (40 ounces, or 1185 ml) low-sodium chicken broth
- 1/4 cup (15 g) fresh, coarsely chopped tarragon leaves
- 4 to 6 whole tarragon sprigs (optional)

LYNETTE'S NOTE

Try to find a light margarine or butter that has the same consistency and flavor as real butter. It may cost a bit more, but there are some good substitutes available.

In a 2-quart (2-L) saucepan, cover the potatoes with water and bring it to a boil. Continue cooking for about 12 minutes, until the potatoes are tender throughout. Remove from the heat and drain in a colander. Set aside.

Cut the green tops away from the leeks and discard them. Split the white portions of the leeks down the middle, leaving just the roots intact, and wash them clean of all sand and grit. Drain in a colander. Slice the leeks into thin half-coins. Discard the roots and set aside.

In a 4-quart (4-L) soup pot, melt the margarine over medium heat. Add the leeks, garlic, and pepper and cook until the leeks are tender, but not brown. Add the broth, potatoes, and tarragon leaves and bring to a simmer over low heat. Cook for about 15 minutes. Remove from the heat and let cool for about 15 minutes. With a slotted spoon, remove three-quarters of the solid ingredients and place in a blender or food processor. Blend until smooth. Return the mixture to the soup pot. Heat and stir to an even consistency. Serve in warmed soup bowls and garnish with the tarragon sprigs (if using).

YIELD: Makes 5 (about 1-cup) servings.

NUTRITIONAL ANALYSIS
Each with: **Calories:** 186.63 **Protein:** 5.24 g **Carbs:** 36.71 g **Total Fat:** 3.05 g **Sat Fat:** 0.51 g **Cholesterol:** 0.00 mg **Sodium:** 96.93 mg **Sugars:** 6.73 g **Fiber:** 4.57 g

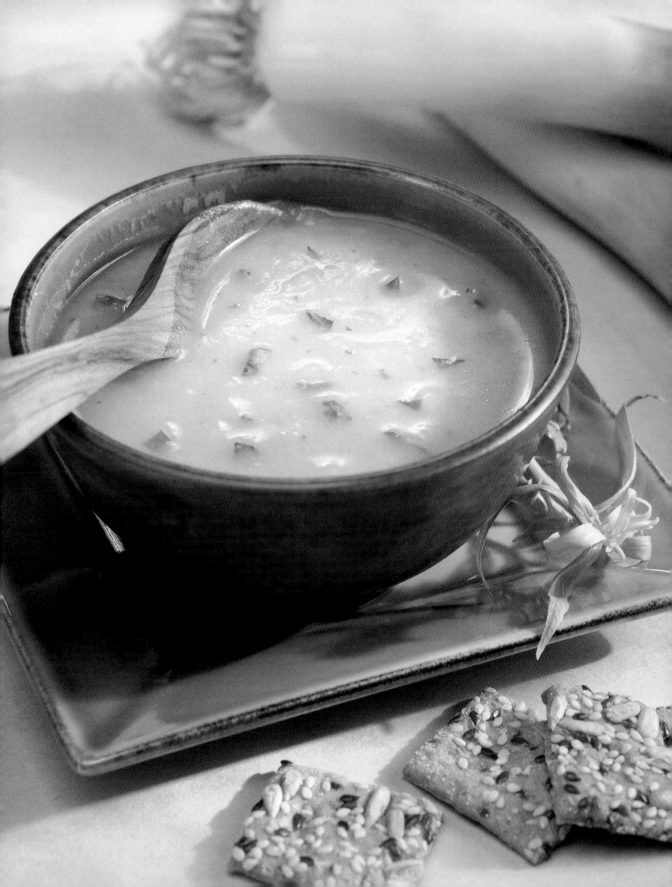

Chicken and Sausage Gumbo

You're going to love this zesty gumbo! It's packed full of flavor and protein.

TEXTURE: Regular

INGREDIENTS

- 1 bag (3^1/$_2$ ounces, or 45 g) boil-in-bag brown rice
- 2 tablespoons (16 g) whole-wheat flour
- 1 tablespoon (15 ml) extra-virgin olive oil
- 1 medium onion, chopped
- 2 medium bell peppers, chopped
- 1 cup (227 g) frozen okra
- 1 cup (100 g) chopped celery
- 2 cloves garlic, chopped
- ^{1}/$_2$ teaspoon dried thyme
- ^{1}/$_4$ teaspoon paprika
- 2 cups (280 g) chopped cooked chicken breast
- 4 ounces (55 g) turkey kielbasa, cut into ^{1}/$_2$-inch (1.25-cm) pieces
- 1 can (14^1/$_2$ ounces, or 411 g) low-sodium diced tomatoes with peppers and onions
- 1 can (14^1/$_2$ ounces, or 440 ml) fat-free, low-sodium chicken broth

Prepare the rice according to the package instructions, minus the salt and fat.

While the rice is cooking, combine the flour and oil in a Dutch oven or large heavy-duty pot. Sauté over medium-high heat, stirring constantly, for 3 minutes. Add the onion, bell peppers, okra, celery, garlic, thyme, and paprika. Cook for about 3 minutes, or until the vegetables are tender.

Stir in the chicken, kielbasa, tomatoes, and broth. Cook for 6 more minutes, or until thoroughly heated. Serve over the brown rice.

YIELD: Makes 6 (about 1-cup) servings.

NUTRITIONAL ANALYSIS
Each with: **Calories:** 265.51 **Protein:** 22.52 g **Carbs:** 24.68 g **Total Fat:** 8.25 g **Sat Fat:** 1.96 g
Cholesterol: 61.61 mg **Sodium:** 613.06 mg **Sugars:** 5.30 g **Fiber:** 3.35 g

Julianna's Kale, Apple, and Lentil Soup

This delicious recipe, from Julianna Pax, Ph.D., shows just how versatile lentils can be. Try this recipe, and the other Lentil Soup, found on page 115, to see which flavor suits your fancy.

TEXTURE: Mechanical Soft

INGREDIENTS

- 1 pound (454 g) green lentils, picked over and rinsed
- 6 cups (1419 ml) low-sodium chicken broth
- 8 cups (1892 ml) water
- 2 cups (320 g) chopped white onion
- 2 cups (260 g) peeled and chopped carrots
- 1¼ cups (111 g) washed and sliced leeks
- 1 teaspoon dried thyme or poultry seasoning
- 4 cups (268 g) chopped kale, stems removed
- 2 tablespoons (30 ml) canola oil
- 3 cups (375 g) peeled and chopped apple
- 1 teaspoon salt
- ½ teaspoon ground black pepper

In a 10-quart (10-L) soup pot, add the lentils, broth, and water. Bring to a boil, then simmer, covered, for 30 minutes. As soon as you have the onions and carrots chopped, add them to the simmering pot. Cover the pot and continue simmering for another 30 minutes.

Add the leeks, thyme or poultry seasoning, and kale to the pot and continue simmering, covered, for 10 to 15 more minutes.

In a separate pan, heat the canola oil over medium-high heat. Add the apples. Season with salt and pepper and sauté for 4 to 5 minutes, or until the apples are golden on all sides. Add the apples to the lentil mixture.

YIELD: Makes 16 (about 1-cup) servings.

NUTRITIONAL ANALYSIS
Each with: **Calories:** 138.22 **Protein:** 7.92 g **Carbs:** 26.78 g **Total Fat:** 0.89 g **Sat Fat** 0.04 g
Cholesterol: 0.00 mg **Sodium:** 338.04 mg **Sugars:** 4.96 g **Fiber:** 6.36 g

Sweet Potato Soup

TEXTURE: Pureed

INGREDIENTS

- 2 quarts (64 ounces, or 2-L) low-sodium chicken or vegetable broth, plus more to thin soup (optional)
- 1 quart (1-L) water
- 4 medium to large sweet potatoes, peeled and cut into approximately 1-inch (2.5-cm) cubes
- 3 cups (480 g) diced large yellow onion (about 2 large)
- 3 medium carrots, peeled and sliced into coins
- 2 large ribs celery, sliced into approximately 1-inch (2.5-cm) pieces
- ¼ cup (60 ml) lemon juice (about 1 lemon)
- 3 teaspoons ground caraway seed
- 3 teaspoons dry mustard
- ½ teaspoon cayenne pepper (optional)
- ¼ cup (15 g) chopped fresh parsley
- ½ teaspoon black pepper
- ½ teaspoon salt
- Nonfat plain yogurt or nonfat sour cream (optional)

Pour the broth and water into a 6-quart (6-L) stockpot or Dutch oven. Add the sweet potato, onion, carrots, and celery. Cover the pot and bring it to a boil. Continue boiling about 25 minutes, until the potatoes are soft. (They should fall apart when speared with a fork.) Remove the pot from the heat and let it stand for about 15 minutes. With a slotted spoon, remove all the solids from the pot and place them in a food processor fitted with a metal S blade or a blender and puree. Reserve the liquid in the pot. (Unless you have an industrial-size processor, this requires more than one batch.) Return the puree to the remaining liquid in the pot. Add the lemon juice, caraway, mustard, cayenne pepper (if using), and parsley. Cover the pot and slowly bring to a simmer. Continue simmering for 20 minutes, stirring often. Check seasonings and adjust with the salt and pepper. If a thinner consistency is desired, add additional chicken or vegetable broth in small amounts until the desired consistency is reached. Serve in warmed bowls and garnish with a dollop yogurt or sour cream (if using).

YIELD: Makes 8 (1½-cup) servings.

NUTRITIONAL ANALYSIS

Each with: **Calories:** 113.68 **Protein:** 3.40 g **Carbs:** 24.55 g **Total Fat:** 0.54 g **Sat Fat:** 0.05 g **Cholesterol:** 0.00 mg **Sodium:** 200.15 mg **Sugars:** 6.87 g **Fiber:** 4.23 g

Vegetarian Vegetable Soup

This is completely vegetarian. When soup is just what you need, you just can't beat a bowl of homemade vegetable soup. This soup can easily be frozen in smaller portions for later enjoyment.

TEXTURE: Soft

INGREDIENTS

- 3 cloves garlic
- Juice of 1 lemon
- $1^{1}/_{2}$ teaspoon cayenne pepper (optional)
- 1 cup (100 g) diced celery
- 1 large carrot, diced
- 1 cup (125 g) diced zucchini
- 1 large yellow onion, diced
- $^{1}/_{2}$ cup (75 g) fresh or frozen peas
- $1^{1}/_{2}$ cups (225 g) peeled, diced fresh tomato (see note)
- 2 quarts (64 ounces, or 2-L) low-sodium vegetable broth (see note)
- 2 medium red potatoes, skinned and diced into $^{1}/_{4}$-inch (6-mm) cubes
- $^{1}/_{2}$ teaspoon black pepper
- $^{1}/_{4}$ teaspoon salt

Place all of the ingredients into a large pot and bring to a rolling (rapid) boil. Reduce heat to a soft boil and continue cooking uncovered about 30 minutes, until the dense vegetables are done. The tomatoes can be added toward the end to hold the form longer.

YIELD: Makes 10 (about $1^{1}/_{2}$-cup) servings.

NUTRITIONAL ANALYSIS
Each with: **Calories:** 70.01 **Protein:** 2.87 g **Carbs:** 14.40 g **Total Fat:** 0.28 g **Sat Fat:** 0.04 g **Cholesterol:** 0.00 mg **Sodium:** 95.85 mg **Sugars:** 3.16 g **Fiber:** 2.45 g

NOTE

To peel the tomatoes, score the bottoms with an X and then blanch them. (Drop them into boiling water just long enough to peel back the skins and remove them from the water.) Let cool to the touch. The skins will come right off.

LYNETTE'S NOTE

If you prefer to make a homemade stock instead of using a store-bought one, and you find the flavor is not to your satisfaction, continue cooking uncovered to reduce the liquid. This will condense your soup and intensify the flavor.

MARGARET'S NOTE

If you're having a hard time getting enough protein into your diet, and this soup is a meal for you, add 2 ounces (55 g) of high-protein powder. (Make sure it's appropriate for hot liquids and add it after heating the soup, just before eating it to preserve the quality of the protein.) This can increase the protein content to more than 20 grams per serving. However, it won't be vegetarian. To keep it strictly vegetarian, or vegan, use a rice or soy protein powder.

CHAPTER 5

Salads

Whole-Wheat Elbow Macaroni Salad

Bring this pasta salad to a potluck or barbecue. Garnish it with fresh tomato wedges.

TEXTURE: Regular

INGREDIENTS

- 1 cup (105 g) dry whole-wheat macaroni
- $^{1}/_{2}$ cup (115 g) nonfat mayonnaise
- 1 teaspoon Dijon mustard
- 1 tablespoon (14 ml) lemon juice
- 1 teaspoon celery salt
- $^{1}/_{2}$ teaspoon black pepper
- $^{1}/_{2}$ cup (80 g) finely chopped red onion
- $^{3}/_{4}$ cup (75 g) finely chopped celery
- $^{1}/_{2}$ cup (70 g) finely chopped red bell pepper
- 1 tablespoon (9 g) sliced black olives
- 1 tablespoon (4 g) chopped fresh parsley
- $1^{1}/_{2}$ teaspoons finely chopped green onion

Cook the macaroni according to package instructions, omitting the salt and oil. Drain the macaroni and cool completely in the refrigerator.

While the macaroni cools, place the mayonnaise, mustard, lemon juice, celery salt, and pepper in a small mixing bowl and stir to combine.

When the pasta is completely cooled, place it in a large mixing bowl along with the onion, celery, bell pepper, olives, parsley, and green onion and pour the dressing over the top. Using a large spoon or rubber spatula, gently stir the pasta until it is completely covered with dressing. Transfer to a serving bowl.

YIELD: Makes about 8 ($^{1}/_{2}$-cup) servings.

NUTRITIONAL ANALYSIS

Each with: **Calories:** 69.92 **Protein:** 2.41 g **Carbs:** 14.32 g **Total Fat:** 0.51 g **Sat Fat:** 0.05 g **Cholesterol:** 0.01 mg **Sodium:** 156.99 mg **Sugars:** 3.14 g **Fiber:** 1.96 g

Classic Spinach Salad
with Apple Cider Vinaigrette

This can be served as a side salad or an entrée. It's perfect for a light summer dinner. Make the dressing at least 20 minutes ahead of time. It's great topped with toasted slivered almonds.

TEXTURE: Regular

INGREDIENTS

- 2 tablespoons (28 ml) olive oil
- 1 tablespoon (14 ml) apple cider vinegar
- 1 tablespoon (14 ml) fresh lemon juice
- 1 medium clove fresh garlic, cut into thin slivers
- $^{1}/_{2}$ teaspoon low-sodium soy sauce
- $^{1}/_{4}$ teaspoon black pepper
- 8 $^{1}/_{8}$-inch- (3-mm-) thick red onion rings
- 8 cups (240 g) fresh baby spinach, washed and thoroughly drained and dried
- 4 strips turkey bacon, cooked crisp and crumbled
- 1 small cucumber, peeled and thinly sliced
- 4 Italian plum tomatoes, cored and cut into 4 wedges each
- 2 hard-boiled eggs, cooled, peeled, and cut into 4 wedges each

In a glass jar with a tightly fitting lid, place the oil, vinegar, lemon juice, garlic, soy sauce, and pepper. Shake vigorously. Set aside.

About 20 minutes before serving, place the onion in the jar of salad dressing to marinate.

In a large mixing bowl, place the spinach, bacon, and cucumber.

Remove the onion from the dressing and set aside. Pour the dressing evenly over the salad and gently toss, just enough to ensure complete coverage. Distribute the dressed salad evenly in the center of 4 entrée plates or 8 side salad plates. Place the tomato wedges leaning against the outer edges of each salad. Place the egg wedges next to the tomato wedges. Top the salads with 1 or 2 onion rings. Serve immediately.

YIELD: Makes 8 ($^{1}/_{2}$-cup) servings or 4 (1 cup) servings.

NUTRITIONAL ANALYSIS
Each with: **Calories:** 90.46 g **Protein:** 3.86 g **Carbs:** 5.79 g **Total Fat:** 6.10 g **Sat Fat:** 1.14 g **Cholesterol:** 65.00 mg **Sodium:** 163.85 mg **Sugars:** 2.11 g **Fiber:** 1.80 g

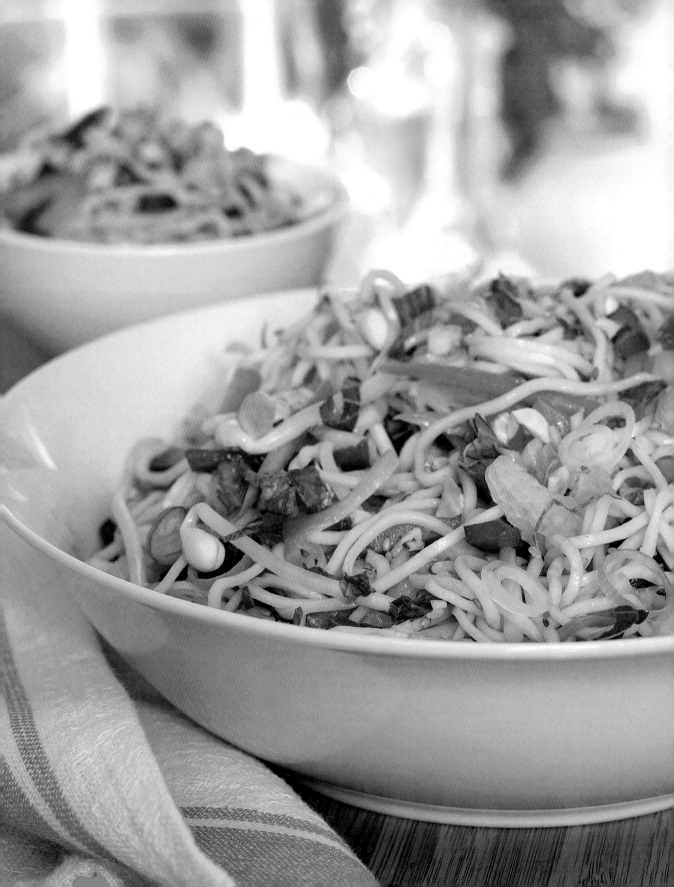

Asian Noodle Salad

This yummy recipe comes from Teresa, a gastric bypass surgery patient in Baltimore.

TEXTURE: Regular

INGREDIENTS

- 1 package (12 ounces, or 210 g) soba noodles or whole-wheat noodles
- 1 teaspoon sesame oil
- 2 tablespoons (30 ml) rice wine vinegar
- 3 tablespoons (45 ml) low-sodium soy sauce
- 1 teaspoon hot chili oil
- 1 tablespoon (16 ml) hoisin sauce
- 3 tablespoons (45 ml) extra-virgin olive oil
- 1 carrot, thinly sliced or julienned
- 2 celery stalks, thinly sliced or julienned
- 5 scallions, white and light green parts, thinly sliced
- 1/2 cup (45 g) thinly sliced napa cabbage
- 1/2 red bell pepper, thinly sliced or julienned
- 1/2 cup (45 g) julienned bok choy
- 1 cup (50 g) bean sprouts, optional
- 3 tablespoons (3 g) fresh cilantro, minced
- 3 tablespoons (24 g) sesame seeds, toasted
- 2 tablespoons (18 g) unsalted peanuts, roughly chopped

In a medium stock pot, cook the noodles according to the package directions. When finished, place the noodles in an ice-water bath to cool. Drain and set aside.

In a medium bowl combine the sesame oil, vinegar, soy sauce, hot chili oil, hoisin sauce, and olive oil. Add the carrot, celery, scallions, cabbage, bell pepper, bok choy, bean sprouts (if using), cilantro, and cooled noodles. Mix to combine. Garnish with sesame seeds and peanuts.

YIELD: Makes 8 (about 1/2-cup) servings.

NUTRITIONAL ANALYSIS
Each with: **Calories:** 280.73 **Protein:** 9.62 g **Carbs:** 37.95 g **Total Fat:** 10.41 g **Sat Fat:** 1.11 g **Cholesterol:** 0.00 mg **Sodium:** 355.33 mg **Sugars:** 5.87 g **Fiber:** 3.50 g

Mandarin Pea Pod Salad

This salad is colorful, nutritious, and wonderful for home entertaining.

TEXTURE: Regular

INGREDIENTS

- 2 packages (10 ounces, 280 g each) prewashed fresh spinach
- 2 cups (475 ml) water
- 2 cups (about 3/4 pound, 340 g) fresh snow peas
- 2 cups (500 g) canned mandarin oranges, drained
- 2 tablespoons (15 g) toasted sesame seeds (optional)
- 2 tablespoons (20 g) thinly sliced shallots
- 1 tablespoon (14 ml) extra-virgin olive oil
- 1/4 cup (60 ml) apple cider vinegar
- 1/4 teaspoon salt
- 1/4 teaspoon black pepper
- 2 tablespoons (28 ml) fresh lime juice (from about 1/2 lime)
- 1 teaspoon lime zest (grated peel of about 1/2 lime)

Cut the stems off of the spinach and shred (with your hands) into about 1-inch (2.5-cm) pieces, arranging evenly on a serving platter.

In a 1 1/2 -quart (1.5-L) saucepan, bring the water to a boil. Remove the stems and strings from the peas.

Prepare an ice bath by filling a medium mixing bowl with ice and just enough cold water to cover. Drop the peas into the boiling water and blanch them for about 45 seconds. With a strainer, remove the peas and immediately place them into the ice bath. (This stops the cooking process and helps to maintain beautiful, bright green color.) After 60 seconds in the ice bath, remove the peas, drain, pat dry with paper towels, and place evenly atop the spinach. Arrange the mandarin oranges evenly over the peas.

In a small plastic container with a lid, combine the sesame seeds (if using), shallots, oil, vinegar, salt, pepper, lime juice, and lime zest. Shake vigorously and/or whisk until the dressing is emulsified. Just prior to serving, pour the salad dressing evenly over the top.

YIELD: Makes 8 (about 3/4-cup) servings.

NUTRITIONAL ANALYSIS
Each with: **Calories:** 102.22 **Protein:** 3.49 g **Carbs:** 17.09 g **Total Fat:** 2.44 g **Sat Fat:** 0.32 g **Cholesterol:** 0.00 mg **Sodium:** 99.57 mg **Sugars:** 11.76 g **Fiber:** 3.72 g

"This salad went over very well with us and our friends. The flavors were a great and refreshing combination."

—Jill and Dan,
gastric banding surgery patients in the Washington, D.C., area

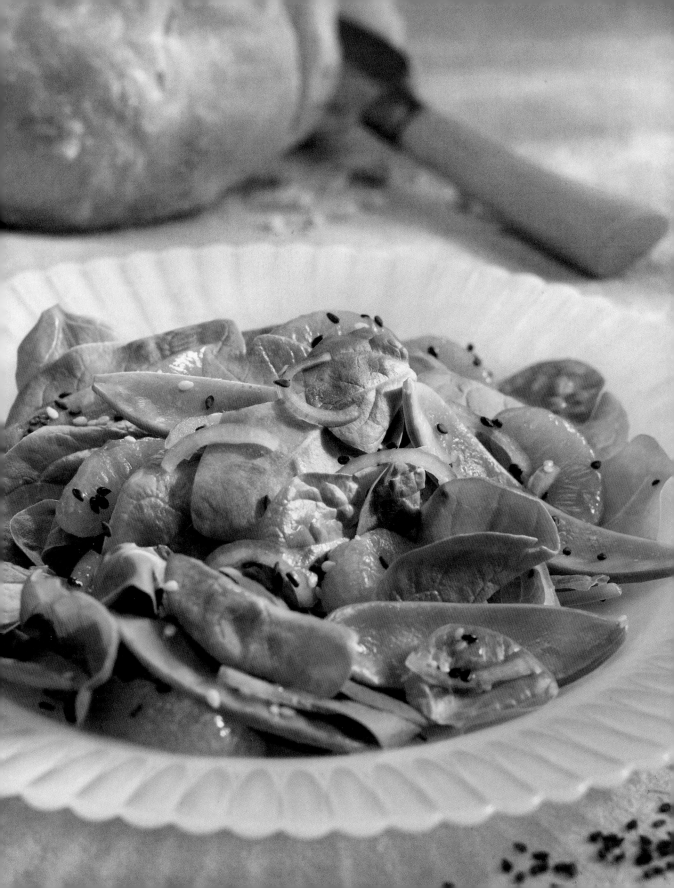

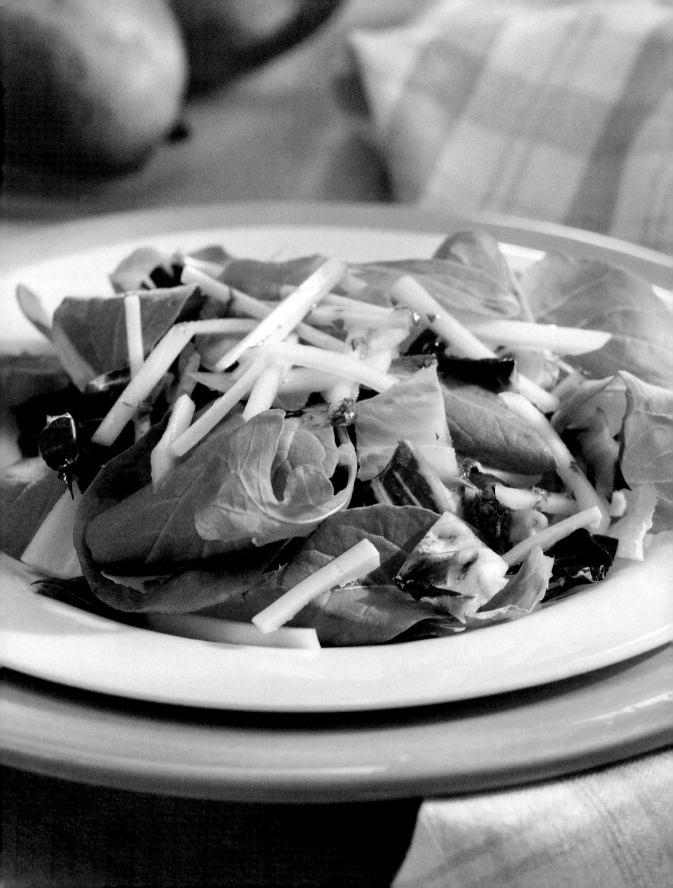

Hearts of Palm Salad
with Arugula and Endive

Try topping this salad with grilled chicken, shrimp, or pork tenderloin cut into thin strips.

TEXTURE: Regular

INGREDIENTS

- Zest and juice of $1/2$ lime
- 1 tablespoon (14 ml) apple cider vinegar
- 1 tablespoon (14 ml) fresh orange juice
- $1/8$ teaspoon fresh minced garlic
- Pinch cayenne pepper (optional)
- 2 tablespoons (28 ml) olive oil
- 3 teaspoons chopped fresh cilantro
- 3 cups (60 g) arugula, washed and dried
- 1 medium Belgium endive, cut into bite-size pieces
- 1 small radicchio, cut into bite-size pieces
- 4 stalks canned hearts of palm, cut into 1-inch (2.5-cm) match sticks
- $1/2$ fresh mango, cut into about 1-inch (2.5-cm) strips

In a small mixing bowl, place the lime zest and lime juice. Add the vinegar, orange juice, garlic, and cayenne pepper (if using). Whisk with a wire whip to combine. Continue whisking while slowly adding the oil until the dressing is emulsified. Add the cilantro and stir. Set aside for the flavors to marry while preparing the salad.

In a salad bowl, place the arugula. Add the endive and radicchio. Top with the hearts of palm and mango. Toss with the dressing just before serving.

YIELD: Makes 6 (about $3/4$-cup) servings.

NUTRITIONAL ANALYSIS
Each with: **Calories:** 87.56 **Protein:** 2.43 g **Carbs:** 9.42 g **Total Fat:** 5.16 g **Sat Fat:** 0.78 g **Cholesterol:** 0.00 mg **Sodium:** 122.06 mg **Sugars:** 3.67 g **Fiber:** 3.93 g

Mexican Shrimp Salad with Jicama

This south-of-the-border salad combines shrimp with jicama, a refreshing flavor with a unique and crunchy texture.

TEXTURE: Regular

INGREDIENTS

- $^1/_3$ cup (35 g) thinly sliced green onions
- $^1/_3$ cup (75 g) nonfat mayonnaise
- $^1/_3$ cup (80 g) nonfat plain yogurt
- 2 teaspoon red pepper sauce
- 1 tablespoon chopped fresh cilantro
- 2 teaspoons prepared horseradish
- 1 teaspoon chili powder
- 1 teaspoon ground cumin
- 2 teaspoons lime juice
- $1^1/_2$ pounds (680 g) precooked medium-size shrimp
- $^1/_2$ medium jicama, skinned and cut into about 1/2-inch (2.5-cm) pieces (about $^3/_4$ cup, or 90 g)
- 4 cups (80 g) hearty salad greens, ready to serve
- 2 tablespoons (28 ml) low-calorie Thousand Island dressing (prepared or on this page)

In a medium mixing bowl, place the green onions, mayonnaise, yogurt, pepper sauce, cilantro, horseradish, chili powder, cumin, and lime juice and stir to combine. Add the shrimp and toss to cover with the dressing. Cover the bowl and refrigerate to marinate for 30 to 60 minutes. Add the jicama and stir to coat. Discard excess marinade.

In another medium mixing bowl, toss the salad greens with the Thousand Island dressing and shrimp. Serve on chilled salad plates.

YIELD: Makes about 6 (1-cup) servings.

NUTRITIONAL ANALYSIS
Each with: **Calories:** 155.42 **Protein:** 24.34 g **Carbs:** 8.22 g **Total Fat:** 2.12 g **Sat Fat:** 0.38 g **Cholesterol:** 172.65 mg **Sodium:** 365.22 mg **Sugars:** 3.48 g **Fiber:** 2.18 g

Thousand Island Dressing

TEXTURE: Pureed

INGREDIENTS

- 1 cup (225 g) nonfat cottage cheese
- 1/3 cup (75 ml) low-fat buttermilk
- 1 teaspoon fresh lemon juice
- 2 tablespoons (30 g) sweet pickle relish
- 1 teaspoon red pepper sauce
- 1 tablespoon (15 g) low-carb ketchup

Place all of the ingredients in a blender or food processor and blend until smooth.

YIELD: Makes 10 (about 2-tablespoon) servings.

NUTRITIONAL ANALYSIS

Each with: **Calories:** 24.20 **Protein:** 2.89 g **Carbs:** 2.81 g **Total Fat:** 0.09 g **Sat Fat:** 0.05 g **Cholesterol:** 1.33 mg **Sodium:** 131.54 mg **Sugars:** 1.62 g **Fiber:** 0.04 g

Chickpea and Tomato Salad

TEXTURE: Regular

INGREDIENTS

- 2 cans (15 ounces, or 425 g each) chickpeas, rinsed and dried
- 4 tomatoes, seeded and chopped
- 2 large hard-boiled eggs, peeled and chopped
- 2 cups (320 g) chopped Vidalia onion
- 3 tablespoons (45 ml) extra-virgin olive oil
- 1/3 cup (80 ml) white wine vinegar
- 1 teaspoon kosher salt
- 1/2 teaspoon black pepper
- 2 tablespoons (9 g) fresh parsley, chopped

Combine the chickpeas, tomatoes, eggs, and onion in a large bowl.

In a smaller bowl, mix the olive oil, vinegar, salt, and pepper. Pour over the salad ingredients. Sprinkle with chopped parsley.

YIELD: Makes 8 (about 1-cup) servings.

NUTRITIONAL ANALYSIS

Each with: **Calories:** 188.98 **Protein:** 7.39 g **Carbs:** 22.35 g **Total Fat:** 8.31 g **Sat Fat:** 1.13 g **Cholesterol:** 53.75 mg **Sodium:** 375.38 mg **Sugars:** 6.16 g **Fiber:** 5.33 g

Marinated Mushroom and Tomato Salad with Dijon Vinaigrette

This salad is a great side dish for beef entrees.

TEXTURE: Regular

INGREDIENTS

- 1 pound (455 g) 1-inch (2.5-cm) button or crimini mushrooms
- 8 large ripe Roma tomatoes
- $1/4$ cup (40 g) thinly sliced red onion
- $1/4$ cup (60 ml) olive oil
- 1 tablespoon (14 ml) balsamic vinegar
- 1 teaspoon sugar
- 1 tablespoon (15 g) Dijon mustard
- 2 tablespoons (6 g) finely chopped fresh chives
- $1/2$ teaspoon sea salt or kosher salt
- $1/4$ teaspoon fresh cracked black pepper
- 2 whole chive stems

Clean the mushrooms with a mushroom brush or paper towels. Cut the end of the stems away and discard. Cut the mushrooms into halves.

Core the tomatoes and cut them in half lengthwise, then slice into $1/4$-inch (6 mm) half-circles.

In a medium mixing bowl, place the mushrooms, tomatoes, and onion and set aside.

In a small mixing bowl, combine the oil, vinegar, sugar, mustard, chopped chives, salt, and pepper and stir vigorously with a wire whisk. Allow the dressing to sit for at least 10 minutes to marry the flavors.

Pour the dressing over the salad and gently toss to ensure complete coverage. Transfer the salad to a serving bowl and garnish with the chive stems in the shape of an X against the rim of the bowl.

YIELD: Makes 12 (about $1/2$-cup) servings.

NUTRITIONAL ANALYSIS

Each with: **Calories:** 73.75 **Protein:** 2.01 g **Carbs:** 5.92 g **Total Fat:** 5.17 g **Sat Fat:** 0.73 g **Cholesterol:** 0.03 mg **Sodium:** 64.00 mg **Sugars:** 3.66 g **Fiber:** 1.44 g

Fresh Mediterranean Salad

TEXTURE: Regular

INGREDIENTS

- 2 tablespoons (30 ml) red wine vinegar
- 2 tablespoons (30 ml) water
- 1 teaspoon dried oregano
- 1 teaspoon black pepper
- 1 teaspoon Dijon mustard
- 1/2 teaspoon kosher salt
- 2 cloves garlic, finely chopped
- 3 tablespoons (45 ml) extra-virgin olive oil

For Salad:

- 2 cups (174 g) sliced fennel bulb
- 1 1/2 (240 g) cups thinly sliced red onion
- 1 cup (160 g) sliced black olives
- 3/4 cup (45 g) fresh parsley, chopped
- 1/2 cup (75 g) crumbled feta cheese
- 1 can (15 1/2 ounces, or 439 g) cannellini beans, rinsed and drained
- 6 plum tomatoes, quartered

To make the vinaigrette: Combine the vinegar, water, oregano, pepper, mustard, salt, and garlic in a bowl. Slowly drizzle in the olive oil while whisking to blend.

To make the salad: Combine the fennel, red onion, olives, parsley, feta cheese, beans, and tomatoes in a large bowl. Toss the salad with the vinaigrette, cover, and chill for at least 1 hour before serving.

YIELD: Makes 12 (about 1/2-cup) servings.

NUTRITIONAL ANALYSIS
Each with: **Calories:** 111.94 **Protein:** 4.45 g **Carbs:** 11.95 g **Total Fat:** 5.54 g **Sat Fat:** 1.16 g
Cholesterol: 1.67 mg **Sodium:** 344.97 mg **Sugars:** 2.48 g **Fiber:** 3.55 g

Greek Salad

This is the perfect accompaniment to Kosher Lamb Souvlaki (page 268)

TEXTURE: Regular

INGREDIENTS

- 2 medium to large cucumbers
- 1 large green bell pepper
- 1 medium red onion, cut into $^1/_4$-inch (6-mm) strips
- 2 tomatoes, cored and diced into 1-inch (2.5-cm) cubes
- $^1/_2$ cup (70 g) whole Greek olives
- $^3/_4$ cup (115 g) feta cheese, cut into $^1/_2$-inch (1.25-mm) cubes, or feta cheese crumbles
- 2 tablespoons (28 ml) olive oil
- 2 teaspoons lemon juice
- 2 teaspoons red wine vinegar
- 2 teaspoons chopped fresh thyme leaves, stems removed
- $^1/_8$ teaspoon salt
- $^1/_8$ teaspoon cracked black pepper
- Bundle fresh thyme

Using a vegetable peeler, remove the cucumber skins and cut the cucumbers in half, lengthwise. Remove the seeds using a spoon to scrape down the middle. Slice the peeled, seeded cucumbers into $^1/_4$- to $^1/_2$-inch (6- to 12-mm) pieces and place them in a large mixing bowl.

Core the bell pepper, remove the membrane, and cut it into $^1/_2$-inch (1.25-cm) pieces and add them to the cucumbers. Add the onion, tomato, olives, and cheese and set aside.

In a medium mixing bowl, combine the oil, lemon juice, vinegar, thyme, salt, and black pepper. Stir vigorously with a wire whip until the dressing is emulsified. Pour the dressing over the salad and mix thoroughly. Place the salad in a serving bowl and garnish it with a bundle of fresh thyme.

YIELD: Makes 8 (about 1-cup) servings.

NUTRITIONAL ANALYSIS
Each with: **Calories:** 116.97 **Protein:** 3.15 g **Carbs:** 6.96 g **Total Fat:** 8.36 g **Sat Fat:** 2.64 g **Cholesterol:** 12.52 mg **Sodium:** 286.38 mg **Sugars:** 4.02 g **Fiber:** 1.60 g

Leftover Salmon Salad

This is a great way to use up leftover salmon. Served on just a small portion of greens, it is ideal for lunch.

TEXTURE: Soft

INGREDIENTS

- 6 ounces (170 g) cold leftover salmon
- 6 small black olives, sliced
- 1 tablespoon (16 g) finely chopped celery
- 1 tablespoon (10 g) finely chopped red bell pepper
- 1^1/$_2$ teaspoons finely chopped red onion
- 1 teaspoon chopped fresh parsley
- 2 cups (40 g) salad greens, washed, drained, and dried with paper towels
- 1^1/$_2$ tablespoons (20 ml) low-fat, low-carb salad dressing (prepared or see pages 152 to 155)
- 1 Italian plum tomato, cored and cut into 4 wedges

Flake the salmon apart with a fork, removing any skin or bones, and place it in a small mixing bowl. Add the olives, celery, pepper, onion, and parsley and mix gently, just enough to combine.

In a small mixing bowl, place the salad greens. Pour the salad dressing over the greens and gently toss to expose all of the surface area to the dressing. Equally distribute the greens onto 2 plates and top with the salmon mixture. Garnish each salad with 2 tomato wedges and serve.

YIELD: Makes 2 (3-ounce salmon, ^{1}/$_2$-cup salad) servings.

NUTRITIONAL ANALYSIS
Each with: **Calories:** 162.99 **Protein:** 17.99 g **Carbs:** 6.21 g **Total Fat:** 7.06 g **Sat Fat:** 0.85 g **Cholesterol:** 46.78 mg **Sodium:** 276.78 mg **Sugars:** 3.53 g **Fiber:** 2.03 g

Home-Style Tuna Salad

TEXTURE: Mechanical Soft

INGREDIENTS

- 2 cans (7 ounces, or 200 g each) white tuna, drained and flaked
- $1/2$ cup (115 g) light mayonnaise
- $1/4$ cup (60 g) sweet pickle relish
- $1/4$ teaspoon dried onion flakes
- 1 teaspoon dried mustard powder
- 1 tablespoon (1 g) dried parsley
- $1^1/2$ teaspoons dried dill weed
- $1^1/2$ teaspoons garlic powder

In a medium bowl, stir together the tuna, mayonnaise, pickle relish, onion flakes, mustard powder, parsley, dill weed, and garlic powder. Mix well. Refrigerate at least 30 minutes before serving.

YIELD: Makes 6 (about $1/2$-cup) servings.

NUTRITIONAL ANALYSIS
Each with: **Calories:** 157.11 **Protein:** 17.00 g **Carbs:** 5.09 g **Total Fat:** 7.12 g **Sat Fat:** 1.15 g
Cholesterol: 26.84 mg **Sodium:** 255.82 mg **Sugars:** 2.87 g **Fiber:** 0.03 g

Tarragon Chicken Salad

Plain old chicken salad can get boring, so try this new twist on the familiar classic.

TEXTURE: Mechanical Soft

INGREDIENTS

- 2 cups (280 g) diced cooked chicken breast
- 1 small apple, cored and diced
- $1/4$ cup (25 g) diced celery
- $1/4$ cup (40 g) diced red onion
- $1/2$ cup (115 g) light mayonnaise
- 1 tablespoon (15 ml) fresh lemon juice
- 2 tablespoons (8 g) fresh tarragon, chopped
- 1 tablespoon (4 g) fresh parsley, chopped
- 1 tablespoon (3 g) fresh chives, chopped
- $1/4$ teaspoon kosher salt
- $1/4$ teaspoon black pepper

In a medium bowl, combine the chicken, apple, celery, and onion.

In a small bowl, combine the mayonnaise, lemon juice, tarragon, parsley, chives, salt, and pepper. Pour the dressing over the chicken mixture and stir to combine. Refrigerate for at least 1 hour before serving.

YIELD: Makes 6 (about $1/2$-cup) servings.

NUTRITIONAL ANALYSIS
Each with: **Calories:** 187.62 **Protein:** 21.76 g **Carbs:** 7.23 g **Total Fat:** 8.23 g **Sat Fat:** 1.24 g **Cholesterol:** 62.59 mg **Sodium:** 581.84 mg **Sugars:** 3.85 g **Fiber:** 1.74 g

Radicchio and Cauliflower Salad with Roasted Walnuts

This colorful, festive salad is great for home entertaining or everyday enjoyment.

TEXTURE: Regular

INGREDIENTS

- 1 tablespoon (8 g) finely chopped walnuts
- 1 large radicchio head, quartered lengthwise, then sliced crosswise into thin strips
- 1 small cauliflower head, cut into small florets
- $1/2$ small red onion, thinly sliced (about $1/3$ cup, or 35 g)
- $1/2$ cup (4 ounces, or 115 g) feta cheese
- 1 clove garlic, minced
- 1 tablespoon (14 ml) balsamic vinegar
- 1 teaspoon Dijon mustard
- 2 teaspoons minced shallot
- 1 teaspoon chopped fresh oregano
- 2 tablespoons (28 ml) olive oil
- $1/8$ teaspoon salt
- 1 pinch freshly ground black pepper

Preheat the oven to 375°F (190°C, or gas mark 5).

Place the walnuts on a sheet pan and bake for about 12 minutes, until the walnuts just begin to brown. Remove the sheet pan from the oven and set aside, allowing nuts to cool completely before adding them to the salad.

In a large bowl, mix the radicchio, cauliflower, and onion. Crumble the feta over the salad.

In a small bowl, whisk together the garlic, vinegar, mustard, shallot, and oregano. Slowly whisk in the oil. Season with the salt and pepper and mix the dressing into the salad. Let the salad sit for 1 hour in the refrigerator and top with toasted walnuts just prior to serving.

YIELD: Makes 6 (about $1/2$-cup) servings.

NUTRITIONAL ANALYSIS
Each with: **Calories:** 109.52 **Protein:** 4.70 g **Carbs:** 5.65 g **Total Fat:** 8.35 g **Sat Fat:** 3.29 g **Cholesterol:** 16.68 mg **Sodium:** 293.74 mg **Sugars:** 3.09 g **Fiber:** 1.55 g

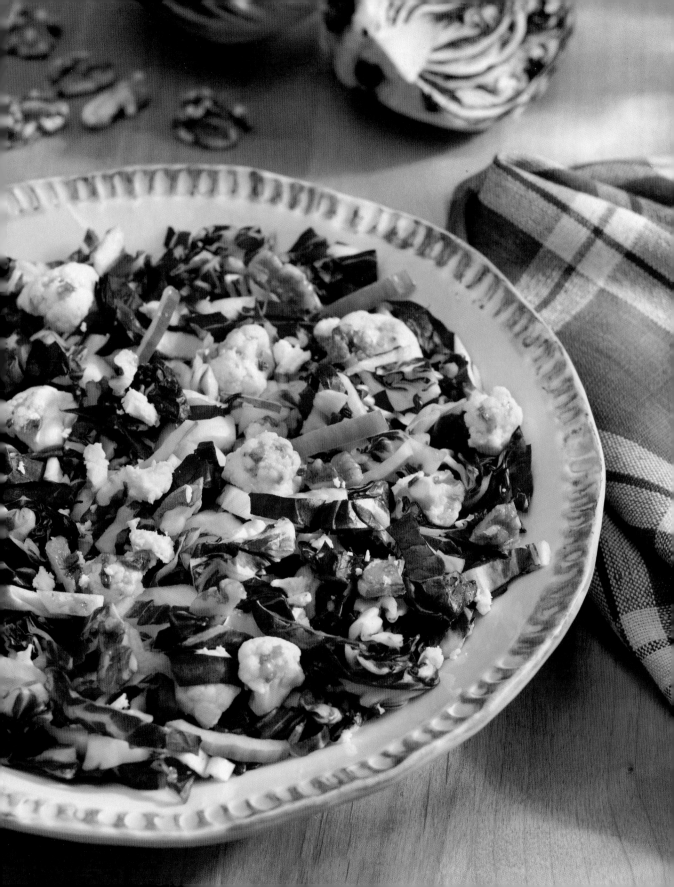

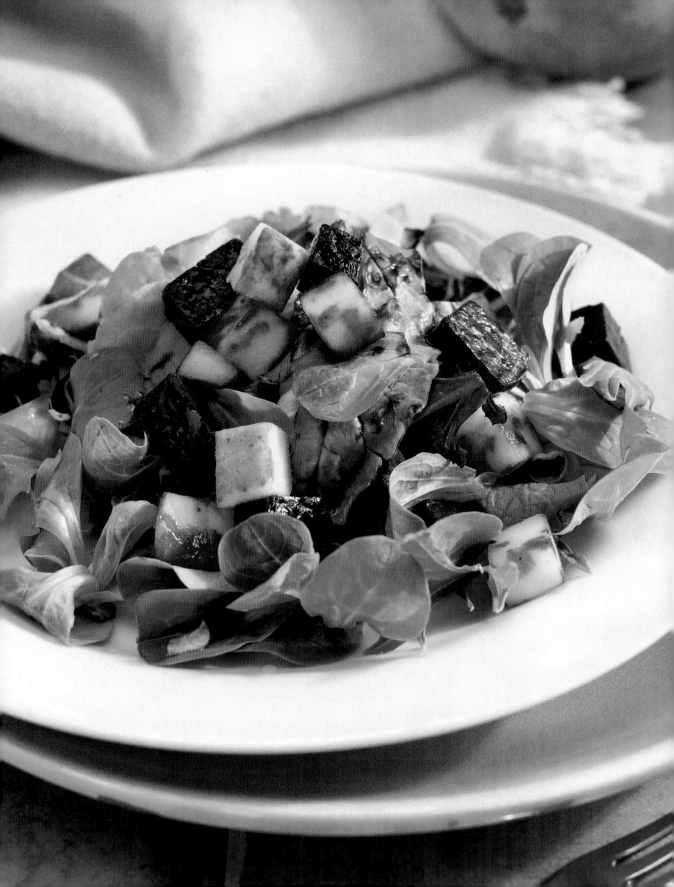

Roasted Beets and Mango Salad

TEXTURE: Regular

INGREDIENTS

- 2 medium beets, peeled and cut into 1-inch (2.5-cm) cubes (about $^3/_4$ pound, or 340 g)
- $^1/_4$ (60 ml) cup 100% orange juice
- 2 tablespoons (28 ml) fresh lime juice
- $^1/_2$ teaspoon black pepper
- 1 tablespoon (15 g) Dijon mustard
- 2 teaspoons extra-virgin olive oil
- $^1/_8$ teaspoon sea salt or kosher salt
- 1 cup (165 g) cubed ripe mango (about 2 mangoes)
- 6 cups (120 g) mixed field greens or gourmet salad mix

Preheat the oven to 425°F (220°C, or gas mark 7).

In a 2-quart (2-L) saucepan, place the beets and cover with water to 1 inch (2.5 cm) above the level of the beets. Boil for 7 minutes, and then drain the beets in a colander.

Spray a $7^1/_2$- x $11^1/_2$-inch (17.5- x 27.5-cm) baking dish with cooking spray. Place the beats in the dish and roast for 30 minutes, until the beets are tender. Place beets in mixing bowl and cool in refrigerator.

In a 1 quart (1-L) mixing bowl, combine the orange juice, lime juice, pepper, mustard, oil, and salt. Mix vigorously with a wire whip or a fork and divide into two equal portions. Add one portion of the dressing to the beets and toss to cover all of the beet surface.

Remove the beets, reserving the remaining dressing. Combine the two portions of the remaining dressing.

In a large mixing bowl, place the salad greens. Pour the dressing over the salad greens. Gently toss to ensure complete exposure of the greens to the dressing.

Add the mangos to the beets and gently fold just enough to disperse beets and mangos evenly.

Divide the salad mixture among six chilled salad plates and top each salad with an equal amount of the beet-mango mixture.

YIELD: Makes 6 (about 1-cup) servings.

NUTRITIONAL ANALYSIS
Each with: **Calories:** 63.92 **Protein:** 1.52 g **Carbs:** 11.88 g **Total Fat:** 1.90 g **Sat Fat:** 0.25 g **Cholesterol:** 0.00 mg **Sodium:** 98.43 mg **Sugars:** 8.67 g **Fiber:** 2.65 g

Marinated Vegetable Salad in Creamy Vinaigrette

TEXTURE: Regular

INGREDIENTS

- $1/4$ cup (60 g) plain nonfat yogurt
- 2 tablespoons (28 ml) white wine vinegar
- 2 teaspoons Dijon mustard
- 1 teaspoon sugar substitute
- 2 teaspoons olive oil
- $1/8$ teaspoon celery salt
- $1/2$ teaspoon cracked black pepper
- $1/4$ teaspoon sea salt or kosher salt
- 2 cups (260 g) sliced carrots (about 2 large)
- 1 cup (100 g) fresh green beans, trimmed and cut into about 1-inch (2.5-cm) pieces
- $1^1/4$ cups (75 g) mushrooms, cut into quarters
- 2 medium tomatoes, cored and cut into 8 wedges each
- 1 small red bell pepper, cut into $1/2$-inch (2.5-cm) pieces
- $1/2$ cup (50 g) thinly sliced green onion

In a small mixing bowl, combine the yogurt, vinegar, mustard, sugar substitute, oil, celery salt, black pepper, and salt and stir vigorously with a wire whip.

In a large mixing bowl, combine the carrots, green beans, mushrooms, tomatoes, red pepper, and onion with the dressing and toss to ensure complete coverage.

YIELD: Makes about 8 ($3/4$-cup) servings.

NUTRITIONAL ANALYSIS
Each with: **Calories:** 66.01 **Protein:** 2.75 g **Carbs:** 10.53 g **Total Fat:** 1.64 g **Sat Fat:** 0.22 g
Cholesterol: 0.16 mg **Sodium:** 156.07 mg **Sugars:** 5.95 g **Fiber:** 3.29 g

Fresh Fruit Salad

This salad is so sweet and satisfying, it could be served as dessert.

TEXTURE: Regular

INGREDIENTS

- 1/2 cup (100 g) nonfat sour cream
- 1 tablespoon (14 ml) lemon juice
- 6 teaspoons brown sugar substitute
- 1/8 teaspoon allspice
- 1/8 teaspoon cinnamon
- 2 fresh peaches, skinned, pitted, and cut into bite-size pieces
- 1 cup (170 g) bite-size honeydew melon pieces
- 1/2 cup (75 g) fresh blueberries
- 1/2 cup (85 g) halved fresh strawberries, stems removed
- 20 seedless grapes, skinned and cut in half

In a medium mixing bowl, combine the sour cream, lemon juice, brown sugar substitute, allspice, and cinnamon. Add the peaches, melon, blueberries, strawberries, and grapes and gently toss to cover with dressing. Refrigerate for 30 minutes before serving in chilled bowls.

YIELD: Makes 6 (about 1/2-cup) servings.

NUTRITIONAL ANALYSIS
Each with: **Calories:** 63.75 **Protein:** 2.03 g **Carbs:** 14.16 g **Total Fat:** 0.24 g **Sat Fat:** 0.04 g **Cholesterol:** 3.33 mg **Sodium:** 22.33 mg **Sugars:** 9.53 g **Fiber:** 1.40 g

Sweet and Sour Marinated Cucumbers

Tangy and delicious, this is a perfect accompaniment to light-textured fish dishes.

TEXTURE: Regular

INGREDIENTS

- ¹/₂ cup (120 ml) white wine vinegar
- 1 teaspoon fresh lemon juice
- ³/₄ cup (25 g) finely chopped green onion
- 6 teaspoons sugar substitute
- 2 tablespoons (8 g) finely chopped fresh parsley
- 1 tablespoon (2 g) chopped fresh dill
- 1 teaspoon poppy seeds
- 1 tablespoon (10 g) minced red onion
- 3 medium cucumbers, peeled

In a small mixing bowl, vigorously stir together the vinegar, lemon juice, green onion, sugar substitute, parsley, dill, poppy seeds, and red onion with a wire whisk. Cover and refrigerate until ready to use.

Cut the cucumbers in half, lengthwise. Using a spoon, scrape out the seeds. Slice the cucumbers into ¹/₂-inch (2.5-cm) pieces. Place the cucumbers into a medium mixing bowl. Pour the marinade over the cucumbers and toss to cover. Cover the bowl. Allow to marinate in the refrigerator for about 20 minutes before transferring to a serving bowl.

YIELD: Makes 6 (about ¹/₂-cup) servings.

NUTRITIONAL ANALYSIS
Each with: **Calories:** 23.73 **Protein:** 0.86 g **Carbs:** 2.99 g **Total Fat:** 0.40 g **Sat Fat:** 0.04 g **Cholesterol:** 0.00 mg **Sodium:** 5.09 mg **Sugars:** 1.64 g **Fiber:** 0.98 g

Asian-Influenced Cabbage Medley

Delicious and refreshing!

TEXTURE: Regular

INGREDIENTS

- 6 cups (540 g) shredded Napa cabbage (Chinese cabbage, about 1 large)
- 1 cup (90 g) shredded red cabbage
- 1 cup (90 g) shredded green cabbage
- $^3/_4$ cup (75 g) chopped daikon radish or white radish
- $^3/_4$ cup (75 g) thinly chopped green onion (chopped diagonally)
- 1 cup (16 g) fresh cilantro leaves
- $^1/_2$ cup (13 g) fresh mint leaves, stems removed
- 1 cup (150 g) fresh or thawed frozen peas
- 2 tablespoons (15 g) toasted sesame seeds
- $^3/_4$ cup (175 g) nonfat mayonnaise
- 3 tablespoons (45 ml) rice wine vinegar
- 1 tablespoon (14 ml) low-sodium soy sauce
- $^1/_2$ teaspoon toasted sesame oil
- $^1/_2$ teaspoon cayenne pepper (optional)

In a large mixing bowl, combine the Napa cabbage, red cabbage, green cabbage, radish, onion, cilantro, mint, peas, and sesame seeds.

In a smaller mixing bowl, combine the mayonnaise, vinegar, soy sauce, sesame oil, and cayenne pepper (if using) and stir with a wire whisk. Add the mayonnaise mixture to the cabbage mixture and toss to combine.

YIELD: Makes 12 (about 1-cup) servings.

NUTRITIONAL ANALYSIS
Each with: **Calories:** 55.45 **Protein:** 3.50 g **Carbs:** 9.25 g **Total Fat:** 0.80 g **Sat Fat:** 0.05 g **Cholesterol:** 0.00 mg **Sodium:** 247.76 mg **Sugars:** 4.90 g **Fiber:** 3.64 g

Watercress Salad with Tarragon and Mint Leaves

This is perfect as an accompaniment to Baked Sea Bass (page 246).

TEXTURE: Regular

INGREDIENTS

- 1 tablespoon (14 ml) olive oil
- 3 tablespoons (45 ml) apple cider vinegar
- 2 teaspoons lemon juice
- $^1/_4$ teaspoon salt
- $^1/_4$ teaspoon black pepper
- 2 cups (70 g) watercress
- $^1/_4$ cup (6 g) fresh spearmint leaves
- $^1/_4$ cup (15 g) fresh tarragon leaves

In a small bowl, combine the oil, vinegar, and lemon juice and whisk briefly until emulsified. Add the salt and pepper.

In a serving bowl, place the watercress, mint, and tarragon. Pour the dressing on top and gently toss with salad tongs, just enough to ensure complete coverage.

YIELD: Makes 4 servings.

NUTRITIONAL ANALYSIS

Each with: **Calories:** 42.44 **Protein:** 1.03 g **Carbs:** 4.96 g **Total Fat:** 3.69 g **Sat Fat:** 0.55 g **Cholesterol:** 0.00 mg **Sodium:** 98.07 mg **Sugars:** 3.10 g **Fiber:** 0.64 g

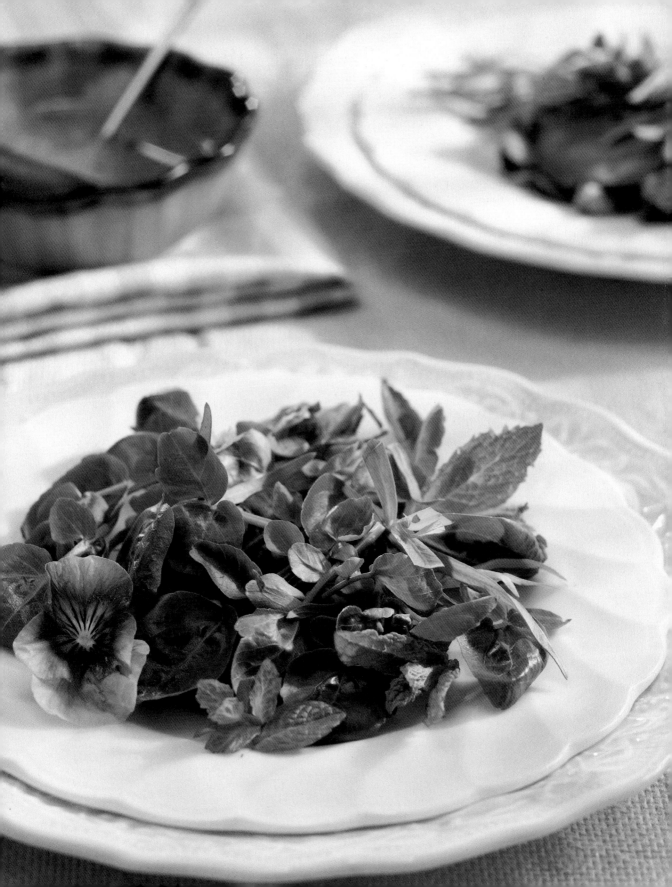

Creamy Lemon Herb Dressing

This low-fat (non-oil-based) salad dressing is the perfect alternative to the same old store-bought flavors. Making delicious salad dressing is really just this simple!

TEXTURE: Pureed

INGREDIENTS

- 1 cup (225 g) nonfat cottage cheese
- 1/3 cup (75 ml) low-fat buttermilk
- 2 teaspoons fresh lemon juice
- 1/2 teaspoon lemon zest
- 1 teaspoon chopped fresh tarragon leaves
- 1 teaspoon chopped fresh parsley
- 1 teaspoon chopped fresh green onion (white and green parts)

Place all of the ingredients in a blender or food processor and blend until smooth.

YIELD: Makes 10 (about 2-tablespoon) servings.

NUTRITIONAL ANALYSIS
Each with: **Calories:** 19.84 **Protein:** 2.90 g **Carbs:** 1.74 g
Total Fat: 0.08 g **Sat Fat:** 0.05 g **Cholesterol:** 1.33 mg
Sodium: 96.71 mg **Sugars:** 1.42 g **Fiber:** 0.03 g

Blue Cheese Dressing

TEXTURE: Pureed

INGREDIENTS

- 1 cup (225 g) nonfat cottage cheese
- 1/3 cup (75 ml) nonfat buttermilk
- 2 tablespoons (15 g) blue cheese crumbles
- 1/2 teaspoon Worcestershire sauce
- 1/2 teaspoon fresh lemon juice
- 1 teaspoon finely chopped fresh parsley
- 1/2 teaspoon black pepper

Place all of the ingredients in a blender or food processor and blend until smooth.

YIELD: Makes 10 (about 2-tablespoon) servings.

NUTRITIONAL ANALYSIS
Each with: **Calories:** 24.88 **Protein:** 3.23 g **Carbs:** 1.76 g
Total Fat: 0.51 g **Sat Fat:** 0.29 g **Cholesterol:** 2.33 mg
Sodium: 115.72 mg **Sugars:** 1.43 g **Fiber:** 0.03 g

Creamy Italian Dressing

TEXTURE: Pureed

INGREDIENTS

- 1 cup (225 g) nonfat cottage cheese
- $1/3$ cup (75 ml) low-fat buttermilk
- 1 teaspoon fresh lemon juice
- $1/2$ teaspoon dried basil
- $1/2$ teaspoon dried oregano
- $1/2$ teaspoon dried thyme
- $1/2$ teaspoon garlic powder

Place all of the ingredients in a blender or food processor and blend until smooth.

YIELD: Makes 10 (about 2-tablespoon) servings.

NUTRITIONAL ANALYSIS
Each with: **Calories:** 20.34 **Protein:** 2.93 g **Carbs:** 1.82 g
Total Fat: 0.08 g **Sat Fat:** 0.05 g **Cholesterol:** 1.33 mg
Sodium: 96.69 mg **Sugars:** 1.44 g **Fiber:** 0.05 g

French Dressing

TEXTURE: Pureed

INGREDIENTS

- 1 cup (225 g) nonfat cottage cheese
- $1/3$ cup (75 ml) low-fat buttermilk
- $1 1/2$ teaspoons paprika
- $1/2$ teaspoon Worcestershire sauce
- 2 teaspoons unsalted tomato juice
- 1 teaspoon onion powder
- $1/2$ teaspoon dry mustard

Place all of the ingredients in a blender or food processor and blend until smooth.

YIELD: Makes 10 (about 2-tablespoon) servings.

NUTRITIONAL ANALYSIS
Each with: **Calories:** 21.80 **Protein:** 3.01 g **Carbs:** 2.05 g
Total Fat: 0.18 g **Sat Fat:** 0.05 g **Cholesterol:** 1.33 mg
Sodium: 97.03 mg **Sugars:** 1.58 g **Fiber:** 0.14 g

Sweet Lemon Poppy Seed Dressing

TEXTURE: Pureed

INGREDIENTS

- 1 cup (225 g) nonfat cottage cheese
- ¹/₃ cup (75 ml) low-fat buttermilk
- 2 teaspoons fresh lemon juice
- ¹/₂ teaspoon lemon zest
- 2 teaspoons honey
- 1 teaspoon poppy seeds

Place all of the ingredients in a blender or food processor and blend until smooth.

YIELD: Makes 10 (about 2-tablespoon) servings.

NUTRITIONAL ANALYSIS

Each with: **Calories:** 25.06 **Protein:** 2.93 g **Carbs:** 2.83 g **Total Fat:** 0.20 g **Sat Fat:** 0.06 g **Cholesterol:** 1.33 mg **Sodium:** 96.65 mg **Sugars:** 2.52 g **Fiber:** 0.04 g

Garden Goddess Dressing

TEXTURE: Pureed

INGREDIENTS

- 1 cup (225 g) nonfat cottage cheese
- ¹/₃ cup (75 ml) low-fat buttermilk
- 1 teaspoon fresh lemon juice
- 2 teaspoons anchovy paste
- 1 tablespoon (4 g) chopped fresh parsley
- 2 teaspoons chopped green onion
- 1 teaspoon chopped fresh oregano leaves (stems removed)

Place all of the ingredients in a blender or food processor and blend until smooth.

YIELD: Makes 10 (about 2-tablespoon) servings.

NUTRITIONAL ANALYSIS

Each with: **Calories:** 21.94 **Protein:** 3.04 g **Carbs:** 1.75 g **Total Fat:** 0.25 g **Sat Fat:** 0.08 g **Cholesterol:** 4.99 mg **Sodium:** 159.49 mg **Sugars:** 1.42 g **Fiber:** 0.07 g

Dill Dressing

TEXTURE: Pureed

INGREDIENTS

- 1 cup (225 g) nonfat cottage cheese
- $\frac{1}{3}$ cup (75 ml) low-fat buttermilk
- 1 teaspoon fresh lemon juice
- $1\frac{1}{2}$ tablespoons (3 g) chopped fresh dill
- $\frac{1}{4}$ teaspoon black pepper
- $\frac{1}{4}$ teaspoon ground celery seed

Place all of the ingredients in a blender or food processor and blend until smooth.

YIELD: Makes 10 (about 2-tablespoon) servings.

NUTRITIONAL ANALYSIS

Each with: **Calories:** 19.87 **Protein:** 2.90 g **Carbs:** 1.70 g **Total Fat:** 0.09 g **Sat Fat:** 0.05 g **Cholesterol:** 1.33 mg **Sodium:** 96.73 mg **Sugars:** 1.40 g **Fiber:** 0.02 g

Horseradish Dressing

This one really packs a punch!

TEXTURE: Pureed

INGREDIENTS

- 1 cup (225 g) nonfat cottage cheese
- $\frac{1}{3}$ cup (75 ml) low-fat buttermilk
- 1 teaspoon fresh lemon juice
- 1 tablespoon (15 g) fresh grated horseradish
- 1 teaspoon chopped fresh parsley
- 1 teaspoon chopped fresh green onion (white parts only)

Place all of the ingredients in a blender or food processor and blend until smooth.

YIELD: Makes 10 (about 2-tablespoon) servings.

NUTRITIONAL ANALYSIS

Each with: **Calories:** 19.72 **Protein:** 2.89 g **Carbs:** 1.71 g **Total Fat:** 0.07 g **Sat Fat:** 0.05 g **Cholesterol:** 1.33 mg **Sodium:** 96.92 mg **Sugars:** 1.41 g **Fiber:** 0.03 g

CHAPTER 6

Protein-Packed Salad Toppers

Crispy Chicken

This is a delicious alternative to your classic fried chicken!

TEXTURE: Regular

INGREDIENTS

- 1 container (6 ounces, or 170 g) plain, low-fat Greek yogurt
- Juice of 1 lemon
- 1 cup (115 g) whole-wheat bread crumbs
- ½ teaspoon garlic powder
- ½ teaspoon kosher salt
- 4 (4-ounce, or 115 g) boneless, skinless chicken breasts
- Cooking spray

Preheat oven to 350°F (180°C, or gas mark 4). Spray a 9 x 13-inch (23 x 33-cm) baking dish with cooking spray, 1 second.

Stir the yogurt in a bowl until smooth. Add the lemon juice and mix thoroughly.

In a separate bowl, combine the bread crumbs, garlic powder, and salt; mix well. Dip each chicken breast in the yogurt mixture, then in the bread-crumb mixture, coating completely.

Place the chicken in the prepared baking dish and bake for 25 minutes to 30 minutes, or until the chicken is cooked through. Let cool for 5 minutes before serving.

YIELD: Makes 6 (4-ounce) servings.

NUTRITIONAL ANALYSIS

Each with: **Calories:** 188.49 **Protein:** 29.20 g **Carbs:** 10.48 g **Total Fat:** 4.10 g **Sat Fat:** 1.14 g **Cholesterol:** 66.13 mg **Sodium:** 321.30 mg **Sugars:** 2.30 g **Fiber:** 2.02 g

Three-Chili Shrimp

This is a spicy treat that will be a great addition to any salad. It can even be served as a side dish for parties or as a filling for wraps and sandwiches.

TEXTURE: Regular

INGREDIENTS

- 1 tablespoon (15 ml) extra-virgin olive oil
- $1/2$ teaspoon paprika
- 1 tablespoon (13 g) sugar
- 1 tablespoon (8 g) chili powder
- 2 teaspoons ancho chili powder
- $1/2$ teaspoon chipotle chili powder
- $1/2$ teaspoon kosher salt
- 2 pounds (910 g) large shrimp, $^{21}/_{25}$ count, peeled and deveined

Heat the olive oil in a medium sauté pan over medium-high heat.

Meanwhile, in a medium bowl, mix together the paprika, sugar, chili powders, and salt. Gently toss the shrimp with the spice blend, coating thoroughly.

Cook the shrimp until cooked through, approximately 3 minutes. Remove from the heat and serve immediately.

YIELD: Makes 8 (about 4-ounce) servings.

NUTRITIONAL ANALYSIS
Each with: **Calories:** 145.11 **Protein:** 23.15 g **Carbs:** 3.14 g **Total Fat:** 3.88 g **Sat Fat:** 0.65 g
Cholesterol: 172.37 mg **Sodium:** 297.69 mg **Sugars:** 1.64 g **Fiber:** 0.33 g

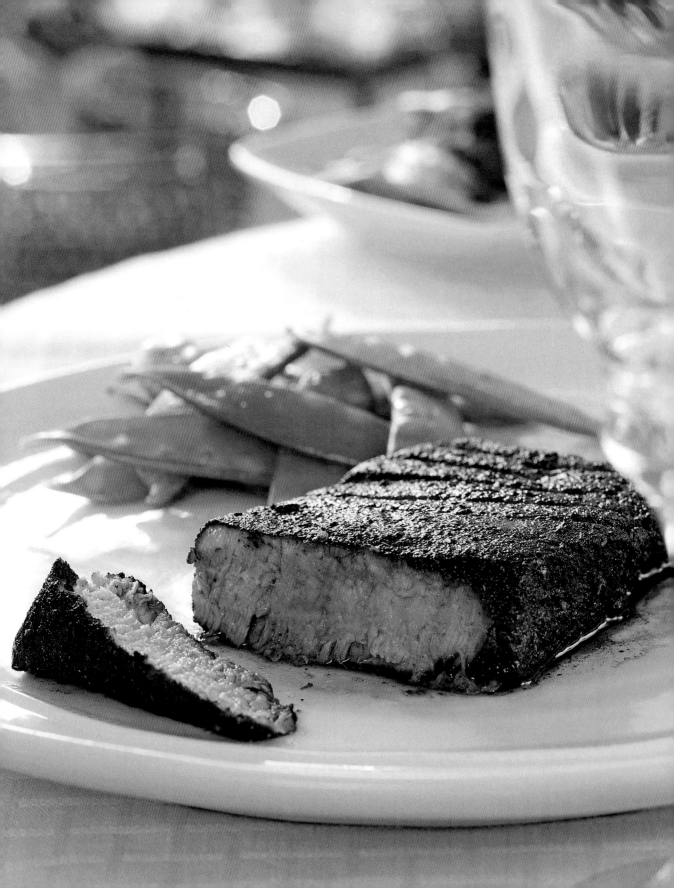

Blackened Tuna Steaks

TEXTURE: Regular

INGREDIENTS

- ¼ cup (59 ml) extra-virgin olive oil
- 2 tablespoons (14 g) paprika
- 1½ tablespoons (8 g) cayenne pepper
- 1½ tablespoons (10 g) onion powder
- 1½ teaspoons kosher salt
- 1½ teaspoons black pepper
- 1½ teaspoons dried thyme
- 1½ teaspoons dried basil
- 1½ teaspoons dried oregano
- 1½ tablespoons (15 g) garlic powder
- 6 (4-ounce, or 115 g) tuna steaks

Heat the olive oil in a medium sauté pan over medium-high heat.

Meanwhile, in a medium bowl, mix together the paprika, cayenne pepper, onion powder, salt, pepper, thyme, basil, oregano, and garlic powder. Coat each tuna steak with the seasoning mix.

Cook the tuna steaks in the pan on one side for 3 minutes, then turn over and cook on the other side for another 3 minutes. Remove from the heat and serve immediately.

YIELD: Makes 6 (about 4-ounce) servings.

NUTRITIONAL ANALYSIS

Each with: **Calories:** 147.16 **Protein:** 17.80 g **Carbs:** 5.75 g **Total Fat:** 6.01 g **Sat Fat:** 1.01 g **Cholesterol:** 35.53 mg **Sodium:** 511.95 mg **Sugars:** 0.43 g **Fiber:** 2.07 g

CHAPTER 7

Appetizers and Entertaining at Home

Vegetable Party Platter

Serve with the delicious Smoked Salmon Dip (page 170) for a festive dish.

TEXTURE: Regular

INGREDIENTS

- 8 whole leaves red leaf lettuce
- 1 red bell pepper, cut into strips
- 1 yellow bell pepper, cut into strips
- 3 Italian plum tomatoes, cored and cut into 4 wedges each
- $^1/_2$ cauliflower head, cut into bite-size florets

On a large serving platter, spread out the lettuce leaves. Arrange the vegetable pieces around the outside of the bowl.

YIELD: Makes 12 (about $^1/_4$-cup) servings.

NUTRITIONAL ANALYSIS

Each with: **Calories:** 25.66 **Protein:** 1.30 g **Carbs:** 5.46 g **Total Fat:** 0.23 g **Sat Fat:** 0.04 g **Cholesterol:** 0.00 mg **Sodium:** 12.80 mg **Sugars:** 3.43 g **Fiber:** 1.95 g

Sweet Corn Relish

Try this zesty relish as a topping for fish or chicken or for a dip with Toasted Pita Chips (page 166).

TEXTURE: Mechanical Soft

INGREDIENTS

- $1^1/_2$ cups (240 g) fresh corn kernels (about 4 large ears, shucked)
- $^1/_2$ medium red bell pepper, cored and finely chopped (about $^1/_2$ cup, or 70 g)
- 2 tablespoons (20 g) finely chopped red onion
- 1 teaspoon finely chopped fresh jalapeno pepper, seeds removed
- 2 teaspoons chopped fresh cilantro
- 1 small clove garlic, minced
- 1 teaspoon salt
- $^1/_4$ teaspoon black pepper

In a small bowl, combine all ingredients and stir to mix. Cover and refrigerate for 30 minutes, stirring once or twice before serving.

YIELD: Makes 8 (about $^1/_4$-cup) servings.

NUTRITIONAL ANALYSIS

Each with: **Calories:** 38.95 **Protein:** 1.25 g **Carbs:** 8.86 g **Total Fat:** 0.43 g **Sat Fat:** 0.06 g **Cholesterol:** 0.00 mg **Sodium:** 42.17 mg **Sugars:** 1.87 g **Fiber:** 1.24 g

Curry Yogurt Dip

Serve with Toasted Pita Chips (page 166) and fresh vegetable sticks. It can be made up to 24 hours ahead of time.

TEXTURE: Pureed

INGREDIENTS

- 1 cup (225 g) nonfat cottage cheese
- 3 tablespoons (45 g) nonfat mayonnaise
- 1 green onion, thinly sliced (white and green parts)
- 3 teaspoons chopped fresh cilantro
- 1^1/$_2$ teaspoons curry powder
- ^{1}/$_8$ teaspoon cayenne pepper (optional)

In a food processor, blend the cottage cheese for about 30 seconds, until smooth.

Using a rubber spatula, scrape the cottage cheese into a small mixing bowl and add the mayonnaise, onion, cilantro, curry powder, and cayenne pepper (if using). Stir to combine, place in a serving bowl, cover, and refrigerate until ready to serve.

YIELD: Makes 8 (about 2-tablespoons) servings.

NUTRITIONAL ANALYSIS

Each with: **Calories:** 25.43 **Protein:** 3.33 g **Carbs:** 2.57 g **Total Fat:** 0.06 g **Sat Fat:** 0.01 g **Cholesterol:** 1.25 mg **Sodium:** 155.32 mg **Sugars:** 1.67 g **Fiber:** 0.19 g

Tzatziki

This is a delicious Greek-style cool and creamy cucumber sauce that will freshen up just about any dish.

TEXTURE: Mechanical Soft

INGREDIENTS

- 2 tablespoons (30 ml) extra-virgin olive oil
- 1 tablespoon (15 ml) white wine vinegar
- 2 cloves garlic, finely minced
- ^{1}/$_2$ teaspoon kosher salt
- ^{1}/$_4$ teaspoon white pepper
- 1 cup (230 g) plain, low-fat Greek yogurt
- 1 cup (230 g) fat-free sour cream
- 2 medium cucumbers, peeled, seeded, and finely chopped
- 1 teaspoon fresh dill, chopped

Combine the olive oil, vinegar, garlic, salt, and pepper in a bowl. Mix well.

Strain the yogurt through a coffee filter set in a strainer in the refrigerator for 2 to 3 hours. After the yogurt has strained, blend it, using a whisk, with the sour cream until smooth.

Next, combine the olive oil mixture with the yogurt mixture. Add the cucumber and dill. Chill for at least 2 hours before serving.

YIELD: Makes about 30 (about ¼-cup) servings.

NUTRITIONAL ANALYSIS

Each with: **Calories:** 24.56 **Protein:** 1.25 g **Carbs:** 2.27 g **Total Fat: 1.20 g Sat Fat:** 0.30 g **Cholesterol:** 1.27 mg **Sodium:** 40.68 mg **Sugars:** 1.32 g **Fiber:** 0.21 g

Fresh Salsa Caliente

TEXTURE: Soft

INGREDIENTS

- 1 cup (180 g) coarsely chopped tomato
- $^1\!/_4$ cup (40 g) coarsely chopped yellow or red onion
- 1 small jalapeno pepper, finely chopped (optional)
- 2 tablespoons (2 g) chopped fresh cilantro
- $^1\!/_4$ teaspoon salt
- $^1\!/_4$ teaspoon cracked black pepper

Place the tomato, onion, and jalapeno pepper (if using) in a food processor fitted with a metal blade. Pulse the mixture just enough to break the pieces down to a bit smaller size. Add the cilantro, salt, and pepper and pulse one or two more times.

YIELD: Makes 6 (about $^1\!/_4$-cup) servings.

NUTRITIONAL ANALYSIS
Each with: **Calories:** 11.98 **Protein:** 0.47 g **Carbs:** 2.62 g **Total Fat:** 0.16 g **Sat Fat:** 0.02 g **Cholesterol:** 0.00 mg **Sodium:** 71.84 mg **Sugars:** 1.39 g **Fiber:** 0.64 g

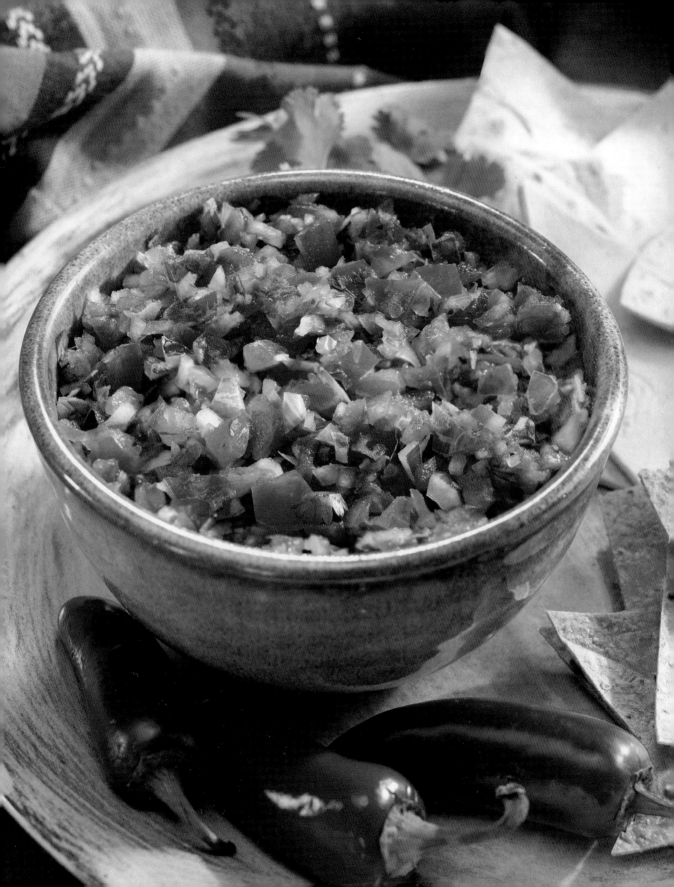

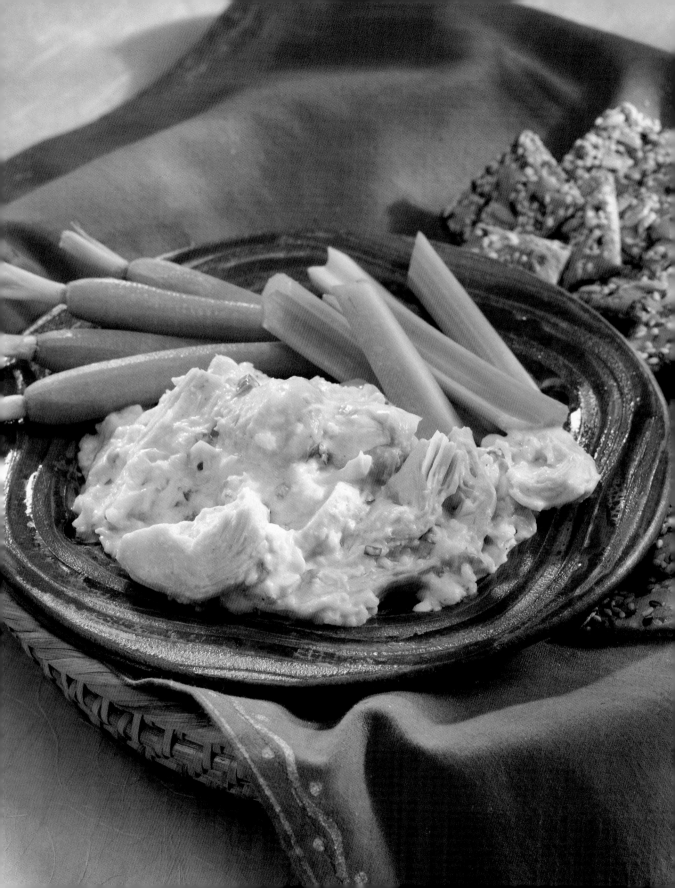

Hot Artichoke Dip

This is a simple, healthy, delicious dip that will get your party started right. I make it for parties, and it's always a hit! For added color and a little more flavor, add 1 tablespoon (10 g) finely chopped red pepper. For a little extra kick, add 1 finely chopped small fresh jalapeno pepper. For more fiber, serve with low-fat, whole wheat crackers.

TEXTURE: Soft (Raw vegetables as pictured: Regular)

INGREDIENTS

- 2 cans (14 ounces, 400 g each) artichoke hearts, drained and cut into quarters
- 1 cup (110 g) shredded low-moisture, part-skim mozzarella cheese
- $^3/_4$ cup (175 g) nonfat mayonnaise
- $^1/_4$ cup (20 g) shredded Parmesan cheese
- $^1/_8$ teaspoon salt
- $^1/_4$ teaspoon black pepper

Preheat the oven to 375°F (190°C, or gas mark 5).

In a 1-quart (1-L) casserole oven-safe dish, place the artichoke hearts. Add the mozzarella cheese, mayonnaise, Parmesan cheese, salt, and pepper. Mix thoroughly with a large spoon, ensuring even distribution. Bake the dip for 15 minutes and serve immediately. (Avoid overheating to ensure the mayonnaise does not separate.)

YIELD: Makes 10 (about $^1/_2$-cup) servings.

NUTRITIONAL ANALYSIS
Each with: **Calories:** 74.47 **Protein:** 4.97 g **Carbs:** 7.30 g **Total Fat:** 2.35 g **Sat Fat:** 1.55 g **Cholesterol:** 7.44 mg **Sodium:** 456.30 mg **Sugars:** 1.87 g **Fiber:** 1.21 g

Toasted Pita Chips

Pita chips are a great alternative to high-fat corn or potato chips and can be flavored in a variety of ways. This recipe is plain and simple to complement the scrumptious flavor of Roasted Garlic below.

TEXTURE: Regular

INGREDIENTS

- 1 tablespoon (14 ml) olive oil
- 6 (6-inch, or 15 cm) whole-wheat pita breads (see note)
- ½ teaspoon celery salt
- ½ teaspoon paprika
- ⅛ teaspoon black pepper

Preheat the oven to 375°F (190°C, or gas mark 5). Using a pastry brush, lightly brush oil onto both sides of each pita. Cut the pitas into 8 wedges each. In a small bowl, combine the celery salt, paprika, and pepper. Place the pitas on a baking sheet and sprinkle one side with the seasoning mixture. Bake the pitas for about 15 minutes, until the chips are beginning to turn golden brown.

YIELD: Makes 48 chips; 1 serving is about 4 pita chips.

MARGARET'S NOTE

You could use low-carb whole-wheat pita bread instead of regular whole-wheat pita to lower the calories and increase the protein of the pita chips.

Roasted Garlic

Roasted garlic is versatile and easy to prepare. (It's also easy on the breath after it's cooked!) In addition to the Toasted Pita Chips (left), try spreading some on a toasted English muffin with scrambled egg substitute for breakfast.

TEXTURE: Puree

INGREDIENTS

- 10 garlic bulbs
- Olive oil

Preheat the oven to 300°F (150°C, or gas mark 2). Peel away the papery skin on the outside of the garlic bulbs, but leave the cloves attached. Rub some olive oil on your hands, then rub the whole bulbs of garlic just enough to give them a slightly shiny appearance. Wrap the bulbs in aluminum foil and place on a sheet pan. Roast the garlic for 1 hour, until the cloves are soft. (You will surely smell it cooking before it's done!) Unwrap the garlic and allow it to cool to the touch before squeezing out the soft, delicious pulp.

YIELD: 12 servings

NUTRITIONAL ANALYSIS

Each with: **Calories:** 100.00 **Protein:** 3.31 g **Carbs:** 18.49 g **Total Fat:** 2.02 g **Sat Fat:** 0.30 g **Cholesterol:** 0.00 mg **Sodium:** 218.61 mg **Sugars:** 0.30 g **Fiber:** 2.46 g

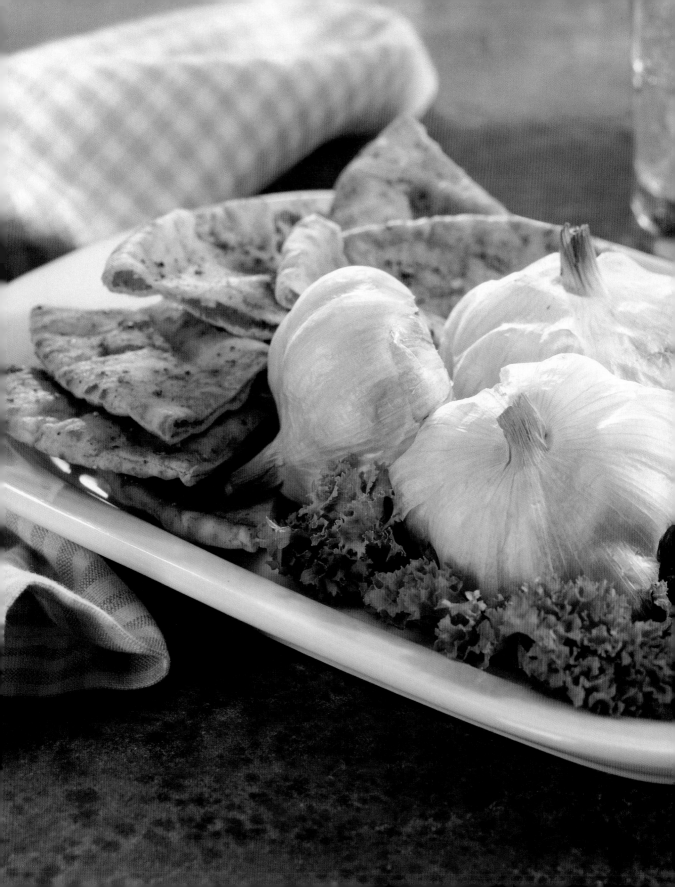

Easy and Delicious Spinach Dip

This dip is great with fresh vegetable sticks or whole wheat pita—a party favorite!

TEXTURE: Soft

INGREDIENTS

- 1 package (10 ounces, or 280 g) frozen, chopped spinach
- $^1/_2$ cup (50 g) chopped green onion
- $^1/_4$ teaspoon garlic powder
- 2 tablespoons (20 g) finely chopped red bell pepper
- $^1/_4$ cup (50 g) water chestnuts, drained and chopped
- 1 cup (200 g) nonfat sour cream
- 1 cup (230 g) nonfat mayonnaise
- 1 tablespoon (14 ml) lemon juice
- $^1/_2$ teaspoon salt
- $^1/_4$ teaspoon black pepper, ground

Thaw and drain the spinach in a colander, pressing all of the excess moisture out.

In a medium mixing bowl, mix the onion, garlic powder, bell pepper, water chestnuts, sour cream, mayonnaise, lemon juice, salt, and black pepper until well incorporated.

YIELD: Makes 14 (about $^1/_4$-cup) servings.

NUTRITIONAL ANALYSIS
Each with: **Calories:** 41.66 **Protein:** 1.85 g **Carbs:** 7.78 g **Total Fat:** 0.10 g **Sat Fat:** 0.01 g **Cholesterol:** 2.86 mg **Sodium:** 250.37 mg **Sugars:** 2.82 g **Fiber:** 0.79 g

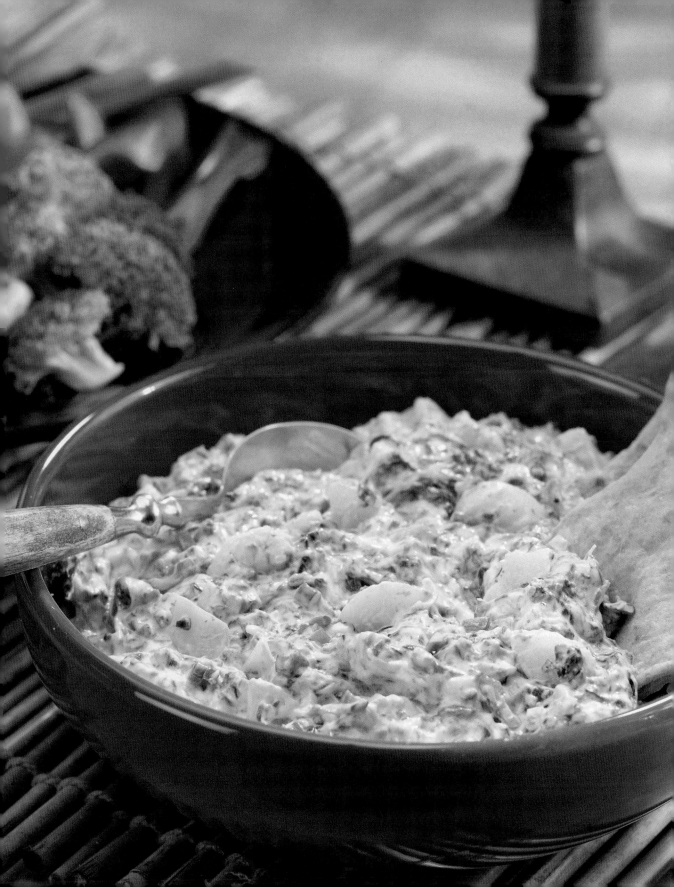

Smoked Salmon Dip

Smoked salmon is always a hit at parties. This dip has tangy kick to it.

TEXTURE: Soft

INGREDIENTS

- 1 cup (225 g) nonfat cottage cheese
- 1/2 cup (100 g) nonfat sour cream
- 3/4 cup (6 ounces, or 170 g) chopped smoked salmon
- 3 large green onions, thinly sliced (white and green parts)
- 2 teaspoons fresh lemon juice
- 1/8 teaspoon cayenne pepper (optional)

In a food processor, blend the cottage cheese for about 30 seconds, until smooth. Using a rubber spatula, scrape the cottage cheese into a medium mixing bowl. Add the sour cream, salmon, onions, lemon juice, and cayenne pepper (if using). Mix well. Place the dip into a serving bowl and refrigerate until ready to serve.

YIELD: Makes about 10 (2-tablespoons) servings.

NUTRITIONAL ANALYSIS

Each with: **Calories:** 54.70 **Protein:** 7.04 g **Carbs:** 3.79 g **Total Fat:** 1.20 g **Sat Fat:** 0.40 g **Cholesterol:** 10.00 mg **Sodium:** 312.08 mg **Sugars:** 1.86 g **Fiber:** 0.07 g

Latkes

This is a great dish for parties.

TEXTURE: Regular

INGREDIENTS

- 3 pounds (1.5 kg) Yukon gold potatoes, skinned and finely grated (see note)
- 1 cup (160 g) finely diced yellow onion
- ³/₄ cup (85 g) finely grated carrot
- ¹/₂ cup (50 g) finely chopped green onion
- ¹/₂ cup (30 g) finely chopped parsley
- ¹/₃ cup (45 g) matzo meal
- ¹/₂ teaspoon baking powder
- 1 cup (235 ml) liquid egg substitute or egg whites
- 1 teaspoon kosher salt
- ¹/₄ teaspoon black pepper
- 2 teaspoons granulated garlic
- ¹/₂ cup (50 g) grated Parmesan cheese
- ¹/₃ cup (75 ml) olive oil

Heat a heavy baking sheet or a large cast-iron skillet in the oven at 450°F (230°C, or gas mark 8).

Drain the potatoes, yellow onion, carrot, green onion, and parsley by pressing them into a fine mesh strainer or by squeezing them in cheesecloth. Once all excess moisture is removed, transfer the grated vegetables to a large (at least 3 quart, or 3-L) mixing bowl. Add the matzo meal, baking powder, egg substitute or egg whites, salt, pepper, garlic, and cheese and mix to incorporate well.

Remove the baking sheet or skillet from the oven. Using a pastry brush, lightly brush it with the oil. Immediately spoon ¼ cup (60 ml) of the latke batter onto the sheet or skillet and return the pan to the oven. Bake for 7 to 10 minutes on each side, until a golden brown color appears. This can be done in batches, making several at a time. Remember to heat the baking sheet then brush it with olive oil just prior to cooking each batch.

YIELD: Makes 50 to 60 (2-inch) latkes, which should serve about 15 people.

NUTRITIONAL ANALYSIS:
2-latkes with: **Calories:** 139.85 **Protein:** 6.17 g **Carbs:** 21.87 g
Total Fat: 3.42 g **Sat Fat:** 1.16 g **Cholesterol:** 1.77 mg
Sodium: 246.62 mg **Sugars:** 2.36 g **Fiber:** 2.87 g

NOTE

You can grate the potatoes by hand or in a food processor fitted with a fine grating disc.

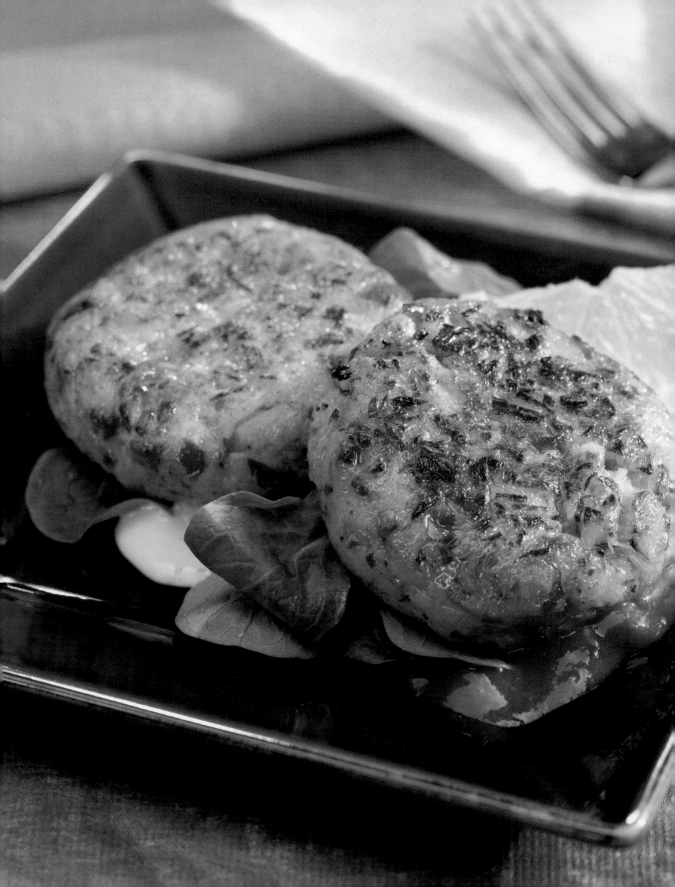

Pacific Dungeness Crab Cakes

These crab cakes contain no bread or flour fillers, just pure, delicious Dungeness crab!

TEXTURE: Soft

INGREDIENTS

- ¹/₂ pound (225 g) Dungeness crabmeat, cooked (any cooked crabmeat may be substituted, except for canned)
- 1 tablespoon (16 g) minced celery
- 2 teaspoons minced red bell pepper
- 2 teaspoons finely chopped fresh cilantro
- 2 tablespoons (30 g) nonfat mayonnaise
- ¹/₈ teaspoon sea salt or kosher salt
- ¹/₈ teaspoon cayenne pepper (optional)
- 2 teaspoons olive oil
- ¹/₂ teaspoon toasted sesame oil
- 2 tablespoons (2 g) gourmet salad greens
- 2 lemon wedges
- 2 tablespoons (30 g) low-fat tartar sauce

NOTE

Two crab cakes equal the portion recommendation for an entrée serving, or one crab cake can be served as an appetizer. A little goes a long way with crabmeat, as it has a very rich flavor and texture.

Place the crabmeat in a strainer or colander and press out excess moisture.

Transfer the crabmeat to a medium mixing bowl, and add the celery, bell pepper, and cilantro.

In a small bowl, combine the mayonnaise, salt, and cayenne pepper (if using) and stir to mix.

Add the mayonnaise mixture to the crabmeat and mix until well incorporated.

Form the mixture into 6 equal patties (about 2 ounces, or 55 g each), pressing firmly enough to hold together, and place on waxed paper on top of a plate. Cover the top of the crab cakes with another sheet of waxed paper and refrigerate for 15 minutes.

In a medium, nonstick skillet, heat the olive oil and sesame oil over medium-high heat and swirl the pan to mix the oils. Gently place the crab cakes in the pan using a thin metal spatula and cook undisturbed for about 6 minutes on each side, until well browned, manipulating them only to avoid burning, then remove the pan from heat.

Place 1 tablespoon (1 g) of the greens in a pile on the center of a plate and place the crab cakes on the pile, leaning off of one side. Place a lemon wedge beside the greens and crab cakes and a teaspoon of the tartar sauce atop each cake.

YIELD: Makes 6 (about 1¹/₂-ounces) crab cakes.

NUTRITIONAL ANALYSIS

Each with: **Calories:** 70.57 **Protein:** 8.49 g **Carbs:** 2.43 g **Total Fat:** 2.68 g **Sat Fat:** 0.29 g **Cholesterol:** 28.73 mg **Sodium:** 269.31 mg **Sugars:** 1.32 g **Fiber:** 0.12 g

Crispy Zucchini Sticks

This recipe is a great and healthy alternative to classic french fries.

TEXTURE: Regular

INGREDIENTS

- Olive oil cooking spray
- $^1/_2$ cup (63 g) whole-wheat flour
- $^1/_2$ cup (63 g) all-purpose flour
- 2 tablespoons (18 g) cornmeal
- $^1/_2$ teaspoon paprika
- 1 teaspoon kosher salt
- $^1/_2$ teaspoon freshly ground black pepper
- $1^1/_2$ pounds (679 g) zucchini, cut into $^1/_2$ x 3-inch (1.25 x 7.5-cm) sticks
- 2 large egg whites, lightly beaten

Preheat oven to 475°F (240°C, or gas mark 9). Coat a large baking sheet with cooking spray.

Combine the whole-wheat flour, all-purpose flour, cornmeal, paprika, salt, and pepper in a large zip-top bag. Dip zucchini sticks in egg whites, then add to the bag and shake to coat.

Arrange the sticks, not touching, on the baking sheet. Bake for 10 minutes, then turn over. Continue to bake until the sticks are golden and tender, about 10 more minutes.

YIELD: Makes 6 (about $^3/_4$-cup) servings.

NUTRITIONAL ANALYSIS
Each with: **Calories:** 113.48 **Protein:** 6.82 g **Carbs:** 21.68 g **Total Fat:** 0.79 g **Sat Fat:** 0.15 g **Cholesterol:** 0.00 mg **Sodium:** 339.87 mg **Sugars:** 0.15 g **Fiber:** 2.94 g

BBQ Turkey Meatballs

This recipe calls for brown sugar substitute; choose one that's suitable in cooking applications (see page 50).

TEXTURE: Soft

INGREDIENTS

- 1 pound (450 g) ground turkey
- 1 cup (160 g) chopped onion
- 3 tablespoons (45 g) liquid egg substitute
- 1/4 cup (60 ml) low-fat milk
- 1/4 cup (30 g) whole-wheat bread crumbs
- 1 teaspoon kosher salt
- 1/4 teaspoon black pepper
- 2 tablespoons (28 ml) extra-virgin olive oil
- 2 cans (8 ounces, or 360 g each) tomato sauce
- 1/4 cup (6 g) brown sugar substitute
- 2 tablespoons (28 ml) vinegar
- 1 teaspoon garlic powder

Combine the turkey, onion, egg substitute, milk, bread crumbs, salt, and pepper in a bowl. Mix thoroughly and shape into 12 meatballs.

Heat the olive oil in a large skillet over medium-high heat, and then brown the meatballs.

In a medium-size bowl, combine the tomato sauce, brown sugar substitute, vinegar, and garlic powder. Pour over the meatballs. Simmer over low heat for 10 to 15 minutes, turning frequently, until the meatballs are well glazed and are cooked through.

YIELD: Makes 12 (about 4-ounce) meatballs.

NUTRITIONAL ANALYSIS

Each with: **Calories:** 120.96 **Protein:** 8.76 g **Carbs:** 10.02 g **Total Fat:** 5.73 g **Sat Fat:** 1.19 g **Cholesterol:** 29.96 mg **Sodium:** 363.20 mg **Sugars:** 4.79 g **Fiber:** 1.86 g

JOE'S TIP

This would also be a great and easy slow cooker recipe that you could bring along to a party. Follow the recipe as it is written, but instead of simmering over low heat for 10 to 15 minutes, pour all the ingredients into the slow cooker and cook on the low setting for 4 to 6 hours, or until the meatballs are cooked through and tender.

Plum Tomatoes with Blue Cheese

This recipe is great as an appetizer for dinner parties. You could substitute feta cheese for the blue cheese and nonfat plain yogurt for the milk.

TEXTURE: Regular

INGREDIENTS

- 2 tablespoons (15 g) blue cheese
- 1 tablespoon (14 ml) nonfat milk
- 1/2 teaspoon hot pepper sauce
- 12 medium Italian plum tomatoes, cored and cut in half lengthwise
- 1 tablespoon (4 g) chopped fresh parsley

In a medium mixing bowl, combine the cheese, milk, and pepper sauce, stirring vigorously to mix. Transfer to a small container, cover, and refrigerate for at least 30 minutes.

Top each tomato half equally with the cheese mixture and sprinkle evenly with parsley. Serve at room temperature.

YIELD: Makes 12 servings.

NUTRITIONAL ANALYSIS
Each with: **Calories:** 29.00 **Protein:** 1.64 g **Carbs:** 2.70 g **Total Fat:** 1.51 g **Sat Fat:** 0.91 g **Cholesterol:** 3.57 mg **Sodium:** 69.93 mg **Sugars:** 1.72 g **Fiber:** 0.80 g

Stuffed Mushrooms

This is another can't miss party favorite or dinner party appetizer and a great source of potassium.

TEXTURE: Soft

INGREDIENTS

- 1 pound (455 g) medium mushrooms (about 18)
- 1 tablespoon (14 ml) olive oil
- 1 clove garlic, minced
- 6 teaspoons finely diced red bell pepper
- $1/4$ cup (40 g) finely diced yellow onion
- 2 tablespoons (15 g) thinly sliced green onion (green and white parts)
- 1 tablespoon (4 g) chopped fresh parsley
- $1/4$ teaspoon dried basil
- $1/4$ teaspoon dried oregano
- $3/4$ cup (75 g) whole-wheat bread crumbs (about $1^1/_2$ slices bread, toasted)
- 2 tablespoons (10 g) grated Parmesan cheese

Preheat the oven to 375°F (190°C, or gas mark 5).

Clean the mushrooms and remove the stems. Finely chop or mince the stems and set aside.

Place the mushroom caps in a 9- x 13-inch (22.5- x 32.5-cm) baking dish.

In a medium nonstick skillet, heat the oil over medium-high heat. Add the mushroom stems and garlic and sauté for about 3 minutes. Add the bell pepper, yellow onion, green onion, parsley, basil, and oregano and continue cooking for about 4 minutes, until the peppers are soft. Remove from heat and add the bread crumbs and cheese. Stir to combine. Fill the mushroom caps with the stuffing mixture and bake for 20 minutes, until the mushrooms are soft.

YIELD: Makes 6 (about $1/_2$-cup) servings.

NUTRITIONAL ANALYSIS
Each with: **Calories:** 75.68 **Protein:** 4.14 g **Carbs:** 7.26 g **Total Fat:** 3.63 g **Sat Fat:** 0.87 g **Cholesterol:** 1.00 mg **Sodium:** 81.86 mg **Sugars:** 2.50 g **Fiber:** 1.59 g

Traditional Hummus

Serve this with cucumber slices, tomato wedges, Greek olives, and pita bread. Note that five Greek olives equals one serving of fat.

TEXTURE: Soft. May be considered pureed in some programs (Olives and cucumbers as pictured: Regular)

INGREDIENTS

- 3–5 cloves fresh garlic, crushed
- 1$\frac{1}{2}$ tablespoons (21 ml) extra-virgin olive oil, divided
- 3 cans (15 ounces, or 430 g each) cooked chickpeas (garbanzo beans), rinsed and drained
- $\frac{1}{4}$ cup (60 g) sesame tahini
- $\frac{1}{2}$ teaspoon toasted sesame oil
- 2 tablespoons (28 ml) cold water
- 2 tablespoons (28 ml) fresh lemon juice
- $\frac{1}{2}$ teaspoon salt
- 2 teaspoons ground cumin

Place the garlic in a food processor with 1$\frac{1}{2}$ teaspoons of the olive oil and process until the garlic is minced, almost paste-like. (You will need to stop the process and scrape down the garlic from the sides of the container a few times.) Add the chickpeas, tahini, sesame oil, water, lemon juice, salt, and cumin, and continue processing. While the puree is still processing, slowly add the remaining olive oil. (The consistency should have a smooth but grainy texture. If a thinner consistency is preferred, add additional water in small increments.)

YIELD: Makes 16 (about $\frac{1}{4}$-cup) servings.

NUTRITIONAL ANALYSIS:

Calories: 111.99 **Protein:** 4.74 g **Carbs:** 13.54 g **Total Fat:** 4.68 g **Sat Fat:** 0.59 g **Cholesterol:** 0.00 mg **Sodium:** 39.90 mg **Sugars:** 2.35 g **Fiber:** 3.89 g

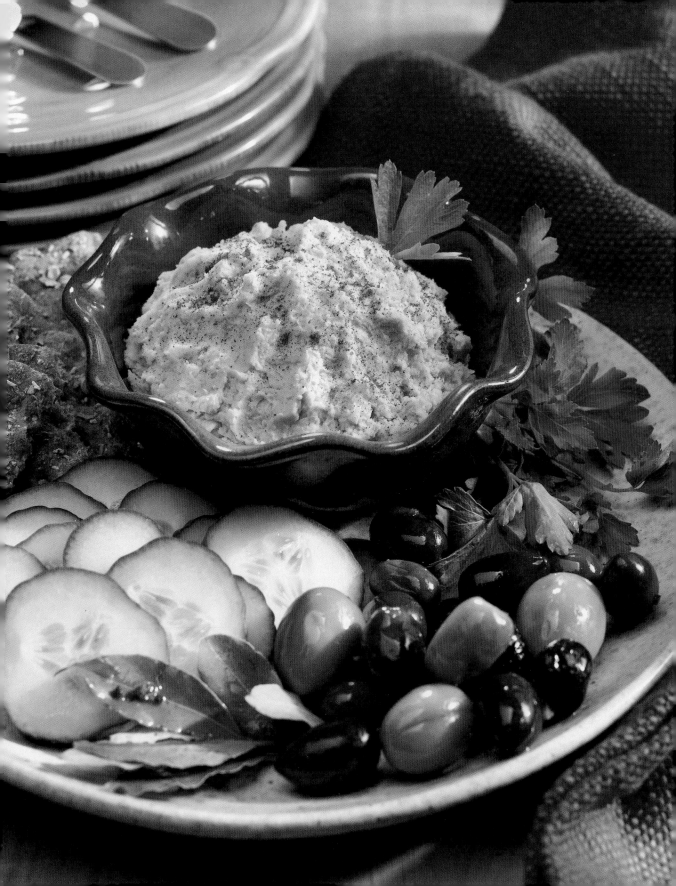

Teresa's Edamame Dip

This dip, using super-healthy green soybeans, comes from Teresa, a gastric bypass surgery patient in Baltimore. You can find shelled edamame in the natural foods freezer section of most grocery stores.

TEXTURE: Puree

INGREDIENTS

- 2 cups (512 g) shelled edamame
- 1 cup (235 ml) water
- 1/2 teaspoon kosher salt, divided
- 2 cloves garlic, finely chopped
- 1 teaspoon lemon or lime zest
- 2 teaspoons lemon or lime juice
- 2 cups (460 g) plain nonfat yogurt
- 1 small cucumber, seeded, peeled, and chopped
- 1 cup (180 g) seeded and diced tomato
- 1/4 cup (20 g) chopped turkey bacon, cooked
- 1/4 cup (30 g) low-fat shredded Cheddar cheese

Bring the edamame, water, 1/4 teaspoon salt, and garlic to a simmer for 15 to 20 minutes. Drain, reserving 1/4 cup (59 ml) of the cooking liquid. Process the edamame until smooth in a food processor or blender. Add the lemon or lime zest and lemon or lime juice and blend. Set aside.

Strain the yogurt through a coffee filter set in a strainer in the refrigerator for 2 to 3 hours. After the yogurt has strained, mix it with the cucumber and remaining 1/4 teaspoon salt.

Spread the edamame mixture on the bottom of a serving plate. Spoon the yogurt mixture over the top, and sprinkle with the tomatoes, turkey bacon, and Cheddar cheese.

YIELD: Makes 16 (about 1/4-cup) servings.

NUTRITIONAL ANALYSIS
Each with: **Calories:** 40.92 **Protein:** 3.92 g **Carbs:** 4.71 g **Total Fat:** 1.10 g **Sat Fat:** 0.11 g **Cholesterol:** 2.19 mg **Sodium:** 126.27 mg **Sugars:** 2.60 g **Fiber:** 0.91 g

Protein-Packed 7-Layer Bean Dip

This is a classic dish for entertaining that is always a big hit. It's also quick and easy to prepare.

TEXTURE: Regular

INGREDIENTS

- 2 cups (476 g) refried beans
- 1 teaspoon chipotle chili powder
- $1/2$ teaspoon ground cumin
- 1 cup (115 g) shredded low-fat Cheddar cheese
- $1/4$ cup (30 g) chopped chile peppers, or canned jalapeños
- 1 avocado, peeled and chopped
- 1 hot-house tomato, seeded and chopped
- $1/3$ cup (77 g) fat-free sour cream
- $1/4$ cup (25 g) sliced black olives
- 2 scallions, sliced

Heat the refried beans in a medium sauté pan over low heat. Stir in enough water to make them creamy. Mix in the chipotle chili powder and cumin.

Once the beans are hot, spread them over the bottom of a warmed serving dish. Immediately add the shredded Cheddar cheese. Layer on the chopped chile peppers (or jalapeños), avocado, tomato, and sour cream. Top with the black olives and sliced scallions. Serve with chips or warmed pita bread for dipping.

YIELD: Makes 8 (about $1/2$-cup) servings.

NUTRITIONAL ANALYSIS
Each with: **Calories:** 173.55 **Protein:** 8.90 g **Carbs:** 18.41 g **Total Fat:** 8.22 g **Sat Fat:** 2.88 g **Cholesterol:** 10.96 mg **Sodium:** 466.05 mg **Sugars:** 2.70 g **Fiber:** 6.53 g

CHAPTER 8

Vegetables and Side Dishes

Easy Broccoli and Cottage Cheese Casserole

TEXTURE: Soft

INGREDIENTS

- 2 cups (475 ml) water
- 3 cups (210 g) fresh broccoli florets
- 16 ounces (455 g) cottage cheese, 1% fat, no added salt
- $^3/_4$ cup (85 g) reduced-fat shredded Cheddar cheese
- 1 cup (160 g) diced yellow onion
- 3 egg whites, plus one whole egg, beaten
- 3 tablespoons (15 g) grated Parmesan cheese

Preheat the oven to 375°F (190°C, or gas mark 5). Coat a 9-inch (22.5-cm) pie pan or a 7- x 9-inch (17.5- x 22.5-cm) casserole dish with cooking spray.

In a 1½-quart (1.5-L) saucepan, bring the water to boil. Boil the broccoli for about 4 minutes, until al dente or still crunchy in the middle. Pour the broccoli into a colander and drain well.

In a medium size mixing bowl, combine the cottage cheese, Cheddar cheese, onion, egg, and Parmesan cheese. Pour the mixture into the pie pan or baking dish and bake for 35 to 45 minutes, until the center of the casserole is set. Allow the casserole to cool for about 10 minutes before serving.

YIELD: Makes 6 (about $^3/_4$-cup) servings.

NUTRITIONAL ANALYSIS
Each with: **Calories:** 149.07 **Protein:** 18.13 g **Carbs:** 7.89 g **Total Fat:** 5.43 g **Sat Fat:** 3.05 g
Cholesterol: 52.35 mg **Sodium:** 229.95 mg **Sugars:** 4.81 g **Fiber:** 0.37 g

Brussels Hash

A delicious and new way to serve delicious Brussels sprouts.

TEXTURE: Regular

INGREDIENTS

- 1 tablespoon (14 ml) olive oil
- 1½ cups (240 g) finely diced white onion
- 1 fresh clove garlic, minced
- 1 pound (455 g) Brussels sprouts, trimmed of stems and minced
- 1 tablespoon (10 g) finely chopped red bell pepper
- ½ cup (120 ml) low-sodium vegetable broth
- ½ teaspoon salt
- ⅛ teaspoon fresh cracked black pepper

In a large skillet, heat the oil over medium heat. Add the onion and sauté, stirring frequently, for 5 minutes until it begins to soften. Add the garlic, Brussels sprouts, and bell pepper. Add the broth and simmer the vegetables, stirring occasionally, 5 to 8 minutes, until the broth has completely evaporated. Stir in the salt and black pepper. Sauté the hash another minute and serve.

YIELD: Makes 6 (about ½-cup) servings.

NUTRITIONAL ANALYSIS
Each with: **Calories:** 68.84 **Protein:** 3.17 g **Carbs:** 6.41 g **Total Fat:** 3.43 g **Sat Fat:** 0.57 g **Cholesterol:** 0.00 mg **Sodium:** 106.79 mg **Sugars:** 3.43 g **Fiber:** 3.96 g

Creamy Polenta with Fresh Oregano and Feta Cheese

Variations

In place of water, use low-sodium chicken broth. In place of oregano and feta cheese, use ¼ cup (25 g) chopped green onion and ⅓ cup (40 g) reduced-fat, shredded Cheddar cheese, or ¼ cup (4 g) chopped fresh cilantro and 2 tablespoons (28 ml) lime juice, or 2 tablespoons (12 g) chopped green chilies and ⅓ cup (40 g) reduced-fat shredded Cheddar cheese. Or add 1 tablespoon (5 g) shredded Parmesan cheese.

Polenta is as versatile as it is easy and delicious. It can be served as a side dish, and it also stands on its own as an entrée when paired with your favorite tomato sauce. Try some of the variations listed (left).

TEXTURE: Soft

INGREDIENTS

- 1 cup (140 g) dry polenta meal (not corn meal)
- 1 cup (235 ml) nonfat milk
- 2½ cups (570 ml) water
- ⅛ teaspoon salt
- 2 tablespoons (8 g) chopped fresh oregano leaves
- ⅓ cup (50 g) feta cheese crumbles

Spray an 8- or 9-inch (20- or 22.5-cm) pie pan, a 7- x 7-inch (17.5- x 17.5-cm) baking dish, or sheet pan with cooking spray.

In a small bowl, place the polenta and pour the milk over the top. Stir the mixture to expose all the polenta to the liquid. (This process will eliminate lumps in the finished product.)

In a 1½-quart (1.5-L) saucepan, bring the water and salt to a soft boil and slowly add the soaked polenta, stirring constantly. Continue cooking, stirring, until the polenta begins to pull away from the sides of the pan. Remove the pan from the heat and stir in the oregano and cheese.

Immediately pour the polenta into the prepared pie pan or baking dish or spoon it free-form into a mound in the center of the sheet pan. Allow the polenta to cool until it sets enough to cut into squares or wedges (if serving from the free-form) and lifts away from the pan in one piece.

YIELD: Makes 8 (about ½-cup) servings.

NUTRITIONAL ANALYSIS
Each with: **Calories:** 125.51 **Protein:** 4.42 g **Carbs:** 23.82 g **Total Fat:** 1.46 g **Sat Fat:** 0.99 g **Cholesterol:** 6.18 mg **Sodium:** 104.50 mg **Sugars:** 1.77 g **Fiber:** 1.12 g

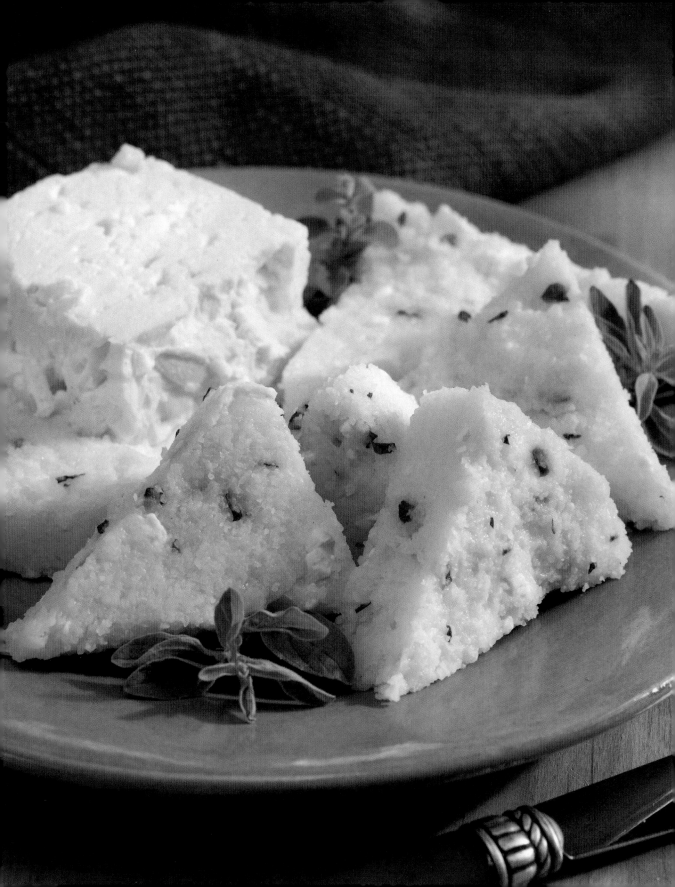

Parmesan Cheese and Green Pea Couscous

Mmm ... this is so good! You have to try it!

TEXTURE: Mechanical Soft

INGREDIENTS

- 1 can (14 ounces, or 425 ml) low-sodium chicken broth
- $1/4$ (60 ml) cup water
- 2 teaspoons extra-virgin olive oil
- 1 cup (175 g) whole-wheat couscous
- $1^1/2$ cups (195 g) frozen peas
- 2 tablespoons (8 g) fresh dill, chopped
- 1 teaspoon fresh lemon zest
- 1 teaspoon kosher salt
- $1/2$ teaspoon black pepper
- $1/2$ cup (50 g) fresh grated Parmesan cheese

Bring the chicken broth, water, and olive oil to a boil in a large saucepan. Stir in the couscous and remove from heat. Cover and allow the couscous to absorb the liquid for 5 minutes.

While couscous is "cooking," cook the peas according to the package directions. Add the cooked peas, dill, lemon zest, salt, and pepper to the couscous. Mix gently and fluff with a fork. Sprinkle with the Parmesan cheese and serve immediately.

YIELD: Makes 8 (about $1/4$-cup) servings.

NUTRITIONAL ANALYSIS
Each with: **Calories:** 144.29 **Protein:** 7.13 g **Carbs:** 22.20 g **Total Fat:** 3.42 g **Sat Fat:** 1.29 g **Cholesterol:** 6.25 mg **Sodium:** 448.74 mg **Sugars:** 0.50 g **Fiber:** 4.15 g

Heather's Ratatouille

This hearty recipe comes from Heather, a gastric bypass surgery patient in the Boston area.

TEXTURE: Regular

INGREDIENTS

- 2 medium eggplants, peeled and cut into $1/2$-inch (1.25-cm) cubes
- 2 medium zucchini, thinly sliced
- $1/2$ teaspoon kosher salt
- 2 tablespoons (30 ml) extra-virgin olive oil
- 2 medium Vidalia onions, chopped
- 1 red bell pepper, seeded and cut into strips
- 1 yellow bell pepper, seeded and cut into strips
- 1 orange bell pepper, seeded and cut into strips
- 3 hot-house tomatoes, seeded and quartered
- 1 clove garlic, crushed
- 2 tablespoons (3 g) dried herbs de Provence
- $1/4$ teaspoon black pepper

Place the eggplant and zucchini in a colander and sprinkle with salt. Let drain for 30 to 60 minutes. Rinse with water then pat dry with a paper towel.

In a large skillet, heat the olive oil over medium heat. Add the onions and cook until translucent, about 6 minutes, stirring occasionally. Remove from the skillet and put in a large bowl.

In turn, cook the eggplant, zucchini, and peppers in the olive oil. When each vegetable is cooked, add it to the bowl. When all the vegetables are cooked, mix them together back in the skillet and add the tomatoes, garlic, herbs de Provence, and black pepper. Heat through and serve.

YIELD: Makes 12 ($3/4$-cup) servings.

NUTRITIONAL ANALYSIS
Each with: **Calories:** 50.07 **Protein:** 1.75 g **Carbs:** 10.05 g **Total Fat:** 1.02 g **Sat Fat:** 0.16 g **Cholesterol:** 0.00 mg **Sodium:** 96.96 mg **Sugars:** 5.14 g **Fiber:** 3.89 g

Roasted Asparagus with Crispy Bacon

TEXTURE: Regular

INGREDIENTS

- 2 slices turkey bacon
- 2 teaspoons olive oil
- 2 teaspoons light butter
- 1/8 cup lemon juice (about 1/2 lemon)
- 1 teaspoon balsamic vinegar
- 1/8 teaspoon minced fresh garlic
- 1 dash salt
- 1/8 teaspoon pepper
- 1 pound (455 g) pencil-thin asparagus
- Lemon wedges (optional)
- Fresh parsley sprigs (optional)

Preheat the oven to 400°F (200°C, or gas mark 6).

In a nonstick pan, cook the bacon until crisp. Drain on paper towels, crumble, and set aside. Wipe out the cooled pan with a paper towel.

In the same pan combine the oil, butter, lemon juice, vinegar, garlic, salt, and pepper. Heat over medium heat until warm.

Rinse the asparagus, pat dry, and cut or snap off the thick, wood-like ends. Add the asparagus to the pan and turn to coat. Transfer the asparagus to a medium (about 7- x 9-inch, or 17.5- x 22.5-cm) baking dish and spread in a single layer. Roast the asparagus on the middle rack for 10 to 12 minutes, until tender. Transfer the asparagus to a plate and garnish with the crumbled bacon. Garnish the serving plate with the lemon and parsley (if using).

YIELD: Makes 6 servings.

NUTRITIONAL ANALYSIS

Each with: **Calories:** 47.32 **Protein:** 2.37 g **Carbs:** 3.57 g **Total Fat:** 3.15 g **Sat Fat:** 0.53 g **Cholesterol:** 3.33 mg **Sodium:** 98.90 mg **Sugars:** 1.66 g **Fiber:** 1.61 g

Green Bean Casserole

This is a delicious way to get your veggies in!

TEXTURE: Soft

INGREDIENTS

- 2 teaspoon extra-virgin olive oil
- 1/4 cup (40 g) diced onion
- 1 tablespoon (6 g) white flour
- 1 cup (235 ml) nonfat milk
- 1/2 cup (55 g) low-fat, shredded Swiss cheese
- 1/4 cup (50 g) nonfat sour cream
- 2 1/4 cups (250 g) fresh green beans, cut in half lengthwise
- 1 large egg white
- 1 tablespoon (14 g) margarine or light butter, melted
- 1 1/2 cups (60 g) seasoned croutons

Preheat the oven to 350°F (180°C, or gas mark 4).

In a 3-quart (3-L) saucepan, heat the oil over medium heat. Add the onion and sauté for approximately 5 minutes, until the onion is tender, but not brown.

In a small mixing bowl, mix the flour and milk with a fork, until all the lumps are gone. Add the flour and milk mixture to the onion and continue cooking, stirring constantly, for 2 to 3 minutes, until the mixture begins to thicken. Stir in the cheese and sour cream. Cook, stirring constantly, for an additional 3 minutes, until the mixture is thick and bubbly.

Spray an 8- x 8-inch (20- x 20-cm) baking dish with cooking spray. Place the green beans in the dish and pour the cheese mixture evenly over the beans.

In a medium bowl, combine the egg white, margarine or butter, and seasoned croutons. Stir the mixture well and pour it evenly over the green beans. Bake for about 25 minutes, until the casserole is thoroughly heated.

YIELD: Makes 8 (1/2-cup) servings.

NUTRITIONAL ANALYSIS

Each with: **Calories:** 97.22 **Protein:** 5.22 g **Carbs:** 10.48 g **Total Fat:** 3.68 g **Sat Fat:** 0.95 g **Cholesterol:** 8.56 mg **Sodium:** 239.62 mg **Sugars:** 4.55 g **Fiber:** 1.60 g

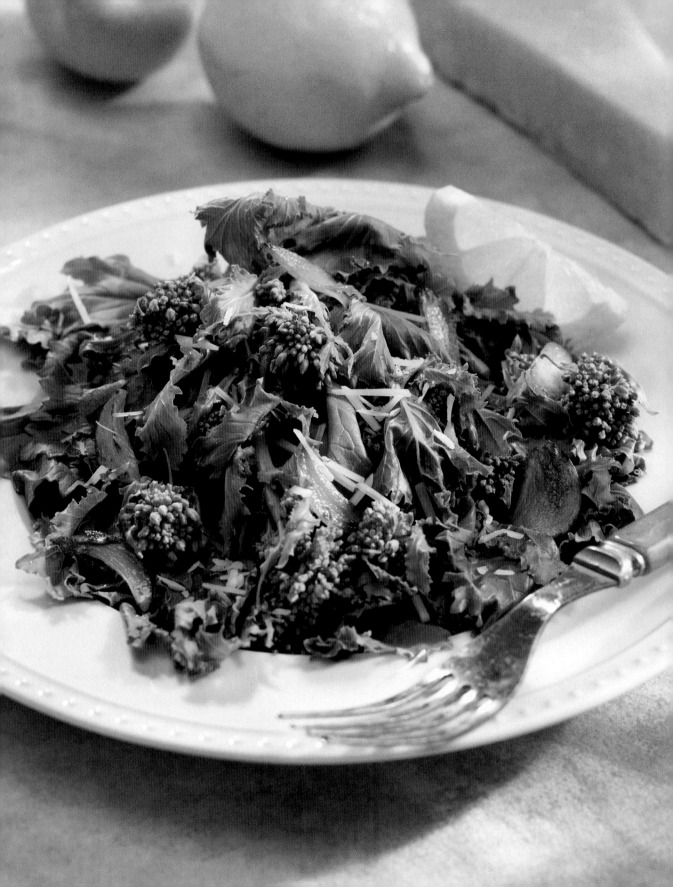

Broccoli Raab

Delicious, simple, and highly nutritious, this vegetable is a wonderful complement to fish or chicken.

TEXTURE: Regular

INGREDIENTS

- 4 cups (1 L) water
- 1 tablespoon (14 ml) extra-virgin olive oil
- 1 clove fresh garlic, cut into thin strips
- 1 pound (455 g) broccoli raab, trimmed
- 2 teaspoons fresh lemon juice
- $\frac{1}{8}$ teaspoon salt
- $\frac{1}{8}$ teaspoon white pepper
- 1 teaspoon reduced-fat butter substitute
- 1 tablespoon (5 g) grated Parmesan cheese

In a 1½-quart (1.5-L) saucepan, bring the water to a boil.

In a medium skillet, heat the oil over medium-high heat. Add the garlic and sauté until it just begins to brown. Immediately remove the garlic from the skillet and place it in a medium mixing bowl.

Add the broccoli raab to the boiling water and cook for 2 to 3 minutes or until broccoli raab is al dente, or still crunchy on the inside.

Place the lemon juice, salt, pepper, butter substitute, and cheese in the mixing bowl along with the garlic. Drain the broccoli raab and add it to the bowl. Gently toss the broccoli raab with the sauce. Serve immediately.

YIELD: Makes 4 (about ½-cup) servings.

NUTRITIONAL ANALYSIS
Each with: **Calories:** 71.08 **Protein:** 4.41 g **Carbs:** 3.74 g **Total Fat:** 5.12 g **Sat Fat:** 1.02 g **Cholesterol:** 0.75 mg **Sodium:** 109.14 mg **Sugars:** 0.45 g **Fiber:** 3.10 g

Channna Dal

This traditional dish from India is so delicious, you'll find yourself craving it after you've made it just once. Serve this in warm bowls with a dollop of plain low-fat yogurt and a sprinkle of fresh cilantro on top and Indian Papadum crackers on the side.

TEXTURE: Soft

INGREDIENTS

- 5 cups (1,175 ml) water
- 2 cups (400 g) channa dal (an Indian bean) or split yellow peas
- 1 medium yellow onion, finely diced
- 1 tablespoon (8 g) fresh grated gingerroot
- 1 tablespoon (10 g) fresh minced garlic (about 3 large cloves)
- 1 teaspoon ground coriander
- 1 teaspoon turmeric
- 1 teaspoon garam masala
- 1 tablespoon (16 g) tomato paste
- 2 tablespoons (28 ml) olive oil
- 2 teaspoons mustard seeds
- 1 teaspoon cumin seeds
- 1 small red chili pepper
- ½ teaspoon sea salt
- ¼ teaspoon white pepper
- 1 tablespoon (14 ml) fresh lemon juice
- 6 fresh cilantro sprigs, chopped

In a 2½-quart (2.5-L) saucepan, bring the water, the channa dal or peas, onion, gingerroot, and garlic to a boil. Reduce the heat to medium-low and stir in the coriander, turmeric, garam masala, and tomato paste. Simmer uncovered for about 15 minutes, stirring occasionally.

When the channa dal is almost done (soft but not paste-like), heat the oil in a medium skillet along with the mustard seeds, cumin seeds, and chili pepper. Cook on medium-high for 1 to 2 minutes, until the seeds begin to crackle. Remove the chili pepper; add the seeds to the dal and stir in the salt, white pepper, and lemon juice. Garnish with cilantro sprigs.

YIELD: Makes 8 (about 1-cup) servings.

NUTRITIONAL ANALYSIS
Each with: **Calories:** 222.10 **Protein:** 12.79 g **Carbs:** 33.72 g **Total Fat:** 4.48 g **Sat Fat:** 0.60 g **Cholesterol:** 0.00 mg **Sodium:** 150.67 mg **Sugars:** 5.30 g **Fiber:** 13.42 g

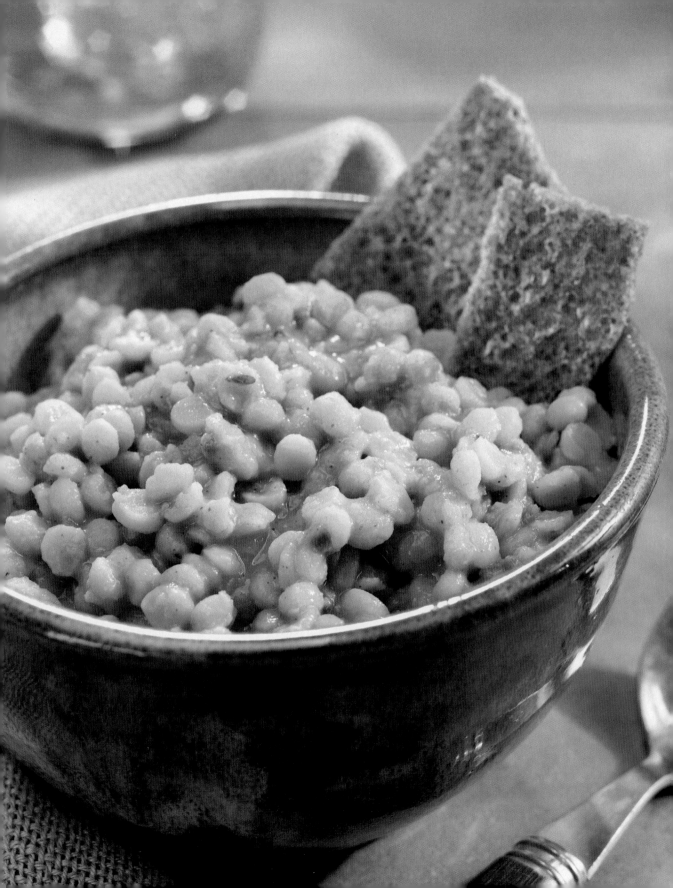

Steamed Asparagus Lemonata

Pure and simple, this is a wonderful complement to meat, fish, poultry, or vegetarian entrées.

TEXTURE: Regular

INGREDIENTS

- 2$^1/_2$ cups (570 ml) water
- 1$^3/_4$ pounds (795 g) fresh "pencil" asparagus
- 1 tablespoon (14 ml) extra-virgin olive oil
- 1 teaspoon light butter
- 2 teaspoons fresh lemon juice
- 1 teaspoon lemon zest
- 1 teaspoon sea salt or kosher salt
- $^1/_8$ teaspoon ground white pepper
- $^1/_8$ teaspoon fresh cracked black pepper
- 2 teaspoons finely chopped fresh parsley

In a 2$^1/_2$-quart (2.5-L) saucepan with a steamer basket, bring the water to a boil.

Meanwhile, wash the asparagus and cut the wood-like ends off and discard. Place the prepared asparagus in the steamer basket and steam for 8 to 10 minutes, until the asparagus turns bright green and is fork-tender just below the tips.

While the asparagus is steaming, in a small saucepan, heat the oil, light butter, lemon juice, lemon zest, salt, white pepper, and black pepper, just until the lemon zest begins to bubble. Add the parsley at the last minute and stir.

Remove the asparagus from the steamer basket and place on a serving dish. Drizzle the oil and lemon mixture evenly over the asparagus and gently rotate for even exposure. Serve immediately.

YIELD: Makes 6 (about $^1/_2$-cup) servings.

NUTRITIONAL ANALYSIS
Each with: **Calories:** 51.77 **Protein:** 2.94 g **Carbs:** 5.37 g **Total Fat:** 2.83 g **Sat Fat:** 0.46 g **Cholesterol:** 0.00 mg **Sodium:** 86.24 mg **Sugars:** 2.54 g **Fiber:** 2.82 g

Mandarin Orange Broccoli

This Asian-influenced dish is fast, easy, and packed with satisfying flavors.

TEXTURE: Regular

INGREDIENTS

- 2 cans (11 ounces, or 310 g each) mandarin orange pieces, drained and liquid reserved
- 1 tablespoon (14 ml) molasses
- 1 tablespoon (14 ml) sugar-free maple syrup
- 1 tablespoon (14 ml) soy sauce
- 1 teaspoon fresh grated gingerroot
- 1$\frac{1}{2}$ teaspoons cornstarch
- 1 teaspoon rice vinegar
- 1 tablespoon (14 ml) peanut oil
- 1 teaspoon sesame oil
- 2 heads fresh broccoli, cut into florets (5-6 cups, or 350–420 g)
- 2 tablespoons (15 g) toasted sesame seeds

In a small mixing bowl, mix together $\frac{1}{4}$ cup (60 ml) of the reserved mandarin orange liquid and the molasses, maple syrup, soy sauce, gingerroot, cornstarch, and vinegar and set aside.

In a wok, heat the peanut oil and sesame oil over medium-high heat. Add the broccoli and one can of the mandarin oranges and cook, stirring briskly, until the broccoli is heated through. (The oranges will almost dissolve.) Stir in the soy-molasses mixture and continue to cook, while stirring the broccoli to coat, for about 3 minutes, until the broccoli is just tender. Remove from the heat and transfer to a serving dish. Sprinkle with the remaining mandarin orange pieces and toasted sesame seeds and serve immediately.

YIELD: Makes 8 (about $\frac{1}{2}$-cup) servings.

NUTRITIONAL ANALYSIS
Each with: **Calories:** 128.60 **Protein:** 2.85 g **Carbs:** 17.38 g **Total Fat:** 5.93 g **Sat Fat:** 0.84 g **Cholesterol:** 0.00 mg **Sodium:** 88.94 mg **Sugars:** 12.13 g **Fiber:** 1.78 g

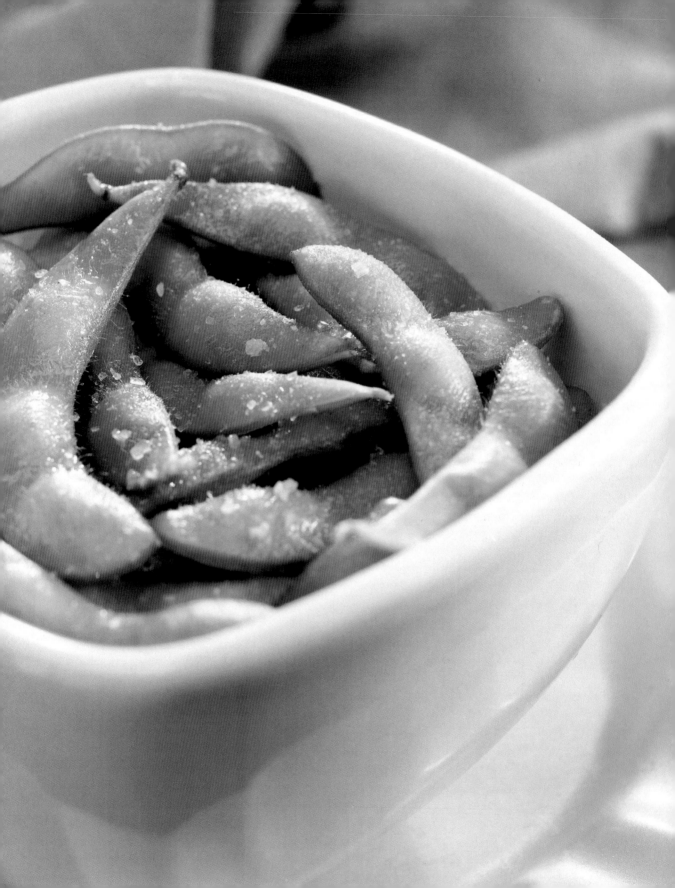

Edamame

Edamame, whole soybeans in the shell, is a simple and nutritious way to get more soy protein in your diet. Pop the shells open and eat the beans inside. You can find them fresh or frozen at your grocer.

TEXTURE: Regular

INGREDIENTS

- 2^1/$_2$ quarts (2.5 L) water
- 1 tablespoon (18 g) salt
- 2 pounds (1 kg) fresh or frozen edamame
- ^{1}/$_8$ teaspoon coarse sea salt

In a 3-quart (3-L) pot, bring the water and table salt to a boil over high heat. Add the edamame, reduce the heat, and simmer for 3 minutes if using fresh beans or 4 minutes if using frozen.

Drain the beans and transfer them to a serving bowl just large enough to hold the edamame. (If the serving container is too large, the beans will cool off too quickly.) Toss the beans with the coarse sea salt and serve immediately.

YIELD: Makes 14 (about 1-cup) servings.

NUTRITIONAL ANALYSIS

Each with: **Calories:** 91.48 **Protein:** 7.62 g **Carbs:** 6.86 g **Total Fat:** 3.81 g **Sat Fat:** 0.38 g **Cholesterol:** 0.00 mg **Sodium:** 29.85 mg **Sugars:** 2.29 g **Fiber:** 3.05 g

Zesty Cajun Black-Eyed Peas

TEXTURE: Regular

INGREDIENTS

- 2 cans (15^1/$_2$ ounces, or 439 g each) black-eyed peas, rinsed and drained
- 2 cups (454 g) canned crushed tomatoes
- 1 cup (235 ml) water
- 1 teaspoon low-sodium chicken bouillon granules, or 1 cube
- 1 large Vidalia onion, chopped
- 2 stalks celery, chopped
- 2 cloves garlic, minced
- ^{1}/$_2$ teaspoon dry mustard
- ^{1}/$_4$ teaspoon ground ginger
- ^{1}/$_4$ teaspoon cayenne pepper
- 1 bay leaf
- ^{1}/$_8$ cup (8 g) roughly chopped fresh parsley

Combine the black-eyed peas, tomatoes, water, bouillon, onion, celery, garlic, mustard, ginger, cayenne pepper, and bay leaf in a large saucepan. Cover and simmer over medium-low heat for 2 hours, stirring occasionally. Add water as necessary to keep peas covered with liquid.

Remove the bay leaf and serve garnished with the parsley.

YIELD: Makes 8 (about 1-cup) servings.

NUTRITIONAL ANALYSIS

Each with: **Calories:** 131.68 **Protein:** 6.13 g **Carbs:** 26.27 g **Total Fat:** 0.17 g **Sat Fat:** 0.04 g **Cholesterol:** 0.03 mg **Sodium:** 685.50 mg **Sugars:** 4.95 g **Fiber:** 5.67 g

Herb and Cheese
Mashed Cauliflower

Try this delicious and unique variation of cauliflower the whole family is sure to love.

TEXTURE: Soft

INGREDIENTS

- 2$\frac{1}{2}$ cups (570 ml) water
- 3 cups (450 g) cauliflower florets (about 1-inch, or 2.5-cm pieces)
- $\frac{2}{3}$ cup (155 ml) nonfat milk
- $\frac{1}{4}$ cup (50 g) nonfat sour cream
- $\frac{1}{2}$ teaspoon salt
- $\frac{1}{8}$ teaspoon ground white pepper
- 2 tablespoons (15 g) finely chopped green onion
- 1 tablespoon (4 g) finely chopped fresh parsley
- 1 tablespoon (14 g) butter substitute

In a 2$\frac{1}{2}$-quart (2.5-L) saucepan with a steamer basket, bring the water to a boil. Place the cauliflower in the steamer basket and steam for about 15 minutes, until the cauliflower is very tender throughout.

Place the cauliflower in a food processor fitted with a metal S blade and puree until smooth.

Add the milk and sour cream and carefully pulse the mixture until smooth. (Pulsate the mixture briefly to avoid the liquids splashing out of the processing bowl.) Add the salt, white pepper, onion, parsley, and butter substitute and continue pulsating until evenly incorporated. Serve warm as a side dish.

YIELD: Makes 4 (about 1-cup) servings.

NUTRITIONAL ANALYSIS

Each with: **Calories:** 88.13 **Protein:** 5.85 g **Carbs:** 14.28 g **Total Fat:** 1.76 g **Sat Fat:** 0.35 g **Cholesterol:** 3.32 mg **Sodium:** 251.67 mg **Sugars:** 7.13 g **Fiber:** 4.41 g

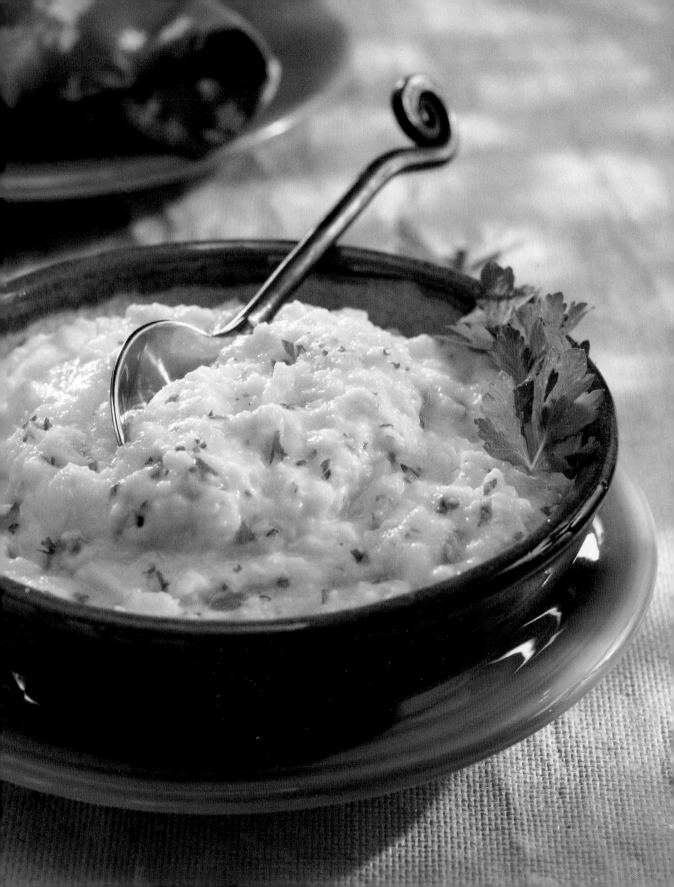

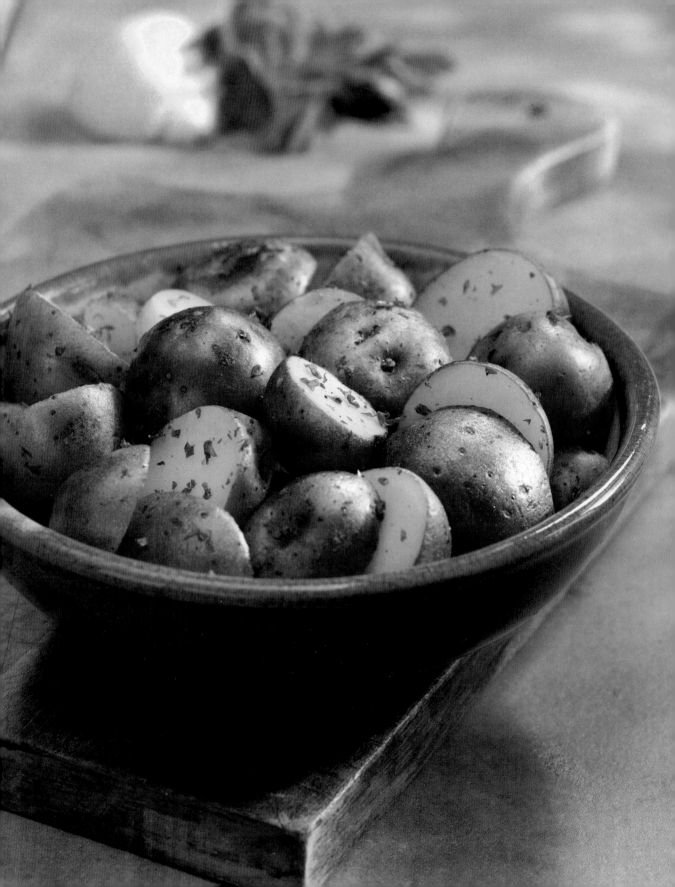

Boiled New Potatoes
with Fresh Parsley

*Pure, unadulterated deliciousness—this is a wonderful complement
to roasted meat dishes.*

TEXTURE: Soft

INGREDIENTS

- 1 pound (455 g) baby red potatoes, washed and halved
- 1 tablespoon (14 g) butter substitute
- 1/4 teaspoon kosher salt
- 1/4 teaspoon fresh cracked pepper
- 1/2 teaspoon fresh lemon juice
- 2 tablespoons (8 g) chopped fresh parsley

In a 2-quart (2-L) saucepan, place the potatoes and enough cold water to cover 1 inch
(2.5 cm) above the level of the potatoes. Bring the water to a boil and cook for about
12 minutes, until the potatoes can be gently speared with a fork when tested. Drain
the potatoes in a colander and transfer them to a medium mixing bowl. While the
potatoes are still hot, add the butter substitute, salt, pepper, lemon juice, and parsley. Gently toss the potatoes to evenly cover with all ingredients. Serve immediately.

YIELD: Makes 4 (about 1/2-cup) servings.

NUTRITIONAL ANALYSIS
Each with: **Calories:** 95.42 **Protein:** 2.23 g **Carbs:** 18.28 g **Total Fat:** 1.67 g **Sat Fat:** 0.28 g
Cholesterol: 0.00 mg **Sodium:** 147.87 mg **Sugars:** 1.17 g **Fiber:** 2.02 g

Sweet Potatoes au Gratin

TEXTURE: Soft

INGREDIENTS

- 1 tablespoon (14 g) light butter
- 1 medium onion, finely diced
- 1 small clove fresh garlic, minced
- 2¹/₂ cups (570 ml) low-sodium vegetable broth
- ¹/₂ cup (50 g) green onions, finely chopped
- ¹/₄ cup (15 g) chopped fresh parsley
- 1 cup (235 ml) nonfat milk
- ¹/₄ teaspoon salt
- ¹/₈ teaspoon ground black pepper
- 3 medium sweet potatoes, peeled and thinly sliced (about 2¹/₂ pounds, 1.25 kg)
- ¹/₂ cup (55 g) shredded reduced-fat Cheddar cheese
- ¹/₄ cup (20 g) shredded Parmesan cheese

Preheat the oven to 375°F (190°C, or gas mark 5). Coat a 9- x 13-inch (22.5- x 32.5-cm) baking dish with cooking spray.

In a 2-quart (2-L) saucepan, melt the butter substitute over medium heat. Add the onion and garlic and sauté until the onion begins to soften, about 5 minutes. Add the broth, green onion, parsley, milk, salt, and pepper and bring to a simmer. Cook until the liquid is reduced to about 2³/₄ cups (650 ml). Add the sweet potatoes and return to a simmer. Continue cooking for an additional 5 minutes.

Pour the mixture into the prepared baking dish and bake for about 35 minutes, until the potatoes are tender, basting the potatoes occasionally with the liquid in the dish. Top the dish evenly with the Cheddar and then the Parmesan and continue to bake for about 20 minutes, until the cheese is bubbly and golden brown.

YIELD: Makes 16 (about ³/₄-cup) servings.

NUTRITIONAL ANALYSIS
Each with: **Calories:** 104.14 **Protein:** 3.96 g **Carbs:** 17.54 g **Total Fat:** 2.03 g **Sat Fat:** 1.03 g **Cholesterol:** 4.37 mg **Sodium:** 116.62 mg **Sugars:** 4.09 g **Fiber:** 2.15 g

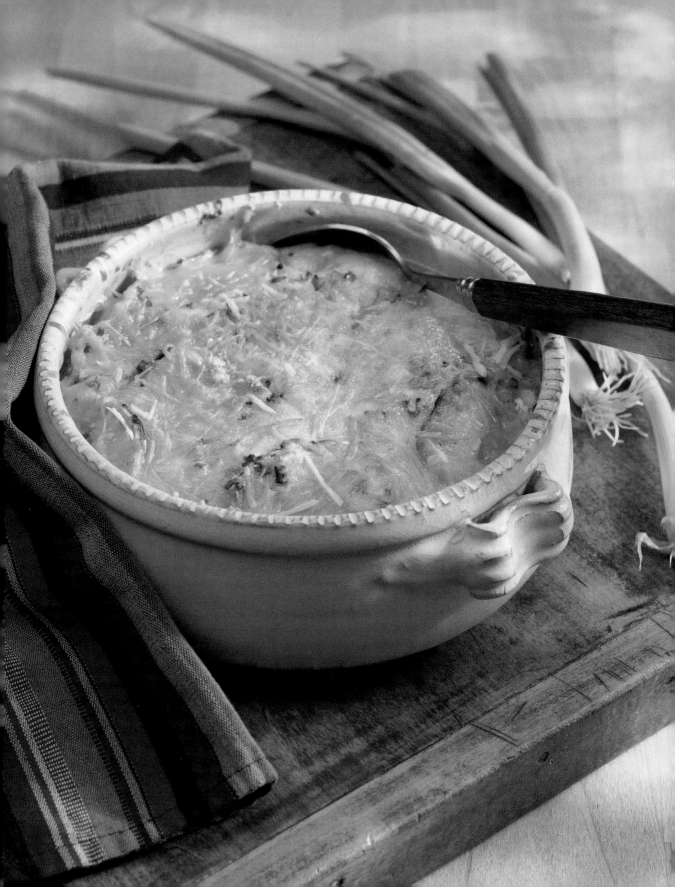

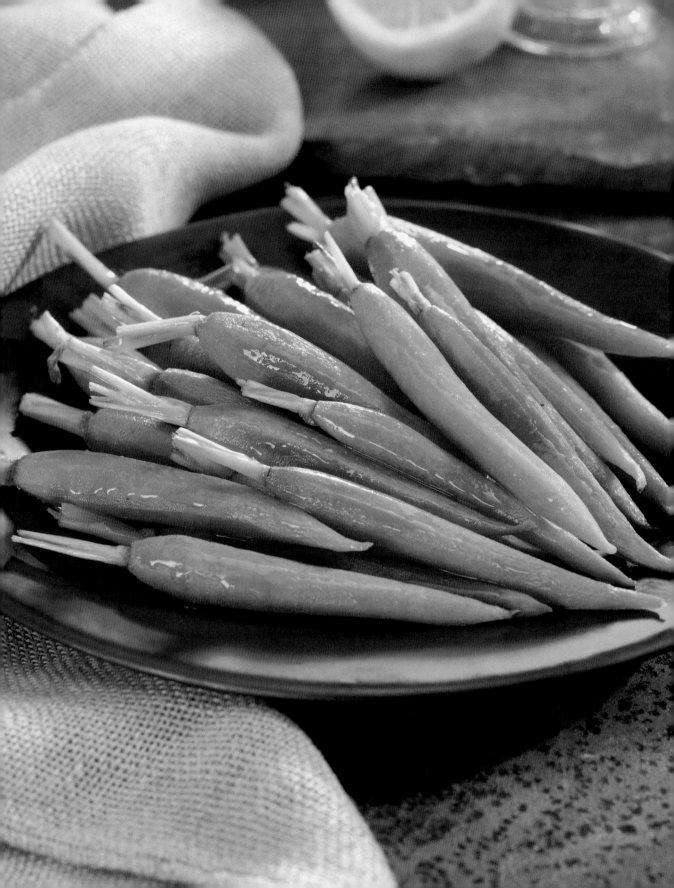

Citrus-Roasted Carrots with Honey

This is a wonderful accompaniment to fish and poultry.

TEXTURE: Soft

INGREDIENTS

- 1 tablespoon (14 ml) olive oil
- 2 teaspoons light butter
- Juice of $1/2$ lemon
- 1 teaspoon honey
- $1/8$ teaspoon sea salt or kosher salt
- $1/8$ teaspoon ground white pepper
- 1 pound (455 g) baby carrots, peeled
- 1 tablespoon (4 g) chopped fresh parsley

Preheat the oven to 375°F (190°C, or gas mark 5). Spray a 7- x 9-inch (17.5- x 22.5-cm) baking dish with cooking spray.

In a medium skillet, heat the oil, butter, lemon juice, honey, salt, and pepper over medium heat. Add the carrots and turn until coated with the mixture.

Transfer mixture to the prepared baking dish. Roast on the medium rack for 20 to 30 minutes, until the carrots are tender and caramelized.

YIELD: Makes 6 (about $1/2$-cup) servings.

NUTRITIONAL ANALYSIS
Each with: **Calories:** 59.93 **Protein:** 0.55 g **Carbs:** 8.07 g **Total Fat:** 3.11 g **Sat Fat:** 0.46 g **Cholesterol:** 0.00 mg **Sodium:** 93.39 mg **Sugars:** 4.74 g **Fiber:** 1.44 g

CHAPTER 9

Dry Rubs for Meats and Poultry

Use dry rubs to add a dynamic flare to meats, fish, poultry, or slices of fresh drained tofu. This is a wonderful way to pack in the flavor. An additional benefit of using dry rubs is that the acids in certain spices will begin to chemically "cook" the product before heat is applied, rendering meats more tender than you might expect. Dry rubs work especially well when cooking on the grill.

Try any of our recommended dry rubs using the following guide: Work the spice mix well into the product, covering entirely. Next, simply let the meat, fish, or poultry stand covered in the refrigerator. Let red meats and pork stand for at least 2 hours, poultry for at least 1 hour, and lighter-textured products such as fish or tofu for at least 30 minutes.

Dill Rub

Try this rub on chicken or fish.

INGREDIENTS

- 2 tablespoons (18 g) onion powder
- 1 teaspoon garlic powder
- 1 tablespoon (2 g) ground sage
- ¹/₂ teaspoon nutmeg
- 1 teaspoon dry mustard
- 2 teaspoons salt-free lemon-pepper seasoning

In a small bowl, combine all of the ingredients.

YIELD: Enough rub for 3 to 4 pounds (1.5 to 2 kg) of chicken or a 5-pound (2.5-kg) roasting hen.

Pork Roast Rub

Full of herbs and spices, this rub will surely leave you feeling satisfied.

INGREDIENTS

- 1 tablespoon (9 g) onion powder
- 2 teaspoons garlic powder
- 2 teaspoons paprika
- 2 teaspoons oregano
- 2 teaspoons ground thyme
- ¹/₈ teaspoon cayenne pepper
- ¹/₈ teaspoon black pepper
- ¹/₂ teaspoon salt

In a small bowl, combine all of the ingredients.

YIELD: Enough rub for a 2- to 3-pound (1- to 1.5-kg) pork loin roast.

Cajun Blackened Rub

This is amazing on fish and shrimp.

INGREDIENTS

- 2 teaspoons ground oregano
- 1 teaspoon ground thyme
- $1/2$ teaspoon cayenne pepper
- $1/2$ teaspoon ground black pepper
- $1/2$ teaspoon ground white pepper
- 1 teaspoon garlic powder
- 1 teaspoon onion powder

In a small bowl, combine all of the ingredients.

YIELD: Enough rub for a 2- pound (1-kg) chicken.

Dry Jamaican Jerk Rub

Try this delicious rub on chicken or pork.

INGREDIENTS

- 1 tablespoon (9 g) onion powder
- 1 teaspoon ground thyme
- 2 teaspoons brown sugar
- 2 teaspoons dried chives
- 1 teaspoon salt
- 2 teaspoons allspice
- 1 teaspoon ground black pepper
- $1/2$ teaspoon ground celery seed

In a small bowl, combine all of the ingredients.

YIELD: Enough rub for $1^1/2$ pounds (700 g) white fish or a 1-pound (455 g) chicken.

Pork Roast Dry Rub

Try this rub and compare it to the Pork Roast Rub on page 206.

INGREDIENTS

- 1 teaspoon black pepper
- ¹/₂ teaspoon salt
- 1 teaspoon sugar
- 1 teaspoon paprika
- ¹/₂ teaspoon dry mustard
- ¹/₈ teaspoon cayenne pepper (optional)

In a small bowl, combine all of the ingredients.

YIELD: Enough rub for a 2-pound (1-kg) pork roast.

Mustard Rub

This rub will definitely put some zing in whatever you're cooking.

INGREDIENTS

- 1 teaspoon black pepper
- ¹/₂ teaspoon salt
- 1 teaspoon sugar
- 1 teaspoon paprika
- 2 teaspoons dry mustard
- ¹/₈ teaspoon cayenne pepper (optional)

In a small bowl, combine all of the ingredients.

YIELD: Enough rub for a 2-pound (1-kg) pork roast.

Tandoori Dry Rub

This rub is especially good with salmon.

INGREDIENTS

- 1 tablespoon (5 g) ground ginger
- 2 teaspoons garlic powder
- 1 tablespoon (7 g) paprika
- 1 teaspoon ground oregano
- 1 teaspoon ground thyme
- ¹/₈ teaspoon cayenne pepper
- ¹/₈ teaspoon black pepper
- ¹/₂ teaspoon salt

In a small bowl, combine all of the ingredients.

YIELD: Enough rub for 1 pound (455 g) chicken or fish.

Curry Dry Rub

This tasty rub would be perfect on chicken or lamb.

INGREDIENTS

- 1 tablespoon (7 g) curry powder
- 2 teaspoons garlic powder
- ¹/₂ teaspoon ground cumin
- ¹/₄ teaspoon ground coriander
- ¹/₈ teaspoon cayenne pepper
- ¹/₄ teaspoon salt

In a small bowl, combine all of the ingredients.

YIELD: Enough rub for 1 pound (455 g) chicken or fish.

Fearsome Garlic Pork Rub

This rub is quite delicious and satisfying. And it's not just great on pork, try rubbing down some chicken.

INGREDIENTS

- 6 cloves fresh garlic, minced
- 2 teaspoons minced fresh parsley
- 1 teaspoon black pepper
- 1 teaspoon salt
- 1 teaspoon paprika
- 2 teaspoons brown sugar

In a small bowl, combine all of the ingredients.

YIELD: Enough rub for a 2–3-pound (1- to 1.5-kg) pork roast.

Ethiopian Spice Mix

This is delicious with sautéed vegetables such as cabbage, carrots, or kale. Try 1 teaspoon of rub per cup of vegetables.

INGREDIENTS

- $1/2$ teaspoon cayenne pepper
- 2 teaspoons paprika
- 1 teaspoon ground cumin
- $1/4$ teaspoon ground cloves
- $1/4$ teaspoon ground fenugreek
- 1 teaspoon salt
- $1/2$ teaspoon ground cardamom
- $1/2$ teaspoon black pepper
- $1/2$ teaspoon ground ginger
- $1/4$ teaspoon cinnamon
- $1/4$ teaspoon ground turmeric

In a small bowl, combine all of the ingredients.

YIELD: Makes about 2 tablespoons

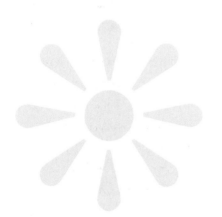

CHAPTER 10

Sauces

Zesty Arrabbiata Sauce

The word arrabbiata *means "angry" in Italian. This zesty, slow cooker sauce would go great on chicken and seafood. It also freezes well.*

TEXTURE: Mechanical Soft

INGREDIENTS

- 2 tablespoons (30 ml) extra-virgin olive oil
- 1 medium Vidalia onion, chopped
- 1 teaspoon minced garlic
- 1 can (8 ounces, or 260 g) tomato paste, no salt added
- 1 can (28 ounces, or 800 g) crushed tomatoes
- $^1/_8$ cup (28 ml) red wine
- $1^1/_2$ teaspoons black pepper
- 1 tablespoon (4 g) crushed red pepper flakes

Heat the olive oil in a medium skillet over medium heat. Add the onion and cook about 5 to 6 minutes, until softened. Add the garlic and sauté for approximately 1 minute.

Add the sautéed onions and garlic to the slow cooker along with the tomato paste, crushed tomato, red wine, black pepper, and crushed red pepper flakes. Cook on the low setting for 3 to 4 hours.

YIELD: Makes 8 (about $^1/_2$-cup) servings.

NUTRITIONAL ANALYSIS
Each with: **Calories:** 97.90 **Protein:** 2.98 g **Carbs:** 13.59 g **Total Fat:** 3.70 g **Sat Fat:** 0.52 g **Cholesterol:** 0.00 mg **Sodium:** 272.55 mg **Sugars:** 7.85 g **Fiber:** 3.16 g

Classic Marsala Sauce

This delicious sauce complements sautéed chicken, pork, and veal.

TEXTURE: Mechanical Soft

INGREDIENTS

- 2 tablespoons (30 ml) extra-virgin olive oil
- 1 package (8 ounces, or 227 g) sliced mushrooms
- ¼ cup (40 g) diced Vidalia onion
- 1 tablespoon (10 g) minced garlic
- 3 tablespoons (23 g) whole-wheat flour
- ½ cup (120 ml) Marsala wine
- 1½ cups (360 ml) low-fat, low-sodium beef stock
- ¼ teaspoon kosher salt
- ¼ teaspoon black pepper

Heat the olive oil in a heavy saucepan over medium-high heat. Add the mushrooms and cook until golden, 5 to 7 minutes. Add the onion and garlic and cook until the onions are translucent. Add the flour and cook for about 1 minute, stirring constantly. Add the Marsala wine and stir until incorporated. Next, add the beef stock and cook until the sauce is thickened. Add the salt and pepper before serving.

YIELD: Makes 6 (about ¼-cup) servings.

NUTRITIONAL ANALYSIS
Each with: **Calories:** 108.41 **Protein:** 2.07 g **Carbs:** 8.41 g **Total Fat:** 5.03 g **Sat Fat:** 0.67 g **Cholesterol:** 1.25 mg **Sodium:** 194.49 mg **Sugars:** 2.73 g **Fiber:** 0.80 g

Classic Pesto Sauce

Vibrant colors and robust basil flavor makes this an amazing addition to just about any dish.

TEXTURE: Puree

INGREDIENTS

- 3 cups (72 g) fresh basil leaves
- 1/2 cup (70 g) pine nuts
- 4 cloves garlic, peeled
- 1/4 cup (25 g) fresh grated low-fat Parmesan cheese
- 1/2 cup (118 ml) extra-virgin olive oil
- 1/4 cup (60 ml) water
- 1/2 teaspoon salt
- 1/4 teaspoon pepper

In a food processor, blend the basil, pine nuts, garlic, and cheese. Pour in the olive oil and water slowly while still processing. Stir in the salt and pepper.

YIELD: Makes 16 (about 1½ -tablespoon) servings.

NUTRITIONAL ANALYSIS
Each with: **Calories:** 67.93 **Sodium:** 1.19 g **Carbs:** 0.87 g **Total Fat:** 6.98 g **Sat Fat:** 0.98 g **Cholesterol:** 1.56 mg **Sodium:** 85.22 mg **Sugars:** 0.16 g **Fiber:** 0.17 g

Easy Mushroom Sauce

This savory sauce would be a great accompaniment for chicken, steak, or even pork.

TEXTURE: Mechanical Soft

INGREDIENTS

- ¹/₂ cup (80 g) chopped yellow onion
- 1¹/₂ cups (105 g) fresh sliced mushrooms
- 2 tablespoons (30 ml) extra-virgin olive oil
- 1 can (103/4 ounces, or 305 ml) reduced-fat condensed cream of chicken soup
- ¹/₃ cup (80 ml) skim milk

Heat the olive oil in a medium saucepan over medium heat. Cook the onions and mushrooms until tender. Stir in the soup and milk. Cook until smooth.

YIELD: Makes 8 (about ¹/₄-cup) servings.

NUTRITIONAL ANALYSIS
Each with: **Calories:** 63.27 **Protein:** 1.40 g **Carbs:** 5.09 g **Total Fat:** 4.30 g **Sat Fat:** 0.81 g **Cholesterol:** 3.25 mg **Sodium:** 186.83 mg **Sugars:** 1.47 g **Fiber:** 0.56 g

White Wine Tarragon Sauce

This easy sauce would be delicious served over salmon, white fish such as cod, or used to steam clams or mussels.

TEXTURE: Puree

INGREDIENTS

- 3 cloves garlic, minced
- 3 tablespoons (30 g) shallots, minced
- 2 tablespoons (28 g) spreadable butter
- 1 teaspoon dried tarragon
- $1/4$ teaspoon kosher salt
- $1/2$ teaspoon white pepper
- $1/4$ cup (60 ml) white wine
- Juice of 1 lemon
- 1 tablespoon (4 g) fresh parsley, chopped

In a medium saucepan over medium-low heat, sweat the garlic and shallots in butter for about 3 minutes. Add the tarragon, salt, and pepper. Raise the heat to medium and stir in the white wine and lemon juice. Bring to a simmer, then whisk for approximately 1 minute. Remove from the heat and sprinkle with the parsley.

YIELD: Makes 6 (about 2-tablespoon) servings.

NUTRITIONAL ANALYSIS
Each with: **Calories:** 49.88 **Protein:** 0.24 g **Carbs:** 2.48 g **Total Fat:** 3.68 g **Sat Fat:** 1.67 g **Cholesterol:** 6.67 mg **Sodium:** 111.21 mg **Sugars:** 0.51 g **Fiber:** 0.39 g

Quick and Easy Low-Sodium Teriyaki Sauce

This would be a great addition to chicken, steak, or shrimp stir-fry. It calls for sugar substitute; choose one that's suitable in cooking applications.

TEXTURE: Puree

INGREDIENTS

- $^1/_3$ cup (80 ml) mirin (Japanese sweet rice wine)
- $^1/_2$ cup (120 ml) low-sodium soy sauce
- $2^1/_4$ cups (600 ml) rice vinegar
- 1 cup (240 ml) orange juice
- $^1/_2$ cup (120 ml) water
- 1 teaspoon sesame oil
- 2 tablespoons (3 g) sugar substitute
- 3 cloves garlic, minced
- $1^1/_2$ teaspoons minced fresh ginger
- $^1/_8$ teaspoon crushed red pepper flakes
- $^1/_8$ teaspoon black pepper

Bring the mirin to a boil in a medium saucepan over high heat. Reduce the heat to medium-low and simmer for approximately 10 minutes. Pour in the soy sauce, rice vinegar, orange juice, water, sesame oil, and sugar substitute. Season with the garlic, ginger, red pepper flakes, and black pepper. Simmer an additional 8 to 10 minutes. Store in a tightly sealed container in the refrigerator.

YIELD: Makes 6 (about $^1/_4$-cup) servings.

NUTRITIONAL ANALYSIS
Each with: **Calories:** 40.25 **Protein:** 1.11 g **Carbs:** 7.43 g **Total Fat:** 0.21 g **Sat Fat:** 0.03 g **Cholesterol:** 0.00 mg **Sodium:** 339.74 mg **Sugars:** 5.46 g **Fiber:** 0.06 g

CHAPTER 11

7 Ingredients or Less

Brussels Sprouts Gratin

This is one cheesy and creamy side dish you're going to love!

TEXTURE: Regular

INGREDIENTS

- 1½ pounds (680 g) Brussels sprouts, trimmed
- 2 tablespoons (30 ml) extra-virgin olive oil
- 3 tablespoons (23 g) whole-wheat flour
- 2 cups (475 ml) skim milk
- ¼ teaspoon kosher salt
- ½ teaspoon black pepper
- 1 cup (100 g) fresh grated low-fat Parmesan cheese

JOE'S TIP

If available at your grocery store, trying purchasing the Brussels sprouts that are on the stalk. They will be packed with more nutrients because they have been on the stalk longer.

Preheat oven to 400°F (200°C, or gas mark 6).

Bring a large pot of water to a boil over medium heat. Add the Brussels sprouts and cook for 5 to 7 minutes. Remove the spouts from the water and transfer them into a bowl of ice water.

To make the sauce, heat the olive oil in a medium saucepan over medium heat. Add the flour and cook, stirring until smooth and bubbling, about 1 minute. Slowly whisk in the milk and continue to cook, whisking frequently, until thick and creamy, about 2 to 3 minutes. Season the sauce with salt and pepper.

Cut the Brussels sprouts in half through the core and put them in an even layer in a 2-quart baking dish. Pour the sauce over the sprouts and sprinkle with the Parmesan cheese evenly over the top. Bake for 10 to 15 minutes, or until the top is brown and bubbling.

YIELD: Makes 8 (about ¾-cup) servings.

NUTRITIONAL ANALYSIS

Each with: **Calories:** 176.30 **Protein:** 11.17 g **Carbs:** 13.27 g **Total Fat:** 8.78 g **Sat Fat:** 3.53 g **Cholesterol:** 16.22 mg **Sodium:** 374.63 mg **Sugars:** 5.75 g **Fiber:** 4.43 g

Creamed Spinach

TEXTURE: Mechanical Soft

INGREDIENTS

- 2 pounds (900 g) fresh baby spinach leaves, washed and dried slightly
- 1 cup (235 ml) skim milk
- 1 teaspoon kosher salt
- $^1/_2$ teaspoon black pepper

In a large pot, heat ¹/₂ cup (120 ml) water over medium-high heat. Wilt the spinach in the hot water.

Drain then spinach and squeeze out as much excess liquid as possible. Roughly chop the spinach and set aside.

In a heavy-bottom pot, over low heat, bring the milk to a simmer and reduce by half, about 4 minutes. Add the spinach and season with salt and pepper. Cook the spinach and milk together for about 1 to 2 minutes.

YIELD: Makes 6 (about ³/₄-cup) servings.

NUTRITIONAL ANALYSIS
Each with: **Calories:** 76.72 **Protein:** 4.96 g **Carbs:** 18.15 g **Total Fat:** 0.04 g **Sat Fat:** 0.02 g **Cholesterol:** 0.82 mg **Sodium:** 577.30 mg **Sugars:** 2.03 g **Fiber:** 7.16 g

Tomato and Feta Chicken

Make this recipe into a meal by pairing it with the Greek Salad on page 138.

TEXTURE: Regular

INGREDIENTS

- Cooking spray
- 4 (4-ounce, or 115 g) boneless, skinless chicken breasts
- 2 tablespoons (30 ml) low-fat Italian salad dressing
- 1 teaspoon dried Italian seasoning
- 2 tomatoes, seeded and sliced
- $^1/_4$ cup (37 g) crumbled feta cheese
- 2 scallions, chopped

Turn the oven onto the broiler setting. Coat a baking sheet with the cooking spray.

Brush the chicken breasts with the Italian dressing and sprinkle with the Italian seasoning. Place the chicken on the baking sheet and broil for 6 to 8 minutes, turning once, or until the chicken is almost finished cooking.

Remove the chicken from the oven and top with the tomatoes, cheese, and scallions. Return the chicken to the oven and broil about 4 inches (10 cm) from the heat for another 2 to 3 minutes, or until the cheese is melted and the chicken is cooked through.

YIELD: Makes 4 (8-ounce) servings.

NUTRITIONAL ANALYSIS
Each with: **Calories:** 223.22 **Protein:** 37.60 g **Carbs:** 3.89 g **Total Fat:** 5.25 g **Sat Fat:** 1.94 g **Cholesterol:** 99.14 mg **Sodium:** 319.33 mg **Sugars:** 2.12 g **Fiber:** 0.76 g

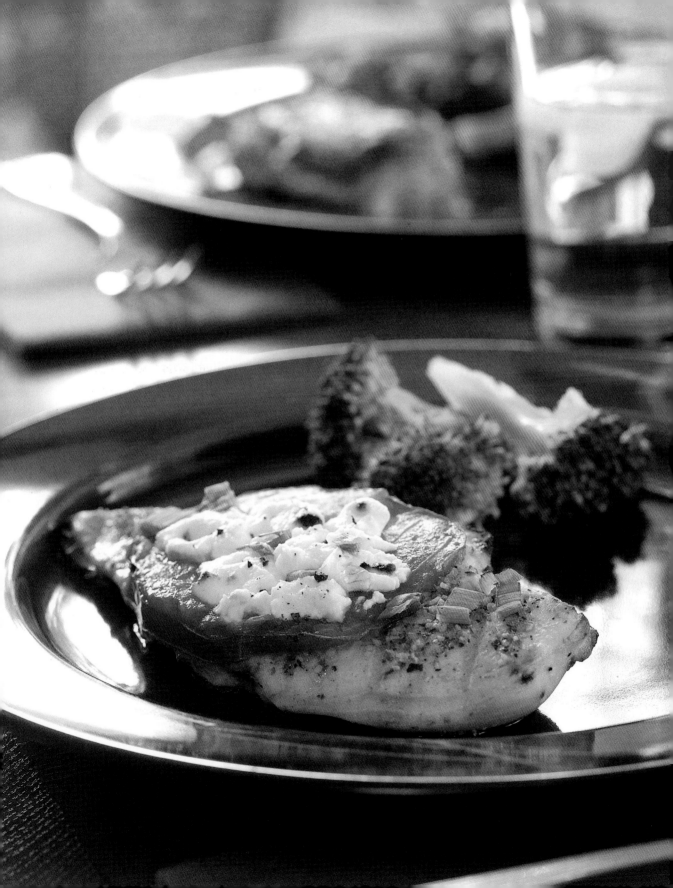

Garlic and Basil Halibut

TEXTURE: Mechanical Soft

INGREDIENTS

- 2 tablespoons (5 g) fresh basil, roughly chopped
- 1 tablespoon (15 ml) extra-virgin olive oil
- 1 garlic clove, minced
- $^1/_2$ teaspoon salt
- $^1/_4$ teaspoon pepper
- 4 (4-ounce, or 115 g) halibut steaks

Turn the oven onto the broiler setting. In a small bowl, combine the basil, olive oil, garlic, salt, and pepper. Brush the mixture over both sides of the halibut.

Place the fish on a sheet pan covered with aluminum foil. Broil about 4 inches (10 cm) from the heat for 8 to 12 minutes, turning once, or until the fish is cooked through.

YIELD: Makes 4 (4-ounce) servings.

NUTRITIONAL ANALYSIS
Each with: **Calories:** 157.85 **Protein:** 23.67 g **Carbs:** 0.34 g **Total Fat:** 6.11 g **Sat Fat:** 0.86 g
Cholesterol: 36.29 mg **Sodium:** 301.39 mg **Sugars:** 0.01 g **Fiber:** 0.05 g

Salmon with Ginger Teriyaki Sauce

This is a great way to use the Quick and Easy Low-Sodium Teriyaki Sauce recipe on page 215. Note that if you do use that sauce for this recipe, the nutritional analysis will be slightly different

TEXTURE: Mechanical Soft

INGREDIENTS

- Cooking spray
- 2 tablespoons (30 ml) low-sodium teriyaki sauce
- 1/2 teaspoon ground ginger
- 2 tablespoons (2 g) roughly chopped fresh cilantro
- 4 (4-ounce, or 115 g) salmon fillets
- 4 slices canned pineapple rings

Preheat the oven to 450°F (230°C, or gas mark 8).

Lightly coat a large shallow baking pan with cooking spray. In a small bowl, combine the teriyaki sauce, ginger, and cilantro; set aside.

Place the salmon and pineapple in the baking pan and brush them with the teriyaki mixture. Bake, uncovered, for 10 to 12 minutes, or until the fish is cooked through. Serve each piece of salmon with a ring of pineapple and extra sauce from the pan on top.

YIELD: Makes 4 (about 6-ounce) servings.

NUTRITIONAL ANALYSIS
Each with: **Calories:** 271.42 **Protein:** 23.66 g **Carbs:** 9.05 g **Total Fat:** 15.26 g **Sat Fat:** 3.46 g
Cholesterol: 62.37 mg **Sodium:** 202.61 mg **Sugars:** 7.00 g **Fiber:** 0.51 g

Baked Cod

Simple and delicious, this is an East Coast favorite.

TEXTURE: Regular

INGREDIENTS

- Cooking spray
- 4 (4-ounce, or 115 g) cod fillets
- 1 tablespoon (15 ml) extra-virgin olive oil
- 1 lemon, cut into 4 wedges
- 2 teaspoons Old Bay Seasoning

Preheat oven to 350°F (180°C, or gas mark 4).

Lightly coat 4 squares of aluminum foil with cooking spray. Place a cod fillet on each piece of foil. Drizzle each fillet with the olive oil. Squeeze a lemon wedge over each fillet, and sprinkle each fillet with ½ teaspoon Old Bay.

Wrap the aluminum foil around the fish and place in the oven; bake until the fish is cooked through, about 10 minutes.

YIELD: Makes 4 (about 4-ounce) servings.

NUTRITIONAL ANALYSIS
Each with: **Calories:** 128.24 **Protein:** 20.20 g **Carbs:** 1.25 g **Total Fat:** 4.26 g **Sat Fat:** 0.64 g
Cholesterol: 48.76 mg **Sodium:** 241.23 mg **Sugars:** 0.50 g **Fiber:** 0.50 g

Greek Yogurt with Honey and Walnuts

TEXTURE: Regular

INGREDIENTS

- 3 cups (690 g) vanilla low-fat Greek yogurt
- 1¹/₂ cups (150 g) walnuts, toasted
- ¹/₂ cup (170 g) honey

Layer ingredients into 6 individual glasses, starting with yogurt and ending with walnuts and honey. Repeat layers.

YIELD: Makes 6 (³/₄-cup) servings.

NUTRITIONAL ANALYSIS

Each with: **Calories:** 228.95 **Protein:** 10.79 g **Carbs:** 30.13 g **Total Fat:** 7.68 g **Sat Fat:** 2.01 g **Cholesterol:** 7.50 mg **Sodium:** 39.65 mg **Sugars:** 25.77 g **Fiber:** 0.56 g

JOE'S TIP

Try mixing up the ingredients by swapping out the walnuts for some of your favorite nuts, as well as using different flavored yogurts and mixing in different berries.

 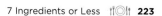

CHAPTER 12

Slow Cooker Recipes

Olé Chicken and Bean Stew

This hearty Mexican-style stew will keep away the chill while giving you tons of the protein you need to stay healthy.

TEXTURE: Mechanical Soft

INGREDIENTS

- 2 teaspoons extra-virgin olive oil
- 1 pound (455 g) boneless, skinless chicken breasts, cut into 1/2-inch (1.25-cm) cubes
- 4 ribs celery, diced
- 2 large bell peppers, sliced
- 2 large yellow onions, diced
- 1/2 cup (120 ml) low-fat, low-sodium chicken stock
- 1 cup (240 ml) water
- 2 cans (15 ounces, or 425 g each) kidney beans, rinsed and drained
- 1 can (15 ounces, or 425 g) black beans, rinsed and drained
- 1 can (15 ounces, or 425 g) cannellini beans, rinsed and drained
- 2 cups (260 g) frozen corn kernels
- 5 tablespoons (38 g) chili powder
- 5 teaspoons (13 g) ground cumin
- 1 teaspoon kosher salt
- 2 teaspoons granulated sugar
- 2 teaspoons red pepper flakes
- 2 teaspoons hot pepper sauce
- 2 tablespoons (2 g) chopped fresh cilantro, plus more for garnish

Heat the olive oil in a large skillet over medium-high heat. When the oil is hot, add the chicken and sear both sides until golden brown. Remove the chicken and put in a slow cooker.

To the hot pan add the celery, bell peppers, and onions, and cook until they have some color, about 8 minutes. Deglaze the pan with chicken stock, then pour the sautéed vegetables into the slow cooker. Add the remaining ingredients, including 2 tablespoons cilantro, to the slow cooker. Cover and cook on the low setting for 4 to 6 hours. Serve with chopped fresh cilantro as garnish.

YIELD: Makes 16 (about 1-cup) servings.

NUTRITIONAL ANALYSIS
Each with: **Calories:** 162.95 **Protein:** 12.69 g **Carbs:** 21.55 g **Total Fat:** 2.79 g **Sat Fat:** 0.41 g **Cholesterol:** 18.14 mg **Sodium:** 319.00 mg **Sugars:** 4.49 g **Fiber:** 5.64 g

JOE'S TIP

Try serving with low-fat Cheddar cheese and a dollop of fat-free sour cream.

Silky Chicken Stroganoff

This chicken stroganoff is so delicious, creamy, and packed with protein. This is one of my own personal favorite recipes.

TEXTURE: Mechanical Soft

INGREDIENTS

- 2 tablespoons (30 ml) extra-virgin olive oil
- 1 1/2 pounds (680 g) boneless, skinless chicken breasts
- 1 container (6 ounces, or 170 g) plain 2% Greek yogurt
- 1 small white onion, diced
- 2 cups (140 g) button mushrooms, sliced
- 1 tablespoon (9 g) chopped garlic
- 1 can ($10^3/_4$ ounces, or 305 g) 98% fat-free condensed cream of mushroom soup
- 1 can ($10^3/_4$ ounces, or 305 g) 98% fat-free condensed cream of chicken soup
- 1/2 cup (115 g) fat-free cream cheese
- 1 teaspoon black pepper
- 1 tablespoon Italian seasoning
- 4 teaspoons (23 g) hot pepper sauce
- 2 teaspoons Worcestershire sauce
- 1 teaspoon kosher salt
- 1 teaspoon red pepper flakes
- 1 tablespoon (1 g) dried parsley

Heat the olive oil in a large skillet over medium-high heat. When the oil is hot, add the chicken and sear both sides until golden brown. Remove the chicken and put in a slow cooker. Add the remaining ingredients to the slow cooker plus 1 cup (235 ml) water. Cover and cook on the low setting for 4 to 6 hours.

YIELD: Makes 8 (about 3/4-cup) servings

NUTRITIONAL ANALYSIS

Each with: **Calories:** 227.70 **Protein:** 25.56 g **Carbs:** 10.53 g **Total Fat:** 8.00 g **Sat Fat:** 1.89 g **Cholesterol:** 63.33 mg **Sodium:** 788.30 mg **Sugars:** 3.23 g **Fiber:** 0.97 g

JOE'S TIP

Try serving this stroganoff over steamed brown rice.

Juicy Caribbean Jerked Chicken

This is a great dish that I've served at dinner parties and as a pulled chicken dish for a Super Bowl party! The chicken is zesty and tender and goes great over rice and stir-fried vegetables. I know this seems to be a very spicy "bird," but it's actually pretty mild. It won't leave you feeling a lot of heat, but rather, more of a subtle "warm" spice. The recipe calls for brown sugar substitute; choose one that's suitable in cooking applications.

TEXTURE: Regular

INGREDIENTS

- ¹/₂ cup (50 g) sliced scallions
- 1 tablespoon (8 g) fresh grated ginger
- 2 tablespoons (2 g) fresh cilantro, roughly chopped
- 2 teaspoons hot pepper sauce
- Juice of 1 lime
- 1¹/₂ teaspoons jerk seasoning
- ¹/₂ teaspoon ground cinnamon
- 1 tablespoon (15 ml) extra-virgin olive oil
- 3 jalapeño peppers, seeded and chopped
- 1 teaspoon freshly cracked black pepper
- ¹/₂ teaspoon kosher salt
- ¹/₂ teaspoon red pepper flakes
- 2 cloves garlic
- 2 tablespoons (3 g) brown sugar substitute
- 1 tablespoon (15 ml) apple cider vinegar
- 1 tablespoon (18 ml) orange juice
- 2 teaspoons Worcestershire sauce
- 4 (4-ounce, or 115 g) boneless, skinless chicken breasts
- 4 (4-ounce, or 115 g) boneless, skinless chicken thighs

Combine the scallions, ginger, cilantro, hot pepper sauce, lime juice, jerk seasoning, cinnamon, olive oil, jalapeños, black pepper, salt, red pepper flakes, garlic, brown sugar substitute, vinegar, orange juice, and Worcestershire sauce in a blender or food processor, and blend until almost smooth. Coat the chicken with the mixture and refrigerate for 12 hours in the ceramic slow cooker insert, wrapped in plastic.

After 12 hours, remove the plastic and cook, covered, on the low setting for 5 to 6 hours, or until the chicken is tender and cooked through.

YIELD: Makes 8 (about ¹/₂-cup) servings.

NUTRITIONAL ANALYSIS
Each with: **Calories:** 146.52 **Protein:** 19.67 g **Carbs:** 1.78 g **Total Fat:** 6.14 g **Sat Fat:** 1.37 g **Cholesterol:** 62.46 mg **Sodium:** 322.21 mg **Sugars:** 0.52 g **Fiber:** 0.30 g

JOE'S TIP

Want more heat in this recipe? Leave in some of the jalapeño seeds.

Pulled Chicken Tacos

I used to make this recipe every week for "taco Tuesdays" with my friends. This is a low-fat, high-protein hit!

TEXTURE: Regular

INGREDIENTS

- 1¹/₂ pounds (680 g) boneless, skinless chicken breasts
- 1 packet (1¹/₄ ounce, or 35 g) low-sodium spicy taco seasoning
- 1 packet (1¹/₄ ounce, or 35 g) low-sodium original taco seasoning
- 1 bottle (12 ounces, or 355 ml) dark beer
- 1 tablespoon (8 g) cornstarch

Combine the chicken and taco seasonings in a slow cooker. In a small bowl, mix the cornstarch thoroughly with the beer, then add to the chicken and combine well. Cook on the low setting for 6 to 8 hours or until the chicken pulls apart.

YIELD: Makes 8 (¹/₄-cup) servings.

NUTRITIONAL ANALYSIS
Each with: **Calories:** 143.96 **Protein:** 18.23 g **Carbs:** 5.68 g **Total Fat:** 2.20 g **Sat Fat:** 0.48 g **Cholesterol:** 54.43 mg **Sodium:** 544.02 mg **Sugars:** 0.00 g **Fiber:** 0.00 g

JOE'S TIP

Try this over a taco salad with chopped greens, tortilla shells, tomatoes, and low-fat cheese. Or just have it as a classic taco with all the fixings.

Silky Smooth Broccoli and Cheddar Soup

This recipe is a classic. Plus, it's full of antioxidants and protein that you and your family are sure to love on those cool fall days.

TEXTURE: Mechanical Soft

INGREDIENTS

- 3 pounds (1365 g) fresh broccoli, chopped, with stems discarded
- 1 tablespoon (15 ml) extra-virgin olive oil
- 1/2 teaspoon black pepper
- 1 teaspoon garlic powder
- 2 cups (475 ml) fat-free milk
- 1/2 cup (58 g) reduced-fat Cheddar cheese, cubed

Place the broccoli, olive oil, black pepper, and garlic powder in a slow cooker and add enough water to cover. Cover, and cook on the high setting for 1 to 2 hours. Add the milk, and continue to cook for 15 minutes. Finally, stir in the cheese and continue cooking until the cheese is melted.

YIELD: Makes 12 (3/4-cup) servings.

NUTRITIONAL ANALYSIS

Each with: **Calories:** 76.27 **Protein:** 5.74 g **Carbs:** 9.72 g **Total Fat:** 2.62 g **Sat Fat:** 0.81 g **Cholesterol:** 4.15 mg **Sodium:** 92.90 mg **Sugars:** 3.95 g **Fiber:** 2.95 g

Brisket with Brown Gravy

This is a great hearty dinner to serve on the coldest of days.

TEXTURE: Regular

INGREDIENTS

- 2 tablespoons (30 ml) extra-virgin olive oil
- 1¹/₂ pounds (680 g) brisket
- 1 teaspoon black pepper
- 1 bunch parsley, stems reserved and leaves chopped
- 2 stalks celery, with leaves, chopped
- 1 bay leaf
- 1 can (14¹/₂ ounces, or 440 ml) low-fat, low-sodium beef broth
- 2 cups (475 ml) red wine
- 2 tablespoons (32 g) tomato paste, no salt added
- 1 packet (1¹/₄ ounce, or 35 g) low-sodium slow cooker pot roast seasoning
- 2 medium onions, chopped
- 2 large carrots, sliced
- 2 packages (8 ounces, or 227 g each) sliced mushrooms
- 1 packet (.87 ounces, or 24 g) low-sodium brown gravy mix
- 1 cup (240 ml) cold water

Heat the olive oil over medium-high heat in a large skillet. Season the brisket on both sides with black pepper, then sear it in the oil until it is browned on both sides.

Add the parsley stems, celery, and bay leaf to the slow cooker, then place the seared brisket on top. In a large bowl, whisk together the broth, wine, tomato paste, and pot roast seasoning. Pour the mixture over the brisket, and top with the onions. Cook on the low setting until the meat is tender, about 4 to 6 hours. About an hour before the brisket is cooked, add the carrots and mushrooms.

When the meat is tender, remove the meat, carrots, and mushrooms from the slow cooker and set aside. Strain out the liquid from the slow cooker into a medium saucepan over medium heat, discarding the parsley stems and bay leaf. In a small bowl, whisk together the gravy mix and the cold water. Whisk in the gravy mixture to the juice on the stove, and cook until thickened, about 2 minutes.

Serve the brisket sliced on a platter, surrounded by the carrots, mushrooms, celery, onions, and gravy. Garnish with the chopped parsley leaves for a splash of color.

YIELD: Makes 14 (about 6-ounce) servings.

NUTRITIONAL ANALYSIS

Each with: **Calories:** 172.22 **Protein:** 17.05 g **Carbs:** 5.50 g **Total Fat:** 5.92 g **Sat Fat:** 1.82 g **Cholesterol:** 20.18 mg **Sodium:** 262.19 mg **Sugars:** 2.31 g **Fiber:** 0.83 g

Super-Sloppy Sloppy Joes

Who doesn't like Sloppy Joes? This recipe is sure to bring you back to your childhood and have you reliving all those happy memories. The recipe calls for brown sugar substitute; choose one that's suitable in cooking applications.

TEXTURE: Mechanical Soft

INGREDIENTS

- 2 tablespoons (30 ml) extra-virgin olive oil
- 1 1/2 pounds (680 g) ground turkey
- 1 pound (455 g) ground turkey sausage
- 1 small yellow onion, chopped
- 1 medium red bell pepper, chopped
- 1 can (8 ounces, or 245 g) low-sodium tomato sauce
- 1/2 cup (120 ml) water
- 1/2 cup (120 g) ketchup
- 1/4 cup (6 g) brown sugar substitute
- 2 tablespoons (30 ml) apple cider vinegar
- 2 tablespoons (22 g) yellow mustard
- 1 tablespoon (8 g) chili powder
- 1 tablespoon (17 g) Worcestershire sauce
- 1/4 cup (31 g) whole-wheat flour
- 10 whole-wheat hamburger buns

Heat the olive oil in a large skillet over medium-high heat. Add the meat and brown, stirring occasionally. Add the onion and bell pepper, and cook, stirring, 10 minutes, or until the meat is cooked. Drain the fat.

Place the meat mixture in a slow cooker. Stir in the tomato sauce, water, ketchup, brown sugar substitute, vinegar, mustard, chili powder, Worcestershire sauce, and flour. Cover and cook on the low setting for 3 to 4 hours, or until the mixture is a sauce-like consistency. Serve over toasted hamburger buns.

YIELD: Makes 10 (1 sandwich) servings.

NUTRITIONAL ANALYSIS
Each with: **Calories:** 295.50 **Protein:** 20.75 g **Carbs:** 31.08 g
Total Fat: 10.45 g **Sat Fat:** 2.30 g **Cholesterol:** 51.76 mg
Sodium: 447.30 mg **Sugars:** 8.83 g **Fiber:** 4.28g

JOE'S TIP

The recipe is also great to cook in a double batch and freeze in individual servings for later.

Easy Baby Vegetable Beef Stew

This is yet another great beef recipe for the crock pot. If you loved Brisket with Brown Gravy (page 229), you will definitely love this one. This recipe is also great to make in large batches and freeze for when you don't have the time to cook.

TEXTURE: Mechanical Soft

INGREDIENTS

- $1/3$ cup (52 g) whole-wheat flour
- 1 teaspoon kosher salt
- 1 teaspoon paprika
- $1/4$ teaspoon black pepper
- $1/4$ teaspoon dried thyme
- $2^1/2$ pounds (1 kg 115g) lean beef, cut into 1-inch (2.5-cm) cubes
- 2 tablespoons (30 ml) extra-virgin olive oil
- 1 package (16 ounces, or 455 g) frozen whole pearl onions, thawed
- 1 package (16 ounces, or 455 g) baby carrots
- $1^3/4$ cups (425 ml) low-fat, low-sodium beef broth
- $3/4$ (175 ml) cup red wine
- 3 tablespoons (48 g) tomato paste, no salt added
- 1 bay leaf
- 2 cloves garlic, chopped
- 1 piece (1 inch, or 2.5 cm) fresh ginger, peeled
- 1 package (8 ounces, or 227 g) sliced button mushrooms

Combine the flour, salt, paprika, black pepper, and thyme in a large zip-top bag and shake well. Add the beef cubes to the bag and toss until the meat is coated.

Heat the oil in a large skillet over medium-high heat. Add the beef to the skillet and brown on all sides. Remove the beef from the skillet and add to the slow cooker; top with the onions and carrots. Add the broth, wine, and tomato paste to the skillet to deglaze, and pour the juices into the slow cooker. Add the bay leaf, garlic, and ginger.

Cook on the low setting for 4 to 6 hours. Add the mushrooms and cook for 1 to 2 more hours, or until the meat is tender. Discard the ginger and bay leaf before serving.

YIELD: Makes 10 (about $3/4$-cup) servings.

NUTRITIONAL ANALYSIS

Each with: **Calories:** 204.56 **Protein:** 21.90 g **Carbs:** 12.91 g **Total Fat:** 6.61 g **Sat Fat:** 2.01 g **Cholesterol:** 50.73 mg **Sodium:** 310.75 mg **Sugars:** 3.29 g **Fiber:** 2.85 g

Rustic Butternut Squash Bread Pudding

This great recipe is perfect for the fall and winter holidays. It's packed full of Vitamins C and E and other antioxidants to help lower the risk for heart disease, cancer, and cataracts. Try this out on the family; they are sure to love it. The recipe calls for brown sugar and sugar substitute; choose ones that are suitable in cooking applications.

TEXTURE: Puree

INGREDIENTS

- Cooking spray
- 5 cups (280 g) whole-wheat bread, cut into approximately 1-inch (2.5-cm) cubes
- 1¹/₂ cups (355 ml) light vanilla soy milk
- ³/₄ cup (191 g) butternut squash puree
- ¹/₄ cup (6 g) brown sugar substitute
- ¹/₄ cup (6 g) sugar substitute
- 1¹/₂ cups (350 g) liquid egg substitute
- 1 container (6 ounces, or 170 g) vanilla 2% Greek yogurt
- ¹/₂ teaspoon kosher salt
- 1 teaspoon ground cinnamon
- ¹/₂ teaspoon ground ginger
- ¹/₈ teaspoon ground allspice
- ¹/₄ teaspoon ground cloves
- ¹/₂ cup (60 g) walnuts, coarsely chopped

Coat the ceramic insert of a slow cooker with cooking spray. Put the cubed bread in the greased slow cooker.

In a separate bowl, whisk together the soy milk, squash puree, sugar substitutes, egg substitute, yogurt, salt, cinnamon, ginger, allspice, and cloves. Pour the liquid ingredients, along with the walnuts, over the bread and mix until combined. Allow the mixture to sit for 5 to 10 minutes. Cover and cook on the medium-high setting for 2¹/₂ hours, or until a toothpick inserted in the middle comes out clean. Remove the cover and cook on the high setting for 10 minutes. Turn off and cover to keep warm. Serve warm.

YIELD: Makes 10 (6-ounce) servings.

NUTRITIONAL ANALYSIS
Each with: **Calories:** 194.55 **Protein:** 12.04 g **Carbs:** 30.05 g **Total Fat:** 5.95 g **Sat Fat:** 0.58 g **Cholesterol:** 1.12 mg **Sodium:** 361.68 mg **Sugars:** 6.93 g **Fiber:** 7.77 g

JOE'S TIP

Try serving with a drizzle of sugar-free maple syrup and low-fat whipped topping.

CHAPTER 13

Dinners

Pork Tenderloin Medallions with Spanish Smoked Paprika

Hearts of Palm with Arugula and Endive Salad (page 133) makes the perfect accompaniment to this delicious and savory dish.

TEXTURE: Regular

INGREDIENTS

- 1 pound (455 g) pork tenderloin roast
- 1 tablespoon (14 ml) olive oil
- 2 tablespoons (28 ml) Worcestershire sauce
- 1 teaspoon Spanish smoked paprika
- 1/8 teaspoon ground white pepper
- 2 teaspoons light butter

Trim off any excess fat from the pork tenderloin and cut it into 1-inch (2.5-cm) medallions.

In a medium mixing bowl, combine the oil, Worcestershire sauce, paprika, and white pepper.

Place the pork in the bowl with the marinade and turn it a few times to coat the medallions evenly.

In a nonstick skillet, heat the butter over medium-high heat. Lay the pork medallions in the pan and cook 4 to 6 minutes, until browned on the first side. Turn and cook an additional 4 to 6 minutes, until the second side is browned. Remove the medallions from the pan and let rest for 5 minutes before serving.

YIELD: Makes 4 (about 3-ounce) servings.

NUTRITIONAL ANALYSIS

Each with: **Calories:** 201.85 **Protein:** 25.01 g **Carbs:** 2.37 g **Total Fat:** 10.87 g **Sat Fat:** 2.51 g **Cholesterol:** 67.15 mg **Sodium:** 65.22 mg **Sugars:** 1.43 g **Fiber:** 0.02 g

Whole Roasted Chicken with Potatoes and Brussels Sprouts

This dinner is easy and elegant, yet packed with flavor from the garlic and white wine.

TEXTURE: Regular

INGREDIENTS

- 1 (5-pound, or 2.5-kg) whole chicken
- 2 teaspoons sea salt or kosher salt
- 1/2 teaspoon black pepper
- 1 teaspoon dried basil
- 4 cloves fresh garlic, halved
- 1/2 cup (120 ml) white wine or chicken stock
- 2 cups (475 ml) water
- 2 tablespoons (28 ml) lemon juice (about 1/2 lemon)
- 12 small to medium baby red potatoes, washed and halved
- 18 Brussels sprouts, washed, trimmed, and halved
- Fresh sprigs parsley

> "I loved this. It was great to take to work the next day."
>
> **—Heather,**
> *a gastric bypass surgery patient in the Boston area*

Preheat the oven to 400°F (200°C, or gas mark 6).

Remove all innards from the chicken. Using kitchen shears or a filet knife, remove all of the skin and trim all of the excess fat.

In a small cup or bowl, combine the salt, pepper, and basil and mix well into a dry rub.

Rub the seasonings evenly on all surface areas of the chicken. Place the chicken breast side down in a 6-quart (6-L) roasting pan with a lid. Add the garlic, wine or stock, water, and lemon juice to the pan. Place the potatoes on one side of the pan, and the Brussels sprouts on the other, along with the chicken.

Cover with the lid and bake for about 1 hour and 15 minutes, basting with the liquid in the pan three or four times. Remove the cover and continue baking for an additional 30 minutes, until a leg can easily be separated from the body when checked with a fork, and the juices from the chicken run clear. (If using a meat thermometer, the internal temperature of the breast should be about 180°F.) Remove the chicken from the pan and let stand for about 5 minutes before carving. For an elegant presentation, serve the chicken, potatoes, and Brussels sprouts on the same serving platter, decorated with fresh parsley sprigs.

YIELD: Makes 6 (about 3–4 ounces chicken, 6 Brussels sprout halves, and 4 potato halves) servings.

NUTRITIONAL ANALYSIS

Each with: **Calories:** 356.93 **Protein:** 29.41 g **Carbs:** 45.76 g **Total Fat:** 4.89 g **Sat Fat:** 0.16 g **Cholesterol:** 76.00 mg **Sugars:** 3.54 g **Sodium:** 464.20 mg

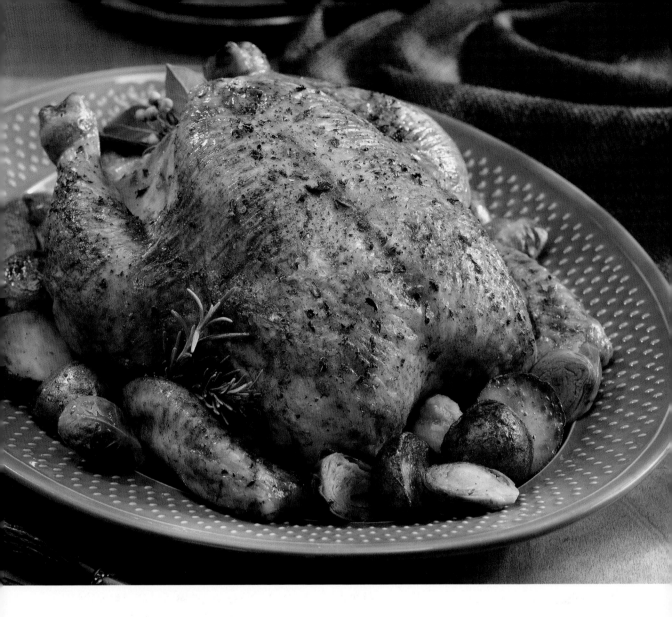

MARGARET'S NOTE

A 5-pound (2.5-kg) chicken will yield approximately 16 ounces (455 g) of white meat and 8 ounces (225 g) of dark meat. The white meat of chicken is lower in fat and cholesterol than the dark meat. You might want to add fat-free gravy or another type of low-fat sauce to make sure it's as moist as possible. The dark meat, with the skin removed, is okay in moderation (about 3 ounces, 85 g, a few times a week), but it's important to avoid the skin to keep the saturated fat and cholesterol down.

Cheddar Chipotle Beer Chicken

TEXTURE: Regular

INGREDIENTS

- 2 tablespoons (28 ml) extra-virgin olive oil
- 2 tablespoons (28 ml) extra-virgin olive oil
- 6 (4-ounce, or 115 g) boneless, skinless chicken breasts
- 1 tablespoon (10 g) chopped garlic
- 1 bottle (12 ounces, or 355 ml) beer of your choosing
- ½ cup (120 ml) skim milk
- 1 tablespoon chipotle powder
- 1 slice (1 ounce, or 15 g) low-fat Cheddar cheese

Heat the olive oil in a medium skillet over medium heat. Sear the chicken until golden brown, about 3 minutes on both sides.

Add the garlic to the pan and sauté for about 1 to 2 minutes. Add the beer, milk, and chipotle powder to the pan. Bring to a simmer, then reduce until the liquid has reached a sauce-like consistency. Remove the pan from the heat and stir in the Cheddar cheese until it is completely incorporated in the sauce.

YIELD: Makes 6 (about 6½-ounce) servings.

NUTRITIONAL ANALYSIS
Each with: **Calories:** 283.05 **Protein:** 37.25 g **Carbs:** 3.91 g **Total Fat:** 9.98 g **Sat Fat:** 2.39 g
Cholesterol: 100.13 mg **Sodium:** 132.32 mg **Sugars:** 1.01 g **Fiber:** 0.00 g

Mediterranean Chicken

This is a colorful, delicious dish that everyone will love.

TEXTURE: Regular

INGREDIENTS

- 4 (3-ounce, or 85 g) boneless, skinless chicken breasts
- $1/2$ teaspoon kosher salt
- $1/4$ teaspoon black pepper
- 2 tablespoons (30 ml) extra-virgin olive oil
- $1/2$ cup (27 g) sun-dried tomatoes, sliced
- $1/4$ cup (25 g) assorted olives, sliced
- $1/2$ cup (120 ml) low-fat, low-sodium chicken broth
- 2 bay leaves
- $1^1/2$ teaspoons Italian seasoning

Preheat the oven to 375°F (190°C, or gas mark 5).

Season the chicken with salt and pepper. In a medium skillet that can go in the oven, heat the olive oil over medium-high heat. Cook the chicken for about 3 minutes on each side. Remove the skillet from the heat, and add the sun-dried tomatoes, olives, chicken broth, bay leaves, and Italian seasoning. Transfer the pan to the oven and bake, uncovered, for 10 to 15 minutes, or until the chicken is completely cooked through.

Remove from the oven and discard the bay leaves before serving.

YIELD: Makes 4 (about 5-ounce) servings.

NUTRITIONAL ANALYSIS
Each with: **Calories:** 187.66 **Protein:** 19.20 g **Carbs:** 4.29 g **Total Fat:** 10.30 g **Sat Fat:** 1.61 g **Cholesterol:** 54.43 mg **Sodium:** 609.57 mg **Sugars:** 2.54 g **Fiber:** 1.10 g

JOE'S TIP

So, you don't like sun-dried tomatoes? Try using freshly diced tomatoes or roasted red peppers instead.

Curried Pork Loin Roast
with Currants, Apples, and Sweet Onions

Begin this a day ahead of time for maximum flavor. The dry rub is also delicious for chicken or beef. Creamy Polenta (the plain with Parmesan cheese version on page 184) makes a lovely accompaniment to this roast. Add Steamed Asparagus Lemonata (page 194) for a complete menu and finish European style with Watercress Salad with Tarragon and Mint Leaves (page 150), for a four-course extravaganza!

TEXTURE: Regular

INGREDIENTS

- 1¹/₂-pound (700 g) pork tenderloin roast
- 1 teaspoon kosher salt
- ¹/₄ teaspoon ground white pepper
- 1 tablespoon (7 g) curry powder
- ¹/₂ teaspoon ground cumin
- ¹/₄ teaspoon cinnamon
- ¹/₄ teaspoon cayenne pepper
- ¹/₈ teaspoon cracked black pepper
- 2 teaspoons olive oil
- 1 teaspoon butter substitute
- 1¹/₂ cups (240 g) diced sweet onion
- 3 tablespoons (20 g) black currants
- ¹/₄ cup (40 g) skinned, cored, and diced green apple
- ¹/₂ cup (120 ml) white wine for cooking or chicken broth

Trim the roast of all excess fat. Place the roast on a piece of parchment or waxed paper.

In a small bowl, combine the salt, white pepper, curry powder, cumin, cinnamon, cayenne pepper, and black pepper and mix together. Distribute the dry rub evenly over the roast and rub it well into the entire surface. Wrap the roast tightly in the parchment or waxed paper, place it in a dish, cover it, and cure it overnight in the refrigerator.

Remove the roast from the refrigerator 20 minutes prior to cooking.

Preheat the oven to 375°F (190°C, or gas mark 5).

In a 7- or 8-inch (17.5- or 20-cm) skillet, heat the oil and butter over medium-high heat. Brown the roast on all sides and place it in a 3-quart (3-L) roasting pan with a lid.

In the same skillet, place the onions, currants, and apple and sauté for 3 to 4 minutes, stirring often to release any brown bits from the bottom of the pan. Add the wine or broth and scrape the bottom of the skillet, incorporating all of the ingredients and absorbing the flavor of the brown bits into the sauté. Continue this process for 1 minute. Pour the sauté mixture over the roast, cover, and bake the roast for 50 to 60 minutes. Uncover and let rest for 10 minutes before carving. Serve the roast on a platter, sliced diagonally, with the onion, apple, and currant mixture over the top.

YIELD: Makes 8 (3-ounce) servings.

NUTRITIONAL ANALYSIS
Each with: **Calories:** 187.72 **Protein:** 24.24 g **Carbs:** 5.07 g **Total Fat:** 6.81 g **Sat Fat:** 2.06 g
Cholesterol: 67.19 mg **Sodium:** 332.38 mg **Sugars:** 3.06 g **Fiber:** 1.07 g

MARGARET'S NOTE

As I mentioned in the Early Postoperative Nutritional Guide (chapter 1), fresh cracked or fresh ground pepper can have a great deal more flavor compared to prepackaged ground pepper. Oil in the peppercorn dehydrates at a much faster rate after it is ground, and so the flavor dissipates as well. Truly fresh black pepper will have a fruity aroma and a hearty bite.

In addition, I find that it's worth researching where your spices come from. Dried spices and seasonings will lose the intensity of flavor as they age. Quality ingredients, including spices and seasonings, can contribute a world of difference to your recipes.

Lobster and Scallop Sauté with Fresh Steamed Green Beans

TEXTURE: Regular

INGREDIENTS

- 1 slice reduced-calorie whole-wheat bread
- 1 cup (100 g) fresh green beans
- Small dash salt
- Small dash pepper
- 2 large sea scallops, sliced in half horizontally
- 2 teaspoons butter substitute
- 1/4 cup (35 g) shelled lobster meat
- 2 tablespoons (28 ml) white wine

Toast the bread, cut it into small cubes, then season it with the salt and pepper.

In a microwave-safe bowl, place the green beans and cover them with water. Place a microwave-safe plate on top of the bowl. Steam the green beans for 4 minutes in the microwave

Coat a 6-inch (15-cm) nonstick omelet pan with cooking spray and heat over high heat. Sear the scallop halves on both sides, transfer to a bowl, and set aside. In the same pan, melt the butter substitute over medium-high heat. Add the lobster, scallops with any juices, and the wine. Cook for about 8 minutes, stirring occasionally, until the wine has reduced a bit and the lobster is cooked. (Lobster is cooked when all translucency has disappeared and the meat is solid white throughout.) Transfer the lobster and scallops to a serving plate or an entrée bowl, top with the croutons and garnish with green beans on one side.

YIELD: Makes about 2 servings

NUTRITIONAL ANALYSIS
Each with: **Calories:** 123.87 **Protein:** 13.24 g **Carbs:** 9.10 g **Total Fat:** 2.76 g **Sat Fat:** 0.43 g **Cholesterol:** 40.39 mg **Sodium:** 442.55 mg **Sugars:** 1.93 g **Fiber:** 2.89 g

Breaded Grouper Fillets

This is sinfully delicious and healthy, too.

TEXTURE: Soft

INGREDIENTS

- 2 tablespoons (30 g) light mayonnaise
- $1/4$ teaspoon lemon zest
- 2 teaspoons water
- 2 teaspoons lemon juice
- $1^1/2$ pounds (700 g) grouper fillets, cut into approximately 4-ounce (115 g) pieces
- 1 cup (100 g) seasoned bread crumbs
- 2 tablespoons (8 g) chopped fresh parsley
- 1 lemon, cut into 6 wedges

Preheat the oven to 375°F (190°C, or gas mark 5). Spray a baking sheet with cooking spray.

In a shallow 2-quart (2-L) mixing bowl, combine the mayonnaise, lemon zest, water, and lemon juice. Place the fillets in the mixture and coat evenly.

Pour the bread crumbs onto a dinner plate. One at a time, lightly coat the fillets in the bread crumbs and place them on the prepared baking sheet. Bake for 15 minutes, until golden and crispy. Place the fillets on a serving plate, sprinkle with the parsley, and garnish with the lemon.

YIELD: Makes 6 (3-ounce) servings.

NUTRITIONAL ANALYSIS
Each with: **Calories:** 198.51 **Protein:** 24.85 g **Carbs:** 14.27 g **Total Fat:** 3.93 g **Sat Fat:** 0.88 g
Cholesterol: 43.82 mg **Sodium:** 445.97 mg **Sugars:** 1.20 g **Fiber:** 1.04 g

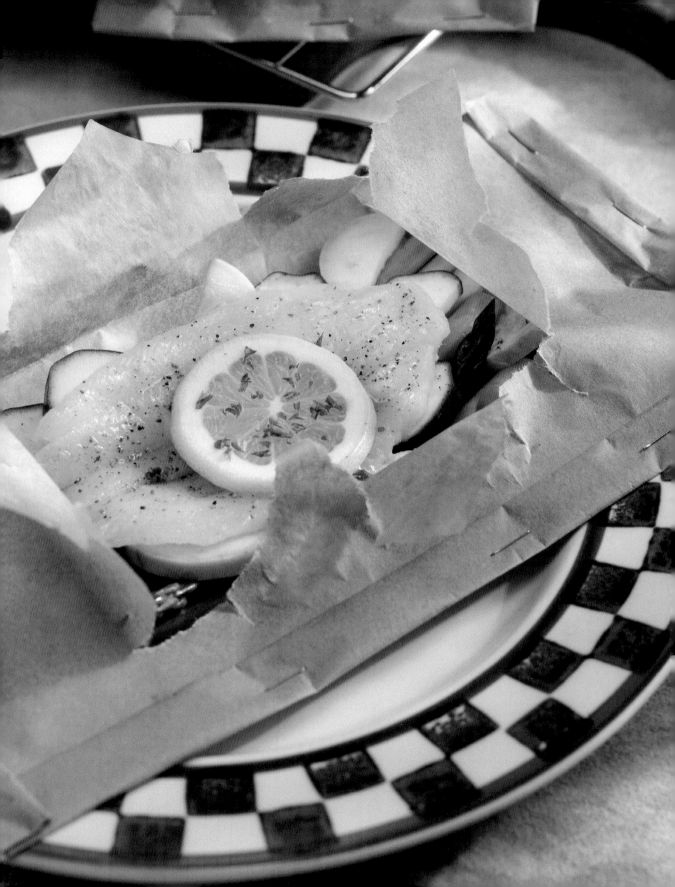

Fillet of Sole with Vegetables Baked in Parchment

So easy and virtually no mess to clean up, these vegetables require very little attention and are cooked to perfection as they steam with the fish in parchment paper.

TEXTURE: Soft

INGREDIENTS

- 4 (5-ounce, or 140 g) sole fillets
- 2 teaspoons olive oil
- 1/8 teaspoon salt
- 1/8 teaspoon ground pepper
- 4 thin lemon slices
- 2 tablespoons (8 g) chopped fresh parsley
- 12 asparagus spears
- 2 small summer squash, stems removed and cut in half, lengthwise

Preheat the oven to 375°F (190°C, or gas mark 5). Cut 4 sheets of parchment paper into 12- x 12-inch (30- x 30-cm) squares and fold each in half.

Open the sheets and place one fillet in the center of the sheet, just below the fold. Rub both sides of each fillet with just enough oil to give a shiny appearance, then sprinkle evenly with the salt and pepper. Place a lemon slice in the center of each fillet and evenly sprinkle with the parsley.

Trim the ends from the asparagus and discard, and then place 3 spears directly under each fillet.

Slice the squash into about 1/4-inch (6 mm) half circles and pile the pieces equally on top of the asparagus. Carefully fold the open three edges of the parchment together tightly, leaving room for air and steam to circulate around the contents of the packet. Staple the folds shut with 2 or 3 staples for each edge and place the 4 packets on a baking sheet. Bake for 15 to 20 minutes. Let stand for about 5 minutes before placing the packets on dinner plates. (You may wish to remove the contents from the parchment entirely before serving, or simply just leave it in the parchment for the individual to deconstruct. That's the fun part! Slice a small incision in the parchment with a small, sharp knife and tear the rest of the way open.)

YIELD: Makes 4 servings (about 4 oz sole, 3 asparagus spears, and 1/2 squash = 1 serving).

NUTRITIONAL ANALYSIS
Each with: **Calories:** 164.79 **Protein:** 26.23 g **Carbs:** 4.25 g **Total Fat:** 5.21 g **Sat Fat:** 0.81 g **Cholesterol:** 70.87 mg **Sodium:** 173.27 mg **Sugars:** 2.37 g **Fiber:** 1.87 g

Fresh Citrus Grilled Shrimp

This is great for a summertime backyard barbecue.

TEXTURE: Regular

INGREDIENTS

- 20 jumbo shrimp, about 1 pound 16/20 count, shelled, cleaned, and deveined
- 1 tablespoon (14 ml) olive oil
- 1 1/2 teaspoons fresh squeezed or pasteurized orange juice
- 1 tablespoon (14 ml) white wine
- Juice from 1/2 lime
- Few sprigs fresh cilantro, chopped
- 1/4 teaspoon fresh minced garlic
- 1/8 teaspoon salt
- 1/8 teaspoon pepper
- 1/4 fresh lime

"The Fresh Citrus Grilled Shrimp was wonderful. The combination of cilantro, garlic, and lime was refreshing and uniquely flavorful. My family commented with each bite on how delicious it was. Prep time was just minutes. As a bariatric lap-band patient, it was very easy to digest. As an aside, I liked this so much that I prepared the recipe again later in the week, replacing the shrimp with scallops, sautéing in a pan."

—**David,** *a gastric banding surgery patient in the Washington, D.C., area*

"This was a great recipe. It was simple, straightforward, and very tasty. We tried this out on our friends, and they loved it. It paired very well with the Mandarin Peapod Salad" (page 130)

—**Jill and Dan,** *gastric banding surgery patients in the Washington, D.C., area*

Rinse, shell, and devein the shrimp, leaving the tails on. Pat the shrimp dry and place them in a medium mixing bowl. Add the oil, orange juice, wine, lime juice, cilantro, garlic, salt, and pepper. Mix to coat all of the shrimp evenly. Cover the bowl with plastic wrap, place it in the refrigerator, and marinate the shrimp for 20 minutes. Remove the shrimp from the refrigerator and bring them to room temperature while preparing the grill.

Prepare the grill for medium-high heat. If using a charcoal barbecue, let the coals burn until they are gray on the entire surface. Using tongs or a long-handled barbecue spatula, place the shrimp on the grill with space in between for even exposure. Cook the shrimp for about 2 to 3 minutes on each side, until they turn opaque orange. Or cook the shrimp indoors in a skillet over medium-high heat for about 2 to 3 minutes on each side, or in the oven at 375°F (190°C, or gas mark 5) for about 8 minutes.

Remove the shrimp from the heat and squeeze the juice from the 1/4 fresh lime over the top.

YIELD: Makes 4 (about 1/2-cup) servings.

NUTRITIONAL ANALYSIS

Each with: **Calories:** 160.04 **Protein:** 23.09 g **Carbs:** 1.80 g **Total Fat:** 5.46 g **Sat Fat:** 0.86 g **Cholesterol:** 172.37 mg **Sodium:** 246.55 mg **Sugars:** 0.33 g **Fiber:** 0.04 g

Fillet of Salmon with Sesame-Orange Glaze

This is such a succulent dish, and it's heart-healthy, too.

TEXTURE: Regular

INGREDIENTS

- 1½ pounds (700 g) wild Atlantic salmon, cut into 6 (4-ounce, or 115-g) pieces
- ¼ teaspoon salt
- ¼ teaspoon black pepper
- 3 tablespoons (45 ml) light soy sauce
- 3 tablespoons (45 ml) fresh or premixed 100% orange juice
- 1 teaspoon orange zest
- ½ teaspoon toasted sesame oil

Preheat the oven to 375°F (190°C, or gas mark 5).

Sprinkle the top and bottom of the salmon with the salt and pepper and set aside for 15 minutes in the refrigerator.

In a small mixing bowl, combine the soy sauce, orange juice, orange zest, and sesame oil. Vigorously whisk with a wire whip or fork. Pour the glaze mixture into a small saucepan and cook over medium-high heat until glaze reduces in volume by one-fourth.

Place the salmon in a 9- x 13-inch (22.5- x 32.5-cm) glass baking dish skin side down and spoon the glaze on top. Bake the salmon fillets using this guide:

MEDIUM RARE:
7 minutes for every 1 inch (2.5 cm) of thickness.

MEDIUM:
12 minutes for every 1 inch (2.5 cm) of thickness.

WELL DONE:
15 minutes for every 1 inch (2.5 cm) of thickness.

EXAMPLE: If your salmon fillets are I-inch (18 mm) thick, for a medium temperature it should cook for 9 minutes (12 minutes x .75 inches).

YIELD: Makes 6 (about 3-ounce) servings.

NUTRITIONAL ANALYSIS
Each with: **Calories:** 176.02 **Protein:** 23.30 g **Carbs:** 2.12 g **Total Fat:** 7.59 g **Sat Fat:** 1.17 g **Cholesterol:** 62.37 mg **Sodium:** 350.32 mg **Sugars:** 1.94 g **Fiber:** 0.05 g

Baked Sea Bass

This is as easy as it is delicious. Impress your friends with this recipe at your next dinner party.

TEXTURE: Soft

INGREDIENTS

- 1¼ pounds (570 g) sea bass
- ½ teaspoon sea salt or kosher salt
- ¼ teaspoon white pepper
- ¼ teaspoon black pepper
- 2 tablespoons (28 ml) extra-virgin olive oil
- 1 tablespoon (3 g) thinly sliced chives
- 2 tablespoons (28 ml) sherry wine for cooking or chicken broth
- 2 teaspoons fresh lemon juice

Cut the fillets into 4 equal servings and place them in a medium baking dish, skin sides down.

In a small bowl, combine the salt and white pepper and lightly coat both sides of the fillets. Sprinkle the top with the black pepper. Cover and let stand in refrigerator for 10 to 15 minutes.

In a small bowl, combine the oil, chives, sherry or broth, and lemon juice and briefly whisk with a fork or wire whisk. Spread the mixture evenly over the fillets and let stand for an additional 10 minutes.

Preheat the oven to 400°F (200°C, or gas mark 6) and bake the fillets about 7 minutes for every inch of thickness, until the center of the fillets are no longer translucent and the outsides of the fillets begin to flake when tested with a fork. Let the fillets stand and cool for about 3 minutes. With a metal spatula, remove the fillets by separating the flesh from the skin and place them in the center of a serving plate.

YIELD: Makes 4 (about 6-ounce) servings.

NUTRITIONAL ANALYSIS

Each with: **Calories:** 207.43 **Protein:** 26.33 g **Carbs:** 0.40 g **Total Fat:** 9.87 g **Sat Fat:** 1.73 g **Cholesterol:** 58.12 mg **Sodium:** 332.99 mg **Sugars:** 0.13 g **Fiber:** 0.14 g

LYNETTE'S NOTE

Colorful garnishes for this plate include fresh, edible flowers, such as nasturtiums, lemon wedges, or fresh herb sprigs.

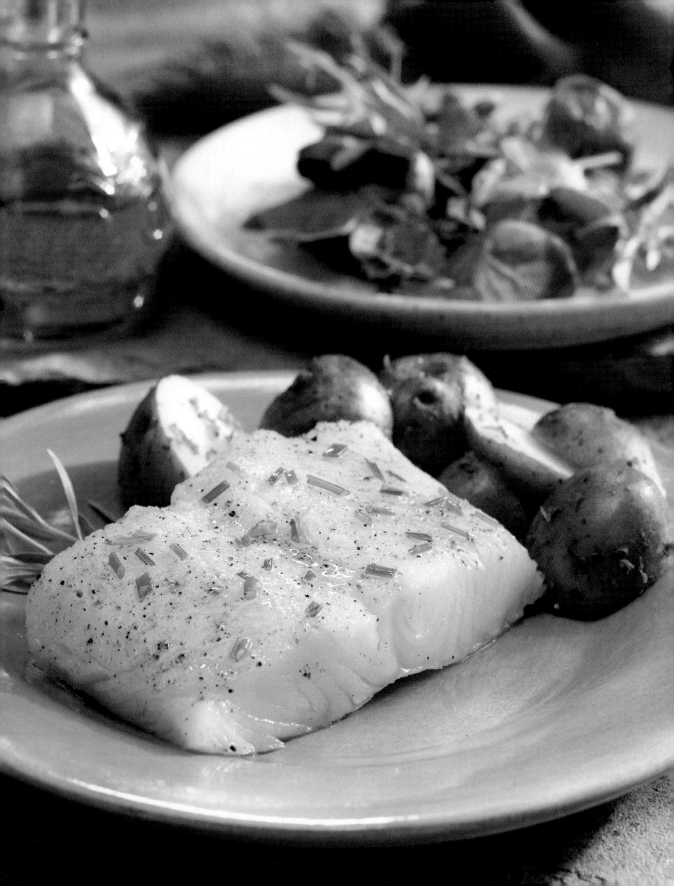

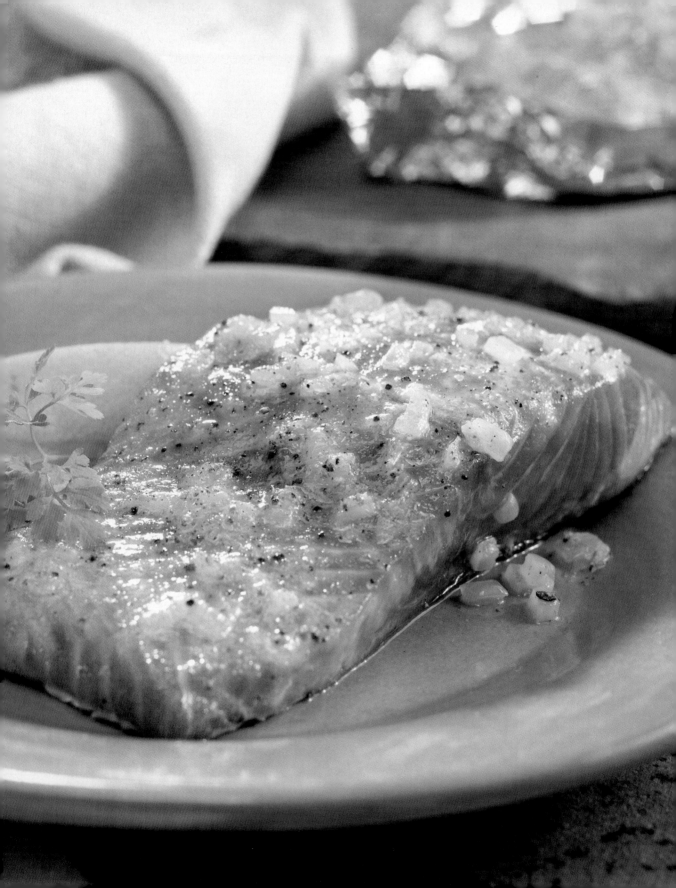

Filet of Salmon à la Herman

We eat a lot of salmon here in the Pacific Northwest. Herman is my dad, and this was his favorite way to cook it. It also gave my mom a break from the kitchen once in a while! My dad used to soak a few small alder branches in a bucket of water for several hours beforehand, and then put them on the grill along with the salmon for that great Pacific Northwest alder smoke flavor.

TEXTURE: Soft

INGREDIENTS

- 1¹/₂ pounds (700 g) wild salmon fillet, cut into 6 (4-ounce, or 115 g) portions
- ¹/₄ teaspoon sea salt or kosher salt
- ¹/₂ lemon, juice and rind (no seeds)
- ¹/₄ cup (55 g) butter substitute
- ¹/₂ large yellow onion, diced
- 1 tablespoon (6 g) fresh cracked black pepper

LYNETTE'S NOTE

This salmon is served perfectly with a garden salad and any of our low-fat dressings on pages 152 to 155.

Prepare the charcoal or gas grill for medium-high heat. Make a "boat" for each of the salmon fillets using heavy aluminum foil by placing the fillet in the center and then folding the edges up around it. Evenly sprinkle the salt over the salmon fillets.

Squeeze the lemon into a small bowl and chop the rind (yellow and white part) into very small pieces, then set aside.

In a small saucepan, melt the butter substitute over medium-high heat. Add the chopped onion and cook until it begins to soften. Add the lemon juice and rind and continue to cook for about 2 minutes, stirring often. Add the pepper, cook for 1 more minute, and remove from the heat. Spoon the sauce over the salmon fillets and place the "boats" on the grill. Cook for about 7 minutes for every inch of thickness of the salmon fillets. When the juice from the salmon begins to appear opaque, it is a good indication of medium-well doneness.

YIELD: Makes 6 (about 4-ounce) servings.

NUTRITIONAL ANALYSIS

Each with: **Calories:** 207.43 **Protein:** 22.90 g **Carbs:** 3.06 g **Total Fat:** 11.21 g **Sat Fat:** 1.78 g **Cholesterol:** 62.37 mg **Sodium:** 204.51 mg **Sugars:** 0.98 g **Fiber:** 0.50 g

Grilled Salmon with Toasted Fennel and Paprika

TEXTURE: Soft

INGREDIENTS

- 1 tablespoon (6 g) fennel seeds
- 2 tablespoons (30 g) packed golden brown sugar
- 3 tablespoons (20 g) Spanish smoked paprika
- 1 tablespoon (19 g) coarse kosher salt
- 2 teaspoons freshly ground black pepper
- 2 teaspoons dried dill weed
- 3-pound (1.5 kg) side of salmon with skin (preferably wild salmon—see Lynette's note)
- 1 tablespoon (14 ml) olive oil
- Several whole fresh parsley sprigs (optional)

LYNETTE'S NOTE

When possible, choose wild salmon over farmed. Farmed salmon contains chemical dyes, antibiotics, growth hormones, and other toxins from being raised in concentrated numbers and unnaturally close proximity to other salmon in the net pens.

Preheat the oven to 350°F (180°C, or gas mark 4).

On a sheet pan, spread out the fennel seeds. Bake them in the oven for about 10 minutes, until the seeds are toasted. (You will smell them when they are done!) Remove the seeds from the oven and let cool. Finely grind the fennel seeds in a spice mill or coffee grinder, then transfer them to a small bowl. Add the sugar, paprika, salt, pepper, and dill weed.

Before lighting the grill, spray the rack with cooking spray. Prepare the barbecue grill for medium-high heat. Brush the salmon lightly on both sides with the oil. Rub the spice mixture generously over the flesh side of the salmon.

Place the salmon skin side down on a heavy-duty sheet of foil, folding the edges of the foil up to form a "boat" for the salmon. Place the "boat" on the grill.

Close the lid on the barbecue and grill for about 8 minutes, just until the juice from the sides of the fillet appears opaque. Open the lid on the grill and continue cooking for about an additional 5 minutes, just until the juice on the top of the fillet begins to appear opaque. (Opaque-colored juice on the top of the salmon indicates a "medium" temperature in the center.)

Remove the salmon from the grill and slide it onto a serving dish. Place the parsley (if using) around the fillet for a beautiful presentation.

YIELD: Makes 10 (about 3½-ounce) servings.

NUTRITIONAL ANALYSIS

Each with: **Calories:** 220.04 **Protein:** 27.57 g **Carbs:** 4.53 g **Total Fat:** 9.68 g **Sat Fat:** 1.48 g **Cholesterol:** 74.84 mg **Sodium:** 438.47 mg **Sugars:** 2.61 g **Fiber:** 1.06 g

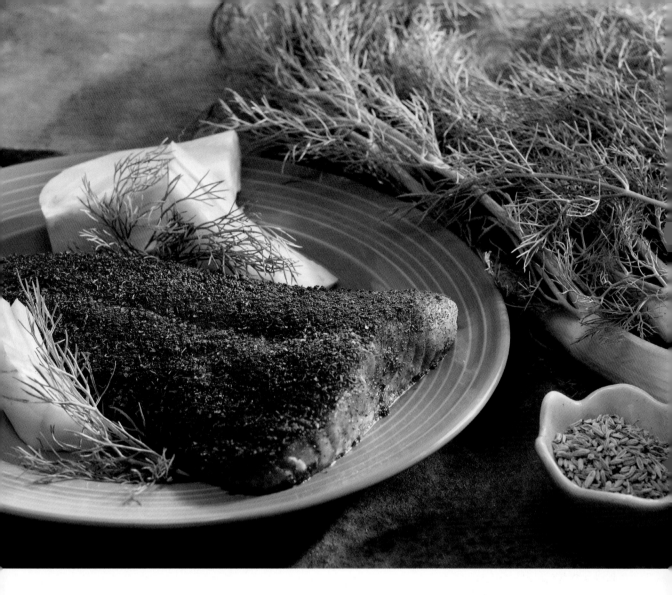

MARGARET'S NOTE

Although this recipe is a bit higher in total fat (40 percent calories from fat compared
with our usual limit of 30 percent of calories from fat), salmon is high in the "good"
fats, like the omega-3-fatty acids and monounsaturated fats, with none of the bad
"trans" fats and very little saturated fat, so it's a heart-healthy meal.

Slow-Cooked Bone-In White Chicken Chili

This dinner literally cooks on its own while you're away at work or play.

TEXTURE: Soft

INGREDIENTS

- 1 pound (455 g) skinless chicken thighs
- 1 pound (455 g) dry Great Northern White beans, rinsed (about 2¹/₂ cups)
- 6 cups (1410 ml) low-fat, low-sodium chicken broth
- 2 tablespoons (30 g) low-sodium tomato paste
- 1 medium green bell pepper, cored and diced (about ³/₄ cup, or 105 g)
- 1 large medium yellow onion, diced (about 1¹/₂ cups, or 240 g)
- 3–6 cloves fresh garlic, chopped
- 1 jalapeño pepper, seeded and minced (optional)
- 1 tablespoon (4 g) dried oregano
- 3 teaspoons ground cumin
- 2 teaspoons paprika
- 1 tablespoon (9 g) chili powder
- ¹/₂ teaspoon cayenne pepper (optional)
- Fresh cilantro sprigs
- Nonfat sour cream

Rinse the chicken and pat them dry with paper towels.

Place the beans in the slow cooker, along with broth and tomato paste. Stir to dissolve the tomato paste and add the chicken, bell pepper, onion, garlic, jalapeño pepper, oregano, cumin, paprika, chili powder, and cayenne pepper (if using). Cook on high for 10 hours. Serve in warm bowls and top each with a sprig of cilantro and a teaspoon of sour cream.

YIELD: Makes 8 (about ³/₄-cup) servings.

NUTRITIONAL ANALYSIS

Each with: **Calories:** 269.78 **Protein:** 25.62 g **Carbs:** 32.44 g
Total Fat: 3.68 g **Sat Fat:** 0.85 g **Cholesterol:** 47.06 mg
Sodium: 111.86 mg **Sugars:** 4.37 g **Fiber:** 11.59 g

Maria and Karen's Zesty Lemon and Caper Chicken

Thanks, Maria and Karen, for creating this ultra-tasty dish.

TEXTURE: Regular

INGREDIENTS

- 1 pound (455 g) boneless chicken breasts cut in half, lengthwise
- $\frac{1}{8}$ teaspoon salt
- $\frac{1}{8}$ teaspoon black pepper
- 1 tablespoon (14 ml) olive oil
- 2 teaspoons light butter
- $\frac{1}{4}$ cup (60 ml) low sodium, nonfat chicken broth
- $\frac{1}{4}$ cup (60 ml) white wine or chicken broth
- 2 tablespoons (20 g) capers, rinsed
- Juice and zest of 1 lemon, (about $\frac{1}{4}$ cup, or 60 ml juice)
- $\frac{1}{4}$ teaspoon garlic powder
- Chopped fresh parsley

"My family and I loved this recipe, and it was really easy to make (and healthy too!). The chicken was very tender and had lots of flavor. We will definitely make this on a regular basis. Thanks so much!"

—**Kim,** *a gastric bypass surgery patient in the Boston area*

Rinse the chicken breasts and pat them dry with paper towels.

Sprinkle the salt and pepper on both sides of the chicken.

In a medium nonstick skillet, heat the oil and butter over medium-high heat. When the oil is hot, just before the butter begins to brown, add the chicken. Brown the chicken on both sides and remove the breasts from the pan and set aside, reserving all that remains in the bottom of the pan. (The chicken is not done in the middle at this point. It will finish cooking in the next phase of the recipe.) Add the wine or broth, capers, lemon juice, and garlic powder to the skillet and return it to a simmer, scraping the bottom of the pan to release all of the browned bits into the sauce. Simmer at least 2 to 3 minutes more, until the sauce is slightly reduced. Return the chicken breasts to the pan along with any exuded juices and cover with a lid. Continue cooking for about 5 minutes, until the chicken is done at its thickest portion.

Place the chicken breasts on a serving platter or onto dinner plates and pour equal amounts of the sauce over each one. For extra zest, grate a small amount of lemon peel (thin yellow skin only) onto the chicken just before serving. A sprinkle of chopped fresh parsley makes an additional and complementary-tasting garnish.

YIELD: Makes 4 (about 3-ounce) servings.

NUTRITIONAL ANALYSIS

Each with: **Calories:** 180.02 **Protein:** 26.35 g **Carbs:** 1.61 g **Total Fat:** 5.91 g **Sat Fat:** 1.04 g **Cholesterol:** 65.77 mg **Sodium:** 371.15 mg **Sugars:** 0.48 g **Fiber:** 0.09 g

Boneless Chicken Breast Cacciatore

This easy and flavorful dish is sure to please your craving for Italian food.

TEXTURE: Regular

INGREDIENTS

- 1¹/₂ pounds (700 g) boneless, skinless chicken breasts (about six 4-ounce, 115 g chicken breasts)
- 1 teaspoon salt
- ¹/₂ teaspoon black pepper, ground
- 1 tablespoon (14 ml) extra-virgin olive oil
- 1¹/₂ large green bell peppers, seeded, membranes removed, and cut into ¹/₂-inch (1.25-cm) strips
- 1 cup (160 g) medium yellow onion, cut into ¹/₂-inch (1.25-cm) strips
- 1³/₄ cups (315 g) diced plum tomatoes or 1 can (14¹/₂ ounces, or 415 g), whole, no salt added, peeled tomatoes
- 2 tablespoons (30 g) low-sodium tomato paste
- 2 tablespoons (28 ml) lemon juice (¹/₂ fresh lemon)
- 1 teaspoon dried oregano
- 1 teaspoon dried basil
- 1 teaspoon dried thyme

Preheat the oven to 375°F (190°C, or gas mark 5). Spray a 9- x 13-inch (22.5- x 32.5-cm) glass baking dish with cooking spray.

Sprinkle both sides of the chicken with the salt and pepper.

Coat a 10-inch (25-cm) skillet with cooking spray. Heat the oil over medium-high heat. Place the chicken in the hot skillet, smoothest side down. Cook for about 4 minutes, until browned on one side only, then place the chicken browned side up into the prepared baking dish.

Return the skillet to the stove and add the peppers and onion. Cook over medium-high heat, until the edges begin to brown. Add the tomatoes, breaking them up slightly with your hands first, along with the juice. Add the tomato paste, lemon juice, oregano, basil, and thyme and then stir with a rubber spatula, loosening any brown bits in the bottom of the pan. Pour all of the mixture over the chicken and bake uncovered for 20 minutes, until the thickest portion of chicken is done. (The juice should run clear when tested in the middle. If using a meat thermometer, the internal temperature should be about 180°F.)

YIELD: Makes 6 (about 3-ounce) servings.

NUTRITIONAL ANALYSIS
Each with: **Calories:** 185.77 **Protein:** 28.23 g **Carbs:** 8.68 g **Total Fat:** 3.94 g **Sat Fat:** 0.74 g **Cholesterol:** 65.77 mg **Sodium:** 321.27 mg **Sugars:** 4.61 g **Fiber:** 2.13 g

"This is a great chicken dish when you are sick of chicken! There is just enough flair to it given by the peppers and onion. I added some fresh herbs that I had on hand, and they were a wonderful addition. I also added some low-fat shredded mozzarella, and it made it almost like low-fat chicken Parmesan, only with very tangy sauce. This took almost no time to make and only two pans to clean up!"

—**Juli,** *a gastric bypass surgery patient in the New Bedford, Massachusetts, areaa*

Chicken, Broccoli, and Mushroom Casserole

This "almost one pot" casserole makes an easy and delicious dinner for the whole family.

TEXTURE: Soft

INGREDIENTS

- 6 (4-ounce, or 115 g) boneless, skinless chicken breasts
- ⅛ teaspoon salt
- ⅛ teaspoon black pepper
- 1 package (10 ounces, or 280 g) frozen broccoli florets
- 2 teaspoons light butter
- ¾ pound (340 g) fresh mushrooms, cleaned and sliced
- 1 can (8 ounces, or 225 g) low-fat condensed cream of celery soup
- 2 teaspoons lemon juice
- ½ cup (120 ml) nonfat milk
- ¼ cup (25 g) sliced green onions (white and green parts)
- ¼ cup (25 g) seasoned bread crumbs
- 2 tablespoons (10 g) grated Parmesan cheese
- 2 tablespoons (8 g) finely chopped fresh parsley

Preheat the oven to 375°F (190°C, or gas mark 5). Spray a medium-large (about 9- x 13-inch, or 22.5- x 32.5-cm) baking dish with cooking spray.

Sprinkle the chicken with the salt and pepper and place them in the prepared baking dish. Bake the chicken for 15 minutes. (It will finish cooking in the following process.) Leave the oven on.

Meanwhile, thaw and drain the broccoli florets.

Remove the chicken from the baking dish, cool in the refrigerator for 15 minutes, and then cut it into 1-inch (2.5-cm) pieces. Place the chicken back into the baking dish. Add the broccoli.

In an 8- or 9-inch (20- or 22.5-cm) nonstick skillet, melt the light butter over medium-high. Sauté the mushrooms for about 8 minutes, until soft, then distribute them evenly along with any juices over the chicken and broccoli.

In a small mixing bowl, combine the soup, lemon juice, milk, and onions and stir to mix. Pour the mixture over the chicken, broccoli, and mushrooms and bake for 25 minutes.

In a small bowl, mix together the bread crumbs, cheese, and parsley.

Remove the casserole from the oven and sprinkle the bread crumb mixture over the top.

Return the dish to the oven and bake for 10 minutes more, until the crumb topping is golden brown.

YIELD: Makes 8 (about 1-cup) servings.

NUTRITIONAL ANALYSIS

Each with: **Calories:** 161.11 **Protein:** 24.19 g **Carbs:** 8.95 g **Total Fat:** 3.38 g **Sat Fat:** 1.10 g **Cholesterol:** 51.67 mg **Sodium:** 386.20 mg **Sugars:** 2.62 g **Fiber:** 2.16 g

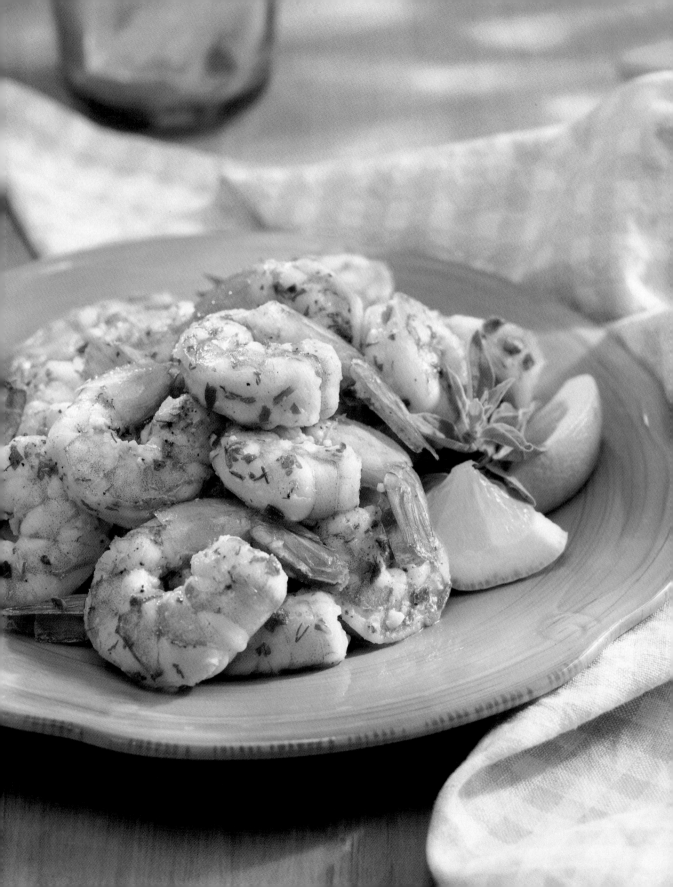

Garlic Shrimp

TEXTURE: Regular

INGREDIENTS

- 3 pounds (1.5 kg) small shrimp, 21/25 count, shelled and deveined
- $^1/_2$ teaspoon sea salt
- $^1/_2$ teaspoon fresh cracked pepper
- 2 cloves fresh garlic, minced
- 2 tablespoons (8 g) chopped fresh parsley
- $^1/_2$ teaspoon chopped fresh thyme
- $^1/_2$ teaspoon chopped fresh oregano
- $^1/_2$ teaspoon crushed red chili flakes (optional)
- 3 tablespoons (45 ml) extra-virgin olive oil
- 2 teaspoons fresh lemon juice
- 2 tablespoons (28 ml) cooking sherry
- Lemon wedges
- Fresh whole sprigs parsley

Sprinkle the shrimp with the salt and pepper and let stand for 10 minutes at room temperature.

In a medium bowl, toss the shrimp with the garlic, chopped parsley, thyme, oregano, and red chili flakes (if using).

In an 8-inch (20-cm) skillet, heat the oil over medium to medium-high heat. Cook the shrimp about 3 minutes on each side, until an opaque orange color appears, then add the lemon juice and sherry. Continue cooking for about 2 minutes. Transfer the shrimp to a serving platter along with all of the liquid in the pan. Garnish the dish with the lemon and parsley sprigs for an elegant presentation. Serve immediately.

YIELD: Makes 12 (about 3$^1/_2$-ounce) servings.

NUTRITIONAL ANALYSIS
Each with: **Calories:** 156.09 **Protein:** 23.11 g **Carbs:** 1.44 g **Total Fat:** 5.48 g **Sat Fat:** 0.87 g **Cholesterol:** 172.37 mg **Sodium:** 224.77 mg **Sugars:** 0.04 g **Fiber:** 0.10 g

Pot Roast à la Sara

This meat, a specialty of my mom's, is so tender it melts in your mouth. You'll love it.

TEXTURE: Regular

INGREDIENTS

- 2 pounds (1 kg) beef bottom round roast
- 1/2 cup (120 ml) red wine or beef broth
- 1/2 cup (120 ml) water
- 4 large cloves garlic
- 1 bay leaf
- 1 teaspoon salt
- 1–2 jalapeño peppers (optional)
- 1 1/2 tablespoons (21 ml) canola oil
- 1/2 pound (225 g) peeled and cubed Yukon Gold or baby red potatoes (cut into 1-inch, or 2.5-cm cubes)
- 1/2 pound (225 g) baby carrots, cleaned and trimmed

Place the beef, wine or broth, water, garlic, bay leaf, salt, and peppers (if using) in a baking dish. Marinate the beef for at least 15 minutes in the refrigerator.

In a 3- or 4-quart (3- or 4-L) heavy-bottomed pot, place the oil over medium-high heat. When the oil is hot, place the beef in the pot, reserving all of the marinade in a separate container. Brown the beef on all sides by allowing it to cook for about 4 to 5 minutes on each side, then rotating it with kitchen tongs or a serving fork. (The object here is to completely brown the entire surface of the roast in order to seal in the juices.) When the roast is nicely browned, add the remaining marinade and reduce the heat to low. Cover with a tight-fitting lid and cook for 1 1/2 hours, until the beef is fork tender. Add the potatoes and carrots. Cook for an additional 1 to 1 1/2 hours, until the potatoes and carrots are tender. Remove the bay leaf before serving.

YIELD: Makes 10 (about 3-ounce meat) servings.

NUTRITIONAL ANALYSIS
Each with: **Calories:** 229.28 **Protein:** 19.56 g **Carbs:** 6.87 g **Total Fat:** 12.60 g **Sat Fat:** 4.29 g **Cholesterol:** 52.62 mg **Sodium:** 183.65 mg **Sugars:** 1.34 g **Fiber:** 1.21 g

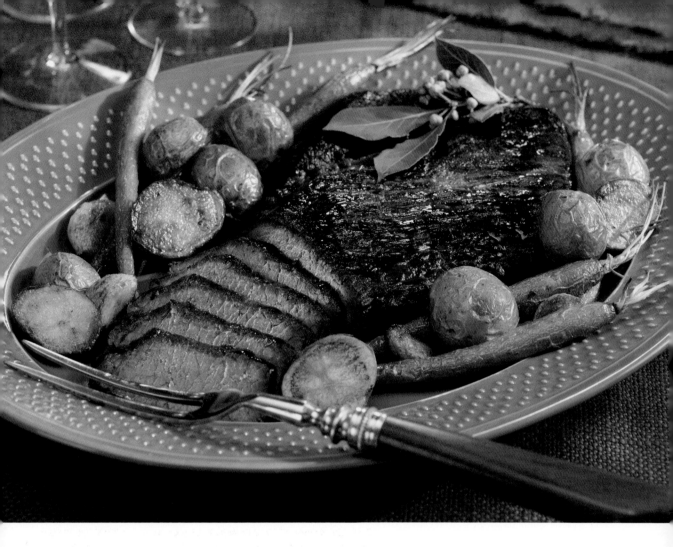

MARGARET'S NOTE

Although this dish is a bit higher in fat than fish or lean chicken, many weight-loss surgery patients may be able to tolerate a 3-ounce serving of this pot roast about 2 or 3 months postop, if not sooner. Eating mindfully (i.e. taking small, pencil-eraser-size bites and chewing at least 15 times prior to swallowing) should allow for better tolerance overall. If you find that meat, even a tender one like this pot roast, is a bit heavier for you, perhaps try only 2 ounces. As always, it's important to stop eating if you feel chest pressure or pain, which is typically your body's signal that you've had enough to eat at a particular sitting.

I hope you enjoy my mom's succulent pot roast dish! Thanks again, Mom!

Oh-So-Easy Shepherd's Pie

TEXTURE: Mechanical Soft

INGREDIENTS

- 2 cups (450 g) prepared mashed potatoes (fresh or boxed)
- $^3/_4$ pound (340 g) lean ground beef
- $^3/_4$ cup (190 g) picante sauce
- $^1/_3$ cup (80 ml) water
- 1 tablespoon (7 g) ground cumin
- 2 teaspoons sugar
- $^1/_2$ teaspoon salt
- $^1/_4$ teaspoon black pepper
- 1 can (15 ounces, or 425 g) kidney beans, drained and rinsed
- $^1/_2$ cup (58 g) extra-sharp Cheddar cheese

Preheat oven to 375°F (190°C, or gas mark 5).

Cook the beef in a large nonstick skillet that can be placed in the oven, over medium-high heat until browned. Stir in the picante sauce, water, cumin, sugar, salt, pepper, and beans; bring to a boil. Reduce heat, and simmer until the mixture thickens.

Remove from the heat. Spoon the mashed potatoes over the meat mixture, covering the meat completely. Sprinkle the top of the mashed potatoes with the cheese, and place the pan in the oven for approximately 10 minutes, or until the potatoes and cheese are slightly golden.

YIELD: Makes 6 (about 1-cup) servings.

NUTRITIONAL ANALYSIS
Each with: **Calories:** 224.59 **Protein:** 19.02 g **Carbs:** 26.17 g **Total Fat:** 5.48 g **Sat Fat:** 2.55 g **Cholesterol:** 38.28 mg **Sodium:** 754.31 mg **Sugars:** 3.43 g **Fiber:** 3.39 g

Pan-Seared Steak Tips with Mushroom Gravy

TEXTURE: Regular

INGREDIENTS

- Cooking spray
- 1 pound (455 g) sirloin steak, cut into ¹/₂-inch (1.25-cm) pieces
- 1 tablespoon (15 ml) extra-virgin olive oil
- 2 tablespoons (20 g) finely minced shallots
- 1 package (8 ounces, or 227 g) baby portabella mushrooms, sliced
- 1 teaspoon garlic, minced
- 1 tablespoon (15 ml) low-sodium soy sauce
- 3 tablespoons (23 g) whole-wheat flour
- 1¹/₂ cups (355 ml) low-fat, low-sodium beef broth
- ¹/₂ teaspoon black pepper
- ¹/₄ teaspoon kosher salt
- ¹/₄ teaspoon dried thyme

Heat a large skillet over medium-high heat. Coat the skillet with the cooking spray and brown the steak on all sides. Remove from the pan, and cover.

Heat the olive oil in the pan and then add the shallots and mushrooms; sauté for approximately 4 minutes, or until the mushrooms and shallots are cooked through. Next, add the garlic and sauté for another 30 seconds. Stir in the soy sauce. Sprinkle the flour over the mushroom mixture, and cook for approximately 1 minute, stirring constantly. Gradually stir in the beef broth. Add the pepper, salt, and thyme, and bring to a simmer. Cook for approximately 4 to 5 minutes, or until the mixture is thickened. Add the beef back to the pan and cook for another minute.

YIELD: Makes 6 (about ³/₄-cup) servings.

NUTRITIONAL ANALYSIS

Each with: **Calories:** 213.38 **Protein:** 24.31 g **Carbs:** 5.52 g **Total Fat:** 9.94 g **Sat Fat:** 3.20 g **Cholesterol:** 46.44 mg **Sodium:** 324.34 mg **Sugars:** 1.67 g **Fiber:** 0.95 g

JOE'S TIP

Try serving this delicious dish with rice or pasta and a side of sautéed vegetables.

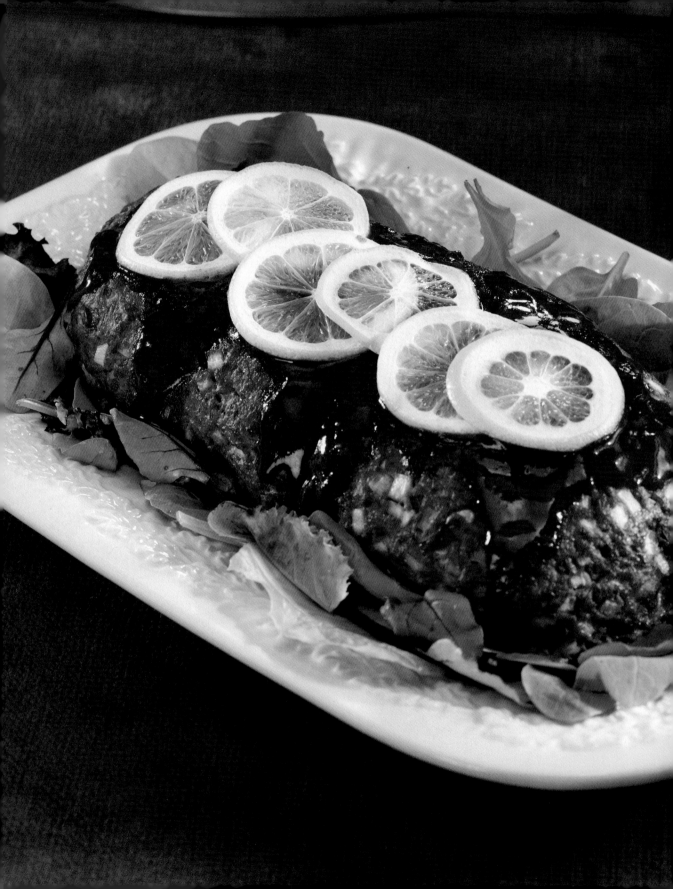

Lemon-Barbecue Meatloaf

This is a great dish for the family, or it can be easy divided and frozen for later.

TEXTURE: Soft

INGREDIENTS

- 2 pounds (1 kg) 95% lean ground beef
- 2 cups (320 g) diced yellow onion (about 1$\frac{1}{2}$ onions)
- 2 tablespoons (28 ml) fresh lemon juice
- 7 tablespoons (105 ml) low-carb barbecue sauce, divided
- 2 tablespoons (30 g) low-sodium tomato paste
- 2 tablespoons (8 g) chopped fresh parsley
- $\frac{1}{4}$ cup (35 g) finely chopped green or red bell pepper
- 1 large egg
- $\frac{1}{4}$ cup (25 g) bread crumbs
- 6 $\frac{1}{8}$-inch (3 mm) thick lemon slices

Preheat the oven to 375°F (190°C, or gas mark 5). Spray a 8$\frac{1}{2}$- x 13$\frac{1}{2}$-inch (22.5- x 32.5-cm) baking dish with cooking spray.

In a large mixing bowl, place the beef, onion, lemon juice, 4 tablespoons (60 ml) of the barbecue sauce, tomato paste, parsley, pepper, egg, and bread crumbs. Mix until well incorporated.

Form the mixture into a loaf and pat it down to condense the consistency. The loaf should touch the width, or short edges of the pan, but leave a few inches of room on both sides of the length.

Bake uncovered for 30 minutes. Remove the loaf from the oven and coat the top with the additional 3 tablespoons (45 ml) barbecue sauce. Place the lemon slices on top of the loaf and return it to the oven. Continue baking for an additional 20 minutes.

YIELD: Makes 12 (about 3-ounce) servings.

NUTRITIONAL ANALYSIS

Each with: **Calories:** 170.19 **Protein:** 22.31 g **Carbs:** 6.04 g **Total Fat:** 5.79 g **Sat Fat:** 2.43 g **Cholesterol:** 75.21 mg **Sodium:** 160.16 mg **Sugars:** 1.91 g **Fiber:** 0.88 g

Savory Ground Turkey Meat Loaf

This is a simple yet delicious dish.

TEXTURE: Soft

INGREDIENTS

- 2 tablespoons (28 ml) olive oil
- 1 medium onion, diced
- 1/2 medium red pepper, cored, seeded, and diced
- 6-8 white mushrooms, cleaned and sliced very thin
- 1/4 cup (60 ml) white wine
- 1 pound (455 g) lean ground turkey (see note)
- 2/3 cup (65 g) Italian bread crumbs
- 1 egg, beaten
- 1/4 teaspoon black pepper
- 1/2 teaspoon seasoning salt
- 1 teaspoon garlic powder
- 1 tablespoon (4 g) chopped fresh parsley
- 1 tablespoon (15 g) ketchup, plus 1 tablespoon (15 g) additional for the top (optional)
- 2 teaspoons yellow or brown mustard, plus 1 teaspoon for the top (optional)

Preheat the oven to 350°F (180°C, or gas mark 4). Spray a 7- x 9-inch (17.5- x 22.5-cm) baking dish with cooking spray.

In a nonstick pan, heat the oil over medium-high heat. When the oil is hot, add the onion, red pepper, and mushrooms. Sauté the vegetables for 4 to 6 minutes, until softened. Add the wine to deglaze pan. Let the vegetables and wine simmer for 2 to 3 minutes to allow the alcohol to evaporate. Place the pan in the refrigerator and cool completely.

In a large mixing bowl, place the turkey, bread crumbs, egg, black pepper, salt, garlic powder, parsley, 1 tablespoon of the ketchup, and 2 teaspoons of the mustard, along with the cooled sauté mixture. With clean, jewelry-free hands, mix thoroughly. When all the ingredients are mixed together, form a rectangular loaf in the prepared baking dish. Add an additional 1 tablespoon ketchup (if using) and 1 teaspoon mustard (if using) to the top and spread evenly over the turkey loaf to seal in the juices and form a tasty crust. Bake for 45 minutes.

YIELD: Makes 6 (about 3-ounce) servings.

NUTRITIONAL ANALYSIS

Each with **Calories:** 220.40 **Protein:** 22.30 g **Carbs:** 14.38 g **Total Fat:** 7.38 g **Sat Fat:** 1.45 g **Cholesterol:** 76.80 mg **Sodium:** 373.71 mg **Sugars:** 3.82 g **Fiber:** 1.80 g

NOTE

You can use ground white breast meat, 99 percent fat-free, but it will be a bit drier.

Heather's Tasty Marinara Sauce

This recipe is from the kitchen of Heather, a gastric bypass surgery patient in the Boston area. To add protein and texture to this sauce, add up to 1 pound (455 g) of browned spicy Italian sausage, without the skin.

TEXTURE: Pureed

INGREDIENTS

- 3 tablespoons (45 ml) extra-virgin olive oil
- 6 cloves garlic, minced
- 1 medium onion, diced (about 1½ cups, or 240 g)
- 4 teaspoons dried basil
- 1 teaspoon crushed red chili flakes (optional)
- 3 cans (14½ ounces, or 415 g each) peeled, crushed low-salt tomatoes

In a 2½-quart (2.5-L) saucepan, heat the oil over medium-high heat. Add the garlic, onion, basil, and chili flakes (if using) and sauté 4 to 6 minutes, until the onion begins to sweat. Add the tomatoes with the liquid and bring the sauce to a boil, stirring occasionally. Reduce the heat to a simmer and continue cooking for at least 30 minutes.

YIELD: Makes 14 (about ½-cup) servings.

NUTRITIONAL ANALYSIS

Each with: **Calories:** 53.16 **Protein:** 1.80 g **Carbs:** 5.37 g **Total Fat:** 3.06 g **Sat Fat:** 0.43 g **Cholesterol:** 0.00 mg **Sodium:** 68.39 mg **Sugars:** 3.00 g **Fiber:** 1.16 g

LYNETTE'S NOTE

This is the kind of sauce that tastes even better the next day. In a proper container, it should last in the refrigerator up to 5 days. Be sure to cool it completely in the refrigerator before placing a lid on it. This helps to avoid creating an environment that can host bacterial growth, which can thrive in warm and moist food products.

Turkey Sausage and Cannellini Bean Casserole

This recipe calls for brown sugar substitute; choose one that's suitable in cooking applications.

TEXTURE: Mechanical Soft

INGREDIENTS

- Cooking spray
- 1 medium onion, chopped
- 1 pound (455 g) turkey sausage, thinly sliced
- 2 garlic cloves, minced
- 1 can (14 ounces, or 425 ml) fat-free, low-sodium chicken broth
- 2 tablespoons (3 g) brown sugar substitute
- 2 tablespoons (32 g) tomato paste, no salt added
- ½ teaspoon dried thyme
- ½ teaspoon freshly ground black pepper
- 3 cans (16 ounces, or 453 g each) cannellini beans, rinsed and drained
- 1 bay leaf
- 2 tablespoons (8 g) fresh parsley, chopped

Preheat oven to 375°F (190°C, or gas mark 5).

Heat a Dutch oven or large heavy-duty pot over medium-high heat and coat it with cooking spray. Add the onions and turkey sausage and sauté for 5 minutes, or until golden brown. Add the garlic, and sauté for 2 minutes more. Deglaze the pan with the chicken broth.

Stir in the brown sugar substitute, tomato paste, thyme, black pepper, cannellini beans, and bay leaf. Bring to a boil; cover, reduce heat, and simmer for 5 minutes. Remove from the burner then bake in the oven until golden brown, about 15 minutes.

Before serving, discard the bay leaf and sprinkle with parsley.

YIELD: Makes 10 (about 1-cup) servings.

NUTRITIONAL ANALYSIS

Each with: **Calories:** 199.17 **Protein:** 17.41 g **Carbs:** 24.24 g **Total Fat:** 3.70 g **Sat Fat:** 0.90 g **Cholesterol:** 34.02 mg **Sodium:** 579.89 mg **Sugars:** 4.17 g **Fiber:** 6.64 g

JOE'S TIP

Try using different-colored beans and different flavors of turkey sausage to play with the look and overall flavor of the dish.

Sausage with Lentils

TEXTURE: Regular

INGREDIENTS

- 2 tablespoons (30 ml) extra-virgin olive oil
- 12 ounces (340 g) chicken sausage, thinly sliced
- 2 medium onions, chopped
- 2 red bell peppers, cored, seeded, and chopped
- 1 orange bell pepper, cored, seeded and chopped
- 1 1/2 cups (290 g) small green lentils, rinsed
- 1 teaspoon dried thyme
- 2 cups (480 ml) low-fat, low-sodium chicken stock
- 1/2 teaspoon kosher salt
- 1/4 teaspoon black pepper
- 4 tablespoons (16 g) fresh parsley, chopped

Heat the olive oil in a large, nonstick skillet over medium-high heat. Add the sausage and cook, stirring frequently, about 10 minutes, or until the sausage is brown.

Pour off the oil from the skillet. Add the onions and bell peppers and cook for about 5 minutes, or until softened. Add the lentils and thyme, and stir until coated with oil.

Stir in the stock, and bring to a boil. Reduce the heat, cover, and let simmer for about 30 minutes, or until the lentils are tender and the liquid has been absorbed; season with salt and pepper.

Return the sausage to the skillet and heat through. Stir in the parsley before serving.

YIELD: Makes 8 (about 1-cup) servings.

NUTRITIONAL ANALYSIS

Each with: **Calories:** 232.47 **Protein:** 16.42 g **Carbs:** 25.82 g **Total Fat:** 7.70 g **Sat Fat:** 1.33 g **Cholesterol:** 31.89 mg **Sodium:** 505.73 mg **Sugars:** 4.52 g **Fiber:** 6.81 g

Kosher Lamb Souvlaki

This is a great dish to bring to a barbecue. Serve it with Yogurt-Cucumber Sauce (next page).

TEXTURE: Regular

INGREDIENTS

- 2 tablespoons (28 ml) extra-virgin olive oil
- 1 tablespoon (10 g) chopped fresh garlic
- 1 teaspoon dried oregano
- 1 teaspoon dried thyme
- 1 teaspoon dried basil
- 2 teaspoons chopped fresh parsley
- ³/₄ teaspoon freshly ground black pepper
- ³/₄ teaspoon kosher salt
- 1 pound (455 g) lamb, cut from the leg into 12 equal-sized cubes
- 2 yellow bell peppers, cored and cut into 1-inch (2.5-cm) strips
- 1 sweet red onion, cut into 8 large pieces
- 16 cherry tomatoes
- 8 (4-inch, or 10-cm) whole-wheat pitas

Begin preparing a minimum of 3 hours ahead of service time to allow the souvlaki to marinate. (The skewers can marinate for up to 24 hours.)

In a small mixing bowl, mix together the first 8 ingredients then set aside.

Distribute the lamb, bell peppers, onion, and tomatoes equally onto 8 skewers. Place the skewers in a large shallow pan and evenly pour the marinade over the skewers. Cover the pan and refrigerate at least 3 hours, rotating the skewers once.

Before lighting the grill, spray the rack with cooking spray. Prepare the grill for medium heat. (If using a charcoal grill, allow the coals to turn a light-ash color.) Place the skewers on the grill and cook 8 to 12 minutes, until the lamb is medium-rare and lightly charred, rotating to cook evenly. Remove the skewers from the grill and let set for 5 minutes. Place one skewer in each pita. Serve immediately.

YIELD: Makes 8 (about 2-ounce) servings.

NUTRITIONAL ANALYSIS
Each with: **Calories:** 225.43 **Protein:** 14.26 g **Carbs:** 21.51 g **Total Fat:** 9.74 g
Sat Fat: 3.76 g **Cholesterol:** 38.56 mg **Sodium:** 274.53 mg **Sugars:** 3.10 g
Fiber: 3.28 g

Greek Yogurt-Cucumber Sauce

TEXTURE: Pureed

INGREDIENTS

- 1 cup (135 g) grated cucumber (Squeeze out excess moisture using paper towels.)
- $1/2$ cup (100 g) nonfat sour cream
- 1 container (7 ounces, or 200 g) 2% Greek yogurt
- 1 clove fresh garlic, minced
- 1 teaspoon lemon juice
- $1/4$ teaspoon salt
- $1/8$ teaspoon ground white pepper
- 1 tablespoon (4 g) chopped fresh parsley

In a medium mixing bowl, stir together the cucumber, sour cream, yogurt, garlic, lemon juice, salt, pepper, and parsley with a wire whip. Serve chilled.

YIELD: Makes 10 (about 1-ounce) servings.

NUTRITIONAL ANALYSIS
Each with: **Calories:** 29.40 **Protein:** 2.61 g **Carbs:** 3.68 g **Total Fat:** 0.43 g **Sat Fat:** 0.30 g **Cholesterol:** 3.00 mg **Sodium:** 45.79 mg **Sugars:** 1.80 g **Fiber:** 0.12 g

Braised" Lamb with Zucchini and Tomatoes

TEXTURE: Regular

INGREDIENTS

- 12 ounces (340 g) lamb chops
- $1/2$ teaspoon kosher salt
- $1/4$ teaspoon black pepper
- 2 tablespoons (30 ml) extra-virgin olive oil
- 1 medium onion, chopped
- 1 garlic clove, minced
- 1 can ($14^1/2$ ounces, or 411 g) diced tomatoes, no salt added
- $1/4$ teaspoon sugar
- 2 medium zucchinis, sliced
- 1 teaspoon dried thyme

Season the lamb chops with salt and pepper. Heat the olive oil in a Dutch oven or large heavy-duty pot over medium-high heat. Add the onion and garlic and sauté for about 5 minutes, or until softened. Add the lamb chops and sear until brown, about 3 minutes on each side.

Stir in the tomatoes with juice, sugar, zucchini, and thyme. Bring to a boil and then turn the heat to medium-low and simmer, stirring occasionally, for 30 to 45 minutes, or until the zucchini and lamb chops are tender. Serve by topping the lamb chops with the vegetables and sauce.

YIELD: Makes 6 (about 6-ounce) servings.

NUTRITIONAL ANALYSIS
Each with: **Calories:** 181.47 **Protein:** 15.97 g **Carbs:** 5.62 g **Total Fat:** 10.14 g **Sat Fat:** 2.95 g **Cholesterol:** 49.33 mg **Sodium:** 214.29 mg **Sugars:** 3.79 g **Fiber:** 1.08 g

Mexican Turkey Skillet Casserole

This is a great dish for the whole family.

TEXTURE: Regular

INGREDIENTS

- ¹/₂ cup (50 g) whole-wheat elbow macaroni
- 1 teaspoon extra-virgin olive oil
- 1 pound (455 g) extra lean ground turkey, 97% fat-free
- 1 teaspoon salt
- 1 tablespoon (9 g) chili powder
- 2 teaspoons paprika
- 2 teaspoons ground cumin
- 2 teaspoons garlic powder
- ¹/₂ teaspoon cayenne pepper (optional)
- 1¹/₂ cups (240 g) diced yellow onion
- 1 can (14¹/₂ ounces, or 415 g) diced tomatoes in juice (no salt added)
- 1 cup (200 g) canned corn (no salt added)
- 4 (8-inch, or 20-cm) low-carb, whole-wheat tortillas
- ¹/₄ cup (50 g) nonfat sour cream
- Fresh sprigs parsley

> "The Mexican Skillet is just so yummy and spicy. It's similar to a nice chili, a sloppy Joe, or just a good, old-fashioned casserole. It makes you forget that it's good for you."
>
> —**Adrienne,** *a BPD surgery patient in the Boston area*

Preheat the oven to 300°F (150°C, or gas mark 2).

Cook the pasta according to package directions, omitting salt and fat.

While the pasta cooks, heat an 8-inch (20-cm) skillet that has been coated with cooking spray and the oil over medium-high heat. Add the turkey, stirring with a large spoon or rubber spatula. Continue cooking about 15 minutes, stirring just enough to break the turkey into crumbles, and until the turkey begins to brown. Add the salt, chili powder, paprika, cumin, garlic powder, and cayenne pepper (if using), and then stir well to incorporate the spices. Add the onion and continue to cook for 4 to 6 minutes, until the onion begins to soften. Add the tomatoes with the juice and the corn, cover the pan, and continue to cook for 5 minutes.

Wrap the tortillas in aluminum foil and bake for 12 minutes. Remove the tortillas from the foil, roll them into cylinders, and place one on the rim of each dinner plate. On the opposite side of each plate, place 1 tablespoon (12 g) of the sour cream. Spoon one serving in the center of each plate and garnish with a fresh parsley sprig.

YIELD: Makes 4 (1-cup) servings

NUTRITIONAL ANALYSIS

Each with: **Calories:** 319.06 **Protein:** 37.19 g **Carbs:** 35.77 g **Total Fat:** 6.00 g **Sat Fat:** 0.78 g **Cholesterol:** 65.00 mg **Sodium:** 667.49 mg **Sugars:** 10.34 g **Fiber:** 14.31 g

MARGARET'S NOTE

This recipe includes 97 percent fat-free ground turkey, but if you can't find this in the market, 93 percent fat-free (no skin) is perfectly acceptable. Enjoy!

One Pot Chicken Dinner in a Pinch

It's fast, easy, and delicious.

TEXTURE: Regular

INGREDIENTS

- 1 tablespoon (14 ml) olive oil
- 2 teaspoons butter alternative
- 4 medium red potatoes, peeled and thinly sliced
- 1 pound (455 g) boneless, skinless chicken breast, cut into bite-size cubes
- 1 cup (70 g) broccoli fresh florets
- 1 cup (150 g) cauliflower fresh florets
- 1 medium onion, diced
- 1 clove fresh garlic, chopped
- 1 can (10 $^3/_4$ ounces, or 290 g) reduced-fat, low-sodium condensed cream of mushroom soup
- $^1/_2$ cup (120 ml) nonfat milk
- 2 whole green onions, chopped
- 2 tablespoons (8 g) chopped fresh parsley
- $^1/_3$ cup (35 g) grated Parmesan cheese

In a 9- or 10-inch (22.5- or 25-cm) skillet, heat the oil and butter alternative over medium-high heat. Add the potatoes and cook for 15 to 20 minutes, until they begin to brown, stirring occasionally. Add the chicken and continue cooking for about 15 minutes, stirring occasionally, allowing the chicken to brown, then reduce the heat to low.

In a microwave-safe bowl, place the broccoli and cauliflower with water to cover the vegetables and microwave on high power for about 5 minutes, until the broccoli and cauliflower are fork tender. Carefully remove the vegetables from the microwave, drain off all liquid, and add them to the chicken and potatoes, along with the onion and garlic. Add the soup, milk, green onions, parsley, and cheese and stir. Cover the skillet and simmer for 12 to 15 minutes, stirring occasionally. Serve in warm bowls for a complete meal.

YIELD: Makes 8 (about 1-cup) servings.

NUTRITIONAL ANALYSIS

Each with: **Calories:** 244.49 **Protein:** 19.54 g **Carbs:** 25.55 g **Total Fat:** 7.46 g **Sat Fat:** 2.33 g **Cholesterol:** 35.93 mg **Sodium:** 160.87 mg **Sugars:** 4.93 g **Fiber:** 3.20 g

Slow-Cooked Sausage and Lentil Stew

Tasty and satisfying, this can be started in the morning and ready at dinnertime.

TEXTURE: Regular

INGREDIENTS

- 1¹/₂ cups (290 g) lentils, soaked in water for 30 minutes
- ¹/₂ cup (50 g) chopped celery
- 2 cups (40 g) chopped fresh spinach, washed and drained
- 3 cloves fresh garlic, coarsely chopped
- 1 cup (160 g) chopped yellow onion
- 4 cups (1 L) water
- 2 tablespoons (30 g) low-sodium tomato paste
- ¹/₂ teaspoon cayenne pepper (optional)
- 1 bay leaf
- Juice of ¹/₂ lemon (about 2 tablespoons, or 28 ml)
- ¹/₂ pound (225 g) light, low-sodium precooked smoked turkey sausage or kielbasa, cut into ¹/₄-inch (6-mm) pieces, skin removed (see note)

In a 3-quart (3-L) slow cooker, place all ingredients and cook on the high setting for 5 hours or on the low setting for 7 hours. Remove the bay leaf before serving.

YIELD: Makes 6 (about 1-cup) servings.

NUTRITIONAL ANALYSIS
Each with: **Calories:** 261.32 **Protein:** 20.45 g **Carbs:** 33.07 g **Total Fat:** 6.01 g **Sat Fat:** 0.09 g **Cholesterol:** 23.33 mg **Sodium:** 371.91 mg **Sugars:** 4.87 g **Fiber:** 15.98 g

NOTE

Removing the skin is essential for easier digestion. Score the sausage lengthwise and peel the skin away from the sausage. The skin will come right off.

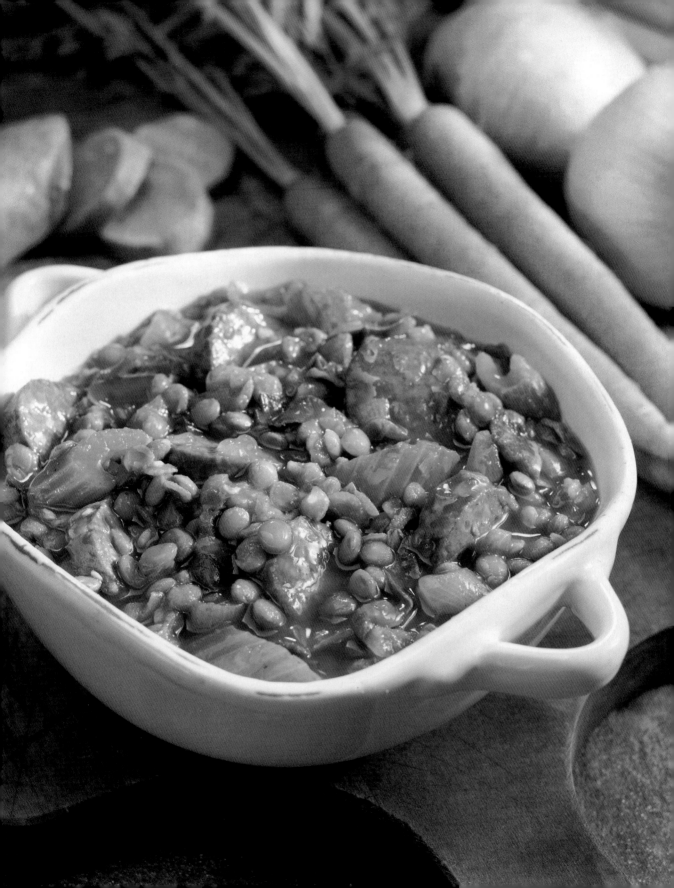

Roasted Veal with Shallots and Fennel

TEXTURE: Soft

INGREDIENTS

- 1 tablespoon (19 g) coarse kosher salt
- 2 teaspoons dried basil
- 1 teaspoon dried oregano
- 1 tablespoon (3 g) chopped fresh thyme
- 1 tablespoon (4 g) chopped fresh parsley
- ½ teaspoon ground white pepper
- 3 pounds (1.5 kg) boneless veal shoulder roast
- 2 tablespoons (28 ml) olive oil, divided
- 2 cups (320 g) thinly sliced shallots
- 2 large bulbs fresh fennel, trimmed and thinly sliced
- ½ cup (120 ml) cooking sherry, beef broth, or veal broth
- Fresh herb sprigs

Preheat the oven to 375°F (190°C, or gas mark 5).

In a small mixing bowl, combine the salt, basil, oregano, thyme, parsley, and white pepper and set aside.

Rub the veal evenly and thoroughly with 1 tablespoon (14 ml) of the oil. Coat the veal evenly with the spice mixture, and let stand for 20 minutes in the refrigerator.

In a large skillet, heat the remaining 1 tablespoon (14 ml) oil to medium-high heat. Place the veal in the pan and cook about 6 minutes on each side, until browned on both sides. Remove the veal from the skillet (reserving the brown bits in the bottom) and place it in a 3- or 4-quart (3- or 4-L) roasting pan. Add the shallots and fennel to the skillet and return to medium-high heat. Continue to cook about 15 minutes, until the onion and shallots are brown. Add the sherry or broth to the pan and stir with a spatula to release the brown bits into the liquid. Continue to cook for 2 minutes, then remove from heat. Pour the shallot mixture over the veal and cover it. Bake the veal for about 20 minutes, until the internal temperature at the thickest portion is 160°F. (If a meat thermometer is not available, make an incision in the thickest portion of the roast to determine doneness. Pink throughout indicates medium to medium rare. Pink in the center indicates medium to medium well.) Let the veal stand for 10 minutes before serving. Transfer the veal to a serving platter and arrange the shallot mixture over the top. Garnish the serving dish with fresh herb sprigs.

YIELD: Makes 12 (about 3-ounces veal) servings.

NUTRITIONAL ANALYSIS
Each with: **Calories:** 159.59 **Protein:** 17.35 g **Carbs:** 5.72 g **Total Fat:** 6.47 g **Sat Fat:** 2.18 g **Cholesterol:** 69.74 mg **Sodium:** 483.42 mg **Sugars:** 0.73 g **Fiber:** 1.02 g

Southwestern Marinated Chicken Breast

TEXTURE: Regular

INGREDIENTS

- 2 tablespoons (28 ml) lime juice (about 2 limes)
- $1/4$ cup (60 ml) low-sodium soy sauce
- 1 tablespoon (14 ml) extra-virgin olive oil
- 1 teaspoon oregano
- $1/2$ teaspoon paprika
- $1^1/2$ teaspoons chili powder
- $1^1/2$ teaspoons cumin seed
- 2 tablespoons (15 g) chopped fresh green onion (white and green parts)
- 3 cloves garlic, minced
- $1^1/2$ teaspoons honey
- $1/4$ cup (60 ml) white wine or lemon juice (optional)
- 2 8-ounce (225 g) whole, boneless, skinless chicken breasts, each cut in half down the middle
- 3 tablespoons (3 g) chopped cilantro leaves
- 1 lime, sliced into 4 slices
- $1/4$ cup (70 g) Fresh Salsa Caliente (page 162) (optional)

In a medium mixing bowl, mix together the lime juice, soy sauce, oil, oregano, paprika, chili powder, cumin, green onion, garlic, honey, and wine or lemon juice. Place the chicken in the bowl and cover all surface area with the marinade. Cover the bowl and place it in the refrigerator for at least 1 hour.

Preheat the oven to 375°F (190°C, or gas mark 5). Coat a 7- x 7-inch (17.5- x 17.5-cm) baking dish with cooking spray.

Spray a medium skillet with cooking spray and heat it over medium-high heat. Place the chicken in the pan, smooth side down and brown one side only.

Place the chicken in the prepared baking dish, browned side up, cover it tightly with aluminum foil, and bake for 15 minutes, until chicken is done at the thickest portion. Transfer the chicken to a platter and slice it on a 45-degree angle. Garnish each serving with the cilantro, lime, and salsa (if using).

YIELD: 4 (about 3-ounce) servings.

NUTRITIONAL ANALYSIS

Each with: **Calories:** 196.09 **Protein:** 27.50 g **Carbs:** 5.87 g **Total Fat:** 5.31 g **Sat Fat:** 0.92 g **Cholesterol:** 65.77 mg **Sodium:** 424.03 mg **Sugars:** 3.47 g **Fiber:** 1.04 g

"This marinade was very easy to make. The dish is not too spicy, but it can be adjusted according to your taste by adding extra chili powder and garlic. I love the mixture of the fresh herbs with the wine and lime juice. This great recipe sure is a keeper!"

—**Juli,** *a gastric bypass surgery patient in the New Bedford, Massachusetts, area*

Easy Oven-Baked "Fried" Chicken

This "fried" chicken is so easy and delicious, you'll want make it several times a week. This dish is packed with zesty flavor, and it goes well with just about any vegetable accompaniments or potato side dishes.

TEXTURE: Regular

INGREDIENTS

- ½ cup (40 g) instant oats
- 1 teaspoon garlic powder
- 1 teaspoon onion powder
- 1 teaspoon ground celery seed
- 1 teaspoon paprika
- 1 teaspoon dried basil
- ½ teaspoon salt
- ½ teaspoon black pepper
- 1 tablespoon (4 g) finely chopped fresh parsley
- 1½ tablespoons (20 g) Dijon mustard
- ½ teaspoon lemon juice
- 4 (4-ounce, or 115 g) boneless, skinless chicken breast halves

Preheat the oven to 375°F (190°C, or gas mark 5). Coat a baking sheet with cooking spray.

In a shallow dish, combine the oats, garlic powder, onion powder, celery seed, paprika, basil, salt, pepper, and parsley and stir to mix.

In a small bowl, combine the mustard and lemon juice. With a pastry brush, coat the chicken with the mustard mixture on both sides. Gently press the chicken into the oat mixture to coat both sides. Place the coated chicken on the prepared baking sheet and bake for 20 minutes, until the chicken is golden brown.

YIELD: Makes 4 (about 3-ounce) servings.

NUTRITIONAL ANALYSIS
Each with: **Calories:** 168.24 **Protein:** 28.09 g **Carbs:** 7.19 g **Total Fat:** 2.55 g **Sat Fat:** 0.52 g **Cholesterol:** 65.88 mg **Sodium:** 271.94 mg **Sugars:** 0.46 g **Fiber:** 1.30 g

Zesty Broiled Marinated Chicken

TEXTURE: Regular

INGREDIENTS

- ¹/₂ cup (8 g) chopped fresh cilantro
- ¹/₄ cup (6 g) fresh spearmint
- 1 teaspoon ground cumin
- ¹/₂ teaspoon cayenne pepper (optional)
- 1 teaspoon chili powder
- 1 tablespoon (14 ml) lime juice
- 1 teaspoon olive oil
- ¹/₄ teaspoon salt
- ¹/₈ teaspoon black pepper
- 3 cloves garlic, coarsely chopped
- 4 (4-ounce, or 115 g) boneless, skinless chicken breasts
- 4 slices lemon
- Fresh sprigs cilantro

"The Zesty Chicken Breasts are easy, spicy, and go easily with a variety of sides… the leftover makes a delightfully yummy sandwich using a low-fat English muffin, a slice of tomato, and low-fat mayonnaise."

—**Adrienne,** *a BPD surgery patient in the Boston area*

"The Zesty Broiled Marinated Chicken was fab! It's easy and very tasty and also great for lunch the next day."

—**Heather,** *a gastric bypass surgery patient in the Boston area*

In a food processor that has been fitted with a metal S blade, place the chopped cilantro, mint, cumin, cayenne pepper (if using), chili powder, lime juice, oil, salt, black pepper, and garlic. Pulsate the ingredients until finely chopped and combined. (It may be necessary to scrape down the sides of the processing container with a rubber spatula.)

In a 2-quart (2-L) mixing bowl, place chicken with the marinade, cover it with plastic wrap, and let stand in the refrigerator for 30 minutes, turning to rotate the chicken once.

Coat the broiler pan with cooking spray. Place chicken breasts on the broiler pan, discarding the remaining marinade. Broil chicken on the center rack for about 8 minutes on each side, until the thickest section of the breasts are done. (To check, make a small incision in the thickest part of the chicken. The juices should run clear. After cooking chicken breasts a few times, you'll soon be able to tell without checking!)

Garnish with the lemon and cilantro sprigs.

YIELD: Makes 4 (about 3-ounce) servings.

NUTRITIONAL ANALYSIS

Each with: **Calories:** 170.60 **Protein:** 26.80 g **Carbs:** 2.35 g **Total Fat:** 5.22 g **Sat Fat:** 0.91 g **Cholesterol:** 65.77 mg **Sodium:** 156.56 mg **Sugars:** 0.15 g **Fiber:** 1.00 g

Spanish Shrimp with Jasmine Rice and Green Beans

TEXTURE: Regular

INGREDIENTS

- 3/4 cup (135 g) dry jasmine rice
- 1 1/2 cups (355 ml) cold water
- 1 pound (455 g) fresh green beans
- 2 cups (475 ml) water
- 1 pound (455 g) medium to large fresh shrimp, peeled and deveined
- 1/2 teaspoon salt
- 1/4 teaspoon black pepper
- 1 tablespoon (14 ml) extra-virgin olive oil
- 1 cup (160 g) julienned sweet onion (cut into 1/4-inch (6-mm) strips
- 2 cloves fresh garlic, minced
- 1 1/2 cups (290 g) quartered plum tomatoes, skins removed
- 1/2 cup (120 ml) sherry or chicken broth or vegetable broth
- 2 teaspoons dried oregano
- 1 teaspoon smoked Spanish paprika
- 1/8 teaspoon cayenne pepper (optional)
- 1/4 cup (15 g) chopped fresh parsley
- 5 lemon wedges

Rinse and drain the rice in cold water, then place it in a 1-quart (1-L) saucepan with the 1 1/2 cups (355 ml) cold water. Bring the rice to a boil and then reduce the heat to a simmer. Continue to cook, loosely covered, for 20 minutes, until the water is absorbed by the rice.

Wash and drain the green beans. Snap off the stems and any remaining strings. In a 2 1/2-quart (2.5-L) saucepan with a steamer basket, place the beans along with the 2 cups (475 ml) water. Cover and bring the water to a boil. Continue to steam the green beans for about 5 minutes, until the desired doneness is reached.

Butterfly the prawns by using a paring knife to score the backside of each one at a depth of about 1/4 inch (6 mm). Place prawns on a plate or sheet pan in a single layer. Sprinkle the salt and pepper on the prawns and set aside.

In an 8-inch (20-cm) skillet, heat the oil over medium-high heat. When the oil is hot, add the onion and garlic and sauté for about 3 minutes, until the onion begins to soften. Add the tomatoes, sherry or broth, oregano, paprika, and cayenne pepper (if using). Reduce the heat to medium-low and continue cooking for 2 minutes. Add the prawns and cook about 5 minutes, until an orange color can be seen throughout each prawn. Remove from the heat.

Divide the rice among five dinner plates. Arrange the prawns around the rice so that the tails are facing upward. Sprinkle each plate with parsley. Arrange the steamed green beans asymmetrically around the prawns. Garnish each plate with a lemon wedge.

YIELD: Makes 5 (about 1-cup) servings.

NUTRITIONAL ANALYSIS

Each with: **Calories:** 296.73 **Protein:** 22.26 g **Carbs:** 34.67 g
Total Fat: 4.76 g **Sat Fat:** 0.74 g **Cholesterol:** 137.89 mg
Sodium: 654.61 mg **Sugars:** 5.89 g **Fiber:** 3.67 g

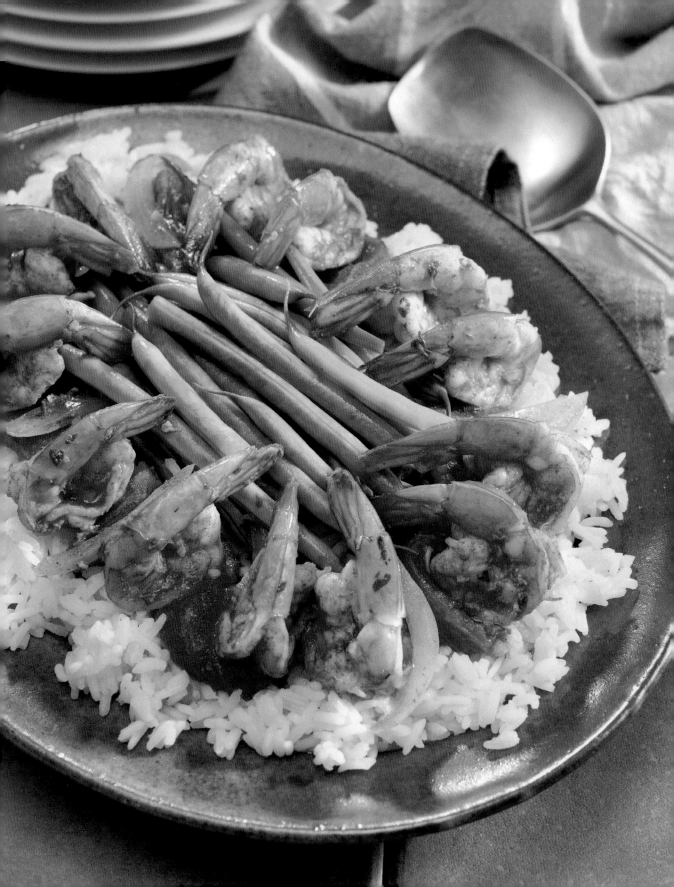

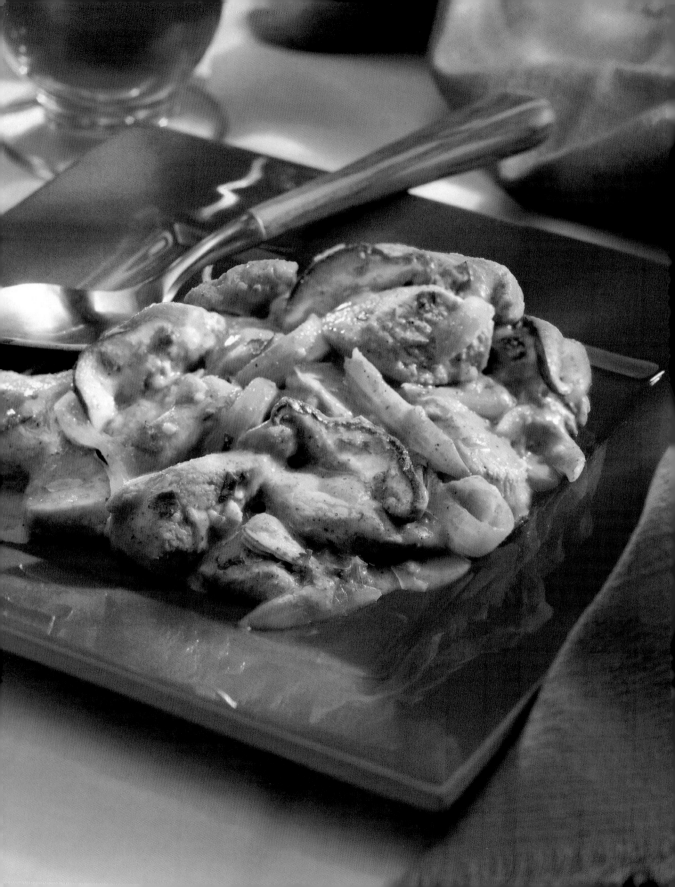

Chicken Curry with Fresh Mint and Shiitake Mushrooms

This dish has a world of complementary flavors!

TEXTURE: Regular

INGREDIENTS

- $\frac{1}{4}$ cup (30 g) curry powder

- $\frac{1}{2}$ teaspoon cayenne pepper (optional)

- 1 cup (235 ml) low-sodium chicken broth, divided

- 1 tablespoon (14 ml) extra-virgin olive oil

- 3 chicken breasts, skinless, boneless, trimmed of excess fat, and cut into bite-size pieces (about 3/4-inch, or 19 mm cubes) (see note)

- 1 medium onion, cut into julienne strips (about $\frac{1}{4}$-inch, or 6-mm thick)

- 5 shiitake mushroom caps, cut into $\frac{1}{8}$-inch (3 mm) strips

- $\frac{1}{4}$ cup white wine or chicken broth or vegetable broth

- 2 cloves fresh garlic, chopped

- 1 tablespoon (8 g) fresh grated gingerroot, peeled

- $\frac{1}{2}$ cup (120 g) plain nonfat yogurt

- 2 tablespoons (2 g) fresh coarsely chopped cilantro, plus additional leaves for garnish

- 1 tablespoon (5 g) chopped fresh mint leaves

In a small bowl, mix the curry powder and cayenne pepper (if using) together with 2 teaspoons of the chicken broth to make a paste and set aside.

Spray a 9-inch (22.5-cm) skillet with cooking spray and heat the oil over medium-high heat.

Add the chicken and sauté 12 to 15 minutes, until it begins to brown. Add the onion and mushrooms and continue to cook 4 to 6 minutes, until the onion begins to soften. Add the curry paste and $\frac{1}{4}$ cup wine or broth and stir until the chicken is evenly covered. Add a little of the remaining chicken broth at a time, until the desired thickness of the curry sauce is reached. Add the garlic and ginger, stir, and reduce heat to a simmer. Cover the skillet and continue simmering for about 5 minutes, until chicken is done. Slowly add the yogurt and stir in to incorporate. Add the cilantro and mint, stirring to mix well, and return the curry to a simmer. Simmer for an additional 2 minutes and then remove from the heat. Garnish with the cilantro leaves.

YIELD: Makes 6 (about 3$\frac{1}{2}$-ounce) servings.

NUTRITIONAL ANALYSIS

Each with: **Calories:** 180.83 **Protein:** 29.52 g **Carbs:** 8.83 g **Total Fat:** 2.00 g **Sat Fat:** 0.48 g **Cholesterol:** 68.86 mg **Sodium:** 421.43 mg **Sugars:** 3.17 g **Fiber:** 1.89 g

NOTE

Fresh shrimp, fresh vegetables, or cubed tofu may be substituted for the chicken.

Baked Chicken Portuguese Style

Creamy Polenta with Fresh Oregano and Feta Cheese (page 184) makes a perfect accompaniment to this extraordinarily tasty chicken dish.

TEXTURE: Regular

INGREDIENTS

- 1¹/₂ pounds (700 g) boneless, skinless chicken breast, cut into 6 (4-ounce, or 115 g) portions
- ¹/₄ teaspoon salt
- ¹/₄ teaspoon black pepper
- 4 tomatoes, skinned and cut into quarters
- 1 cup (160 g) sliced yellow onion
- 1 cup (140 g) sliced red bell pepper
- ¹/₂ cup (70 g) large pitted black olives or pitted Kalamata olives
- 4 cloves fresh garlic, coarsely chopped
- 1 cup (235 ml) red wine for cooking
- 1¹/₂ cups (355 ml) water
- ¹/₄ cup (60 ml) fresh lemon juice (about 1 lemon)

Preheat the oven to 375°F (190°C, or gas mark 5).

Season the chicken with the salt and pepper and let stand for 10 to 15 minutes at room temperature.

Spray a 10-inch (25-cm) skillet with cooking spray and heat it over medium-high heat. Place the chicken in the hot pan and brown one side only. Transfer the chicken to a 7¹/₂- x 11¹/₂ -inch (17.5- x 27.5-cm) baking dish, with the browned sides facing up.

Add the tomatoes, onions, bell pepper, olives, garlic, red wine, water, and lemon juice so that the ingredients are evenly dispersed over the chicken. Bake for approximately 20 minutes, until the chicken is cooked throughout. (Make a small incision in the thickest portion of the chicken. The juice should run clear.)

YIELD: Makes 6 (about 3-ounce) servings.

NUTRITIONAL ANALYSIS
Each with: **Calories:** 314.39 **Protein:** 31.16 g **Carbs:** 34.55 g **Total Fat:** 6.01 g **Sat Fat:** 0.70 g **Cholesterol:** 65.77 mg **Sodium:** 339.83 mg **Sugars:** 19.66 g **Fiber:** 8.93 g

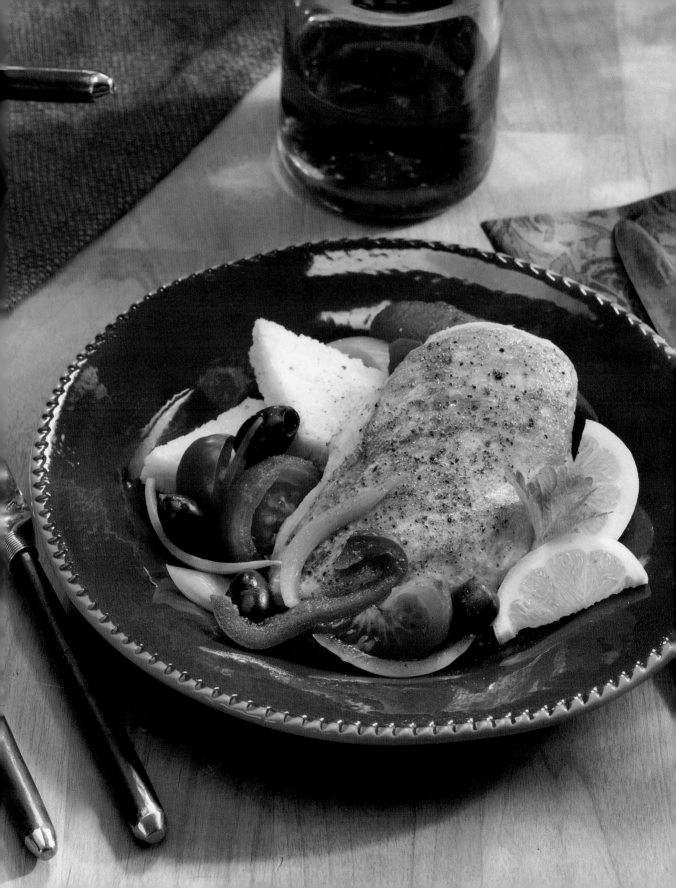

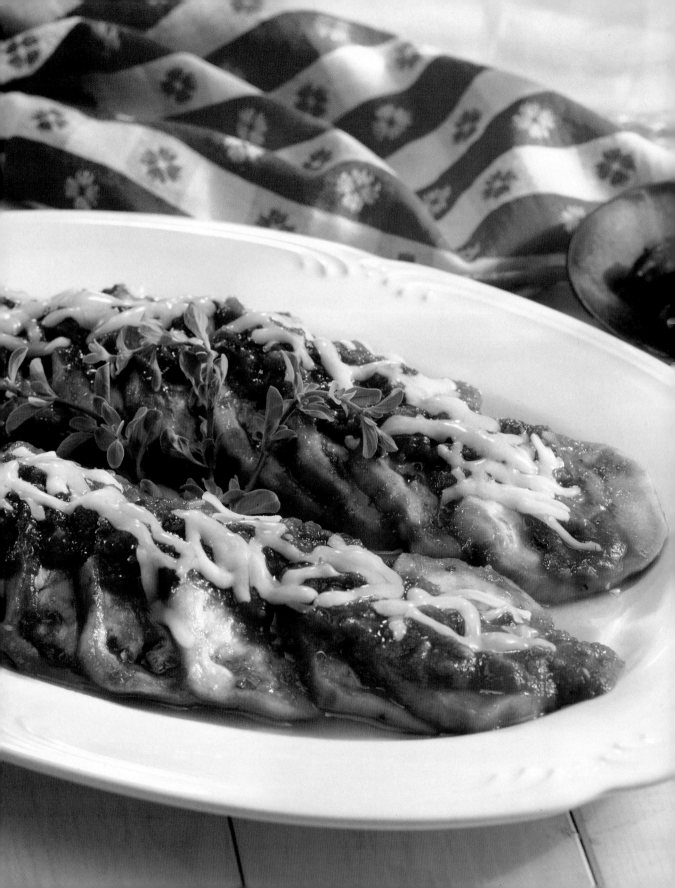

Eggplant Parmesan

TEXTURE: Soft

INGREDIENTS

- 1 large eggplant (about 1¹/₄ pounds, or 570 g)
- ¹/₂ teaspoon salt
- 1 tablespoon (14 ml) olive oil
- ¹/₂ cup (80 g) diced yellow onion
- 2 cans (11 ounces, or 310 g each) tomato sauce, no salt added
- 1 teaspoon dried basil
- 1 teaspoon dried oregano
- ¹/₄ cup (15 g) chopped fresh parsley
- 1 teaspoon dried thyme
- 1 cup (110 g) part skim-milk mozzarella cheese
- 1 tablespoon (5 g) grated Parmesan cheese

Preheat the oven to 375°F (190°C, or gas mark 5). Spray a 9- x 13-inch (22.5- x 32.5-cm) baking dish with cooking spray.

Remove the skin and stem from the eggplant with a vegetable peeler or a small kitchen knife.

Cut the eggplant into ¹/₄-inch (6-mm) circles and arrange them overlapping in the prepared baking dish. Evenly sprinkle the eggplant slices with the salt. Drizzle the oil on top of the eggplant. Distribute the onions evenly on top of the eggplant. Pour the tomato sauce evenly on top of the eggplant, allowing it to disperse throughout the slices. Evenly sprinkle the basil, oregano, parsley, and thyme on top of the sauce. Spread the mozzarella and Parmesan over the top. Bake for 30 to 40 minutes, until the cheese is bubbly and golden brown.

YIELD: Makes 6 (about 1-cup) servings.

NUTRITIONAL ANALYSIS
Each with: **Calories:** 138.58 **Protein:** 6.85 g **Carbs:** 14.72 g **Total Fat:** 6.01 g **Sat Fat:** 2.55 g **Cholesterol:** 10.73 mg **Sodium:** 233.87 mg **Sugars:** 7.16 g **Fiber:** 5.03 g

Spaghetti Squash with Pomodoro Sauce

This is a wonderful substitute for pasta in a delicious sauce.

TEXTURE: Mechanical Soft

INGREDIENTS

- 1 medium spaghetti squash (enough to yield 2 cups, or 310 g cooked)
- 1¹/₂ cups (570 ml) water
- 1 can (14 1/5 ounces, or 415 g) diced tomatoes in juice, no salt added
- 2 cloves garlic, minced
- 6 tablespoons (3 ounces, or 90 ml) white wine or chicken broth or vegetable broth
- ¹/₂ teaspoon kosher salt
- ¹/₂ teaspoon ground white pepper
- 1 tablespoon (14 ml) extra-virgin olive oil
- 1 tablespoon (5 g) grated Parmesan cheese
- Fresh parsley sprigs

Preheat the oven to 375° (190°C, or gas mark 5).

Cut the squash in half lengthwise and scrape out and discard the seeds. Place the halves in a baking dish, skin sides up. Add the water to the baking dish and bake about 40 minutes, until the squash will gently peel away from the skin with a fork.

In a 1- or 2-quart (1- or 2-L) saucepan, place the tomatoes with juice, garlic, wine or broth, salt, white pepper, and oil, cover, and bring to a simmer. Once a simmer is reached, remove the cover and continue cooking for 20 minutes.

For a smoother consistency, an emersion blender can be used to slightly puree the sauce.

Remove the cooked spaghetti squash by gently peeling away from the skin with a fork. Arrange in 1-cup (155 g) mounds on serving plates or in serving bowls as you would pasta and top with the sauce. Garnish with the cheese and parsley.

YIELD: Makes 4 (about ³/₄-cup) servings.

NUTRITIONAL ANALYSIS
Each with: **Calories:** 96.47 **Protein:** 1.80 g **Carbs:** 10.21 g **Total Fat:** 4.01 g **Sat Fat:** 0.69 g **Cholesterol:** 0.25 mg **Sodium:** 274.69 mg **Sugars:** 4.29 g **Fiber:** 2.09 g

MARGARET'S NOTE

This delicious dish provides almost half of your vitamin C for the day. If you'd like to make a complete meal out of this, add about 3 ounces (85 g) shredded part-skim mozzarella cheese or shredded vegetarian (soy) cheese.

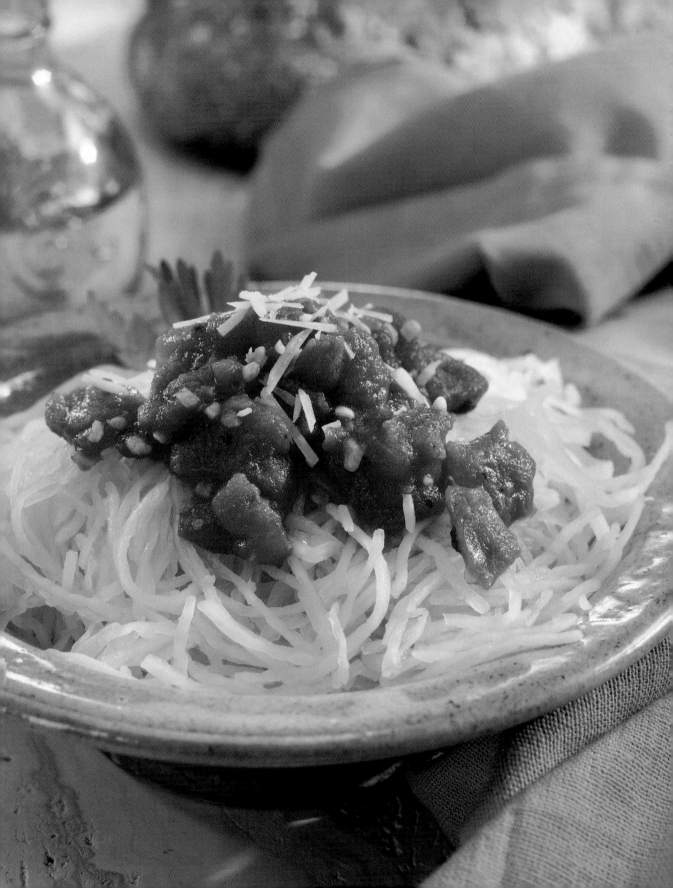

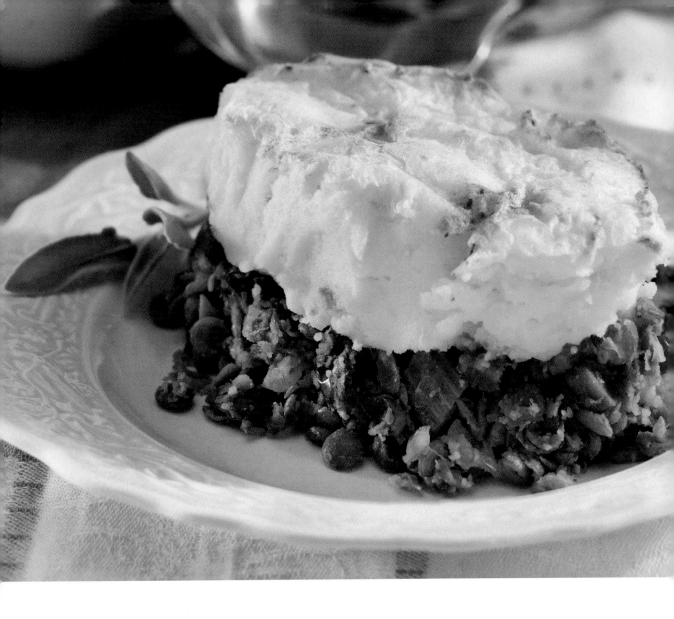

MARGARET'S NOTE

You could add ¾ cup of soy or vegetarian cheese to this recipe. Add it while making
the potato topping or grate it on top of the finished dish. Also, you could substitute
adzuki beans or green or yellow split peas instead of all, or some, of the lentils.

Vegetarian Shepherd's Pie

Lentils make this dish high in fiber, hearty, and delicious.

TEXTURE: Soft

INGREDIENTS

- 1¹/₂ cups (290 g) green or brown lentils
- 1¹/₂ pounds (700 g) russet potatoes
- 3 tablespoons (45 g) light butter, divided
- 1 small yellow onion, diced (about ³/₄ cup, or 120 g)
- ¹/₂ cup (65 g) chopped carrot (about 1 medium)
- 1 medium celery rib, halved lengthwise and thinly sliced
- 2 cloves garlic, chopped
- 1 teaspoon salt
- ¹/₂ teaspoon black pepper
- 1 teaspoon dried basil
- 1 teaspoon dried oregano
- 1 teaspoon dried thyme
- ¹/₄ teaspoon cayenne pepper (optional)
- ¹/₄ cup (15 g) chopped fresh parsley
- 2 medium tomatoes, cored and diced
- 2 tablespoons (28 ml) soy milk, unsweetened
- ³/₄ cup (85 g) soy Cheddar cheese (optional)
- ¹/₂ teaspoon paprika

In a bowl with water, soak the lentils for 30 minutes.

Peel and dice the potatoes into about 1-inch (2.5-cm) cubes. Place the potatoes in a 2¹/₂ -quart (2.5-L) saucepan with cold water to cover about 1 inch (2.5 cm) above the level of the potatoes.

Bring the potatoes to a boil and continue cooking for about 12 minutes, until the potatoes are tender throughout and will mash easily with a fork. Drain the potatoes in a colander and set aside.

In a 2-quart (2-L) saucepan, place the lentils with 3 cups (705 ml) of cold water and bring them to a boil. Reduce the heat to a simmer, loosely cover the pot, and continue cooking for about 30 minutes, or until all the liquid is absorbed and the lentils are tender.

Preheat the oven to 350°F (180°C, or gas mark 4). Coat a 2-quart (2-L) deep baking dish with cooking spray.

In a 9- or 10-inch (22.5- or 25-cm) skillet, melt 1 tablespoon (14 g) of the butter alternative over medium-high heat. Add the onion, carrots, celery, garlic, salt, pepper, basil, oregano, thyme, and cayenne pepper (if using) and sauté for about 5 minutes, until the carrots begin to soften, stirring occasionally. Add the parsley and tomatoes and continue to cook for about 3 minutes. Remove from the heat.

Mash the cooked lentils slightly with a large serving spoon and add them to the vegetable mixture, stirring just enough to incorporate. Spread the mixture evenly in the prepared baking dish and set aside.

Mash the potatoes together with 2 tablespoons (28 g) of the butter alternative, the soy milk, and soy cheese. Distribute the mashed potatoes over the lentil-vegetable mixture and bake in the oven for 30 minutes, until the top appears golden brown. Serve hot and garnish with the paprika.

YIELD: Makes 8 (about 1-cup) servings.

NUTRITIONAL ANALYSIS
Each with: **Calories:** 235.36 **Protein:** 13.11 g **Carbs:** 41.55 g **Total Fat:** 3.06 g **Sat Fat:** 0.49 g **Cholesterol:** 0.00 mg **Sodium:** 214.17 mg **Sugars:** 5.04 g **Fiber:** 14.63 g

Tasty Baked Tofu
with Sautéed Spinach

Delicious vegetarian meals don't come easier than this.

TEXTURE: Soft

INGREDIENTS

- 2 tablespoons (28 ml) light soy sauce
- 1/8 teaspoon toasted sesame oil
- 2 tablespoons (28 ml) apple cider vinegar
- 1 clove garlic, minced
- 1 package (16 ounces, 455 g) firm tofu, drained and cut into cubes or cutlets
- 10 cups (200 g) fresh spinach
- 2 teaspoons extra-virgin olive oil
- 1 clove garlic, sliced into thin strips
- Juice of 1 lemon
- 1/2 teaspoon black pepper

In a 7- or 8-inch (17.5- or 20-cm) baking dish, place the soy sauce, sesame oil, vinegar, and minced garlic. Add the tofu. Marinate for 1 hour, turning the tofu once to expose all sides to the marinade.

Preheat the oven to 350°F (180°C, or gas mark 4).

Drain the excess marinade from the tofu and discard. Bake the tofu for approximately 30 minutes.

Meanwhile, wash, drain, and chop the spinach into 1-inch (2.5-cm) strips. (If using baby spinach, leave it in whole leaves.) Pat the spinach dry with a paper towel.

In an 8-inch (20-cm) skillet, heat the oil over medium heat. Add the sliced garlic and sauté just enough to sweat the garlic. (Do not brown.) Add the spinach, lemon juice, and pepper. Cook for about 4 to 6 minutes, stirring often, until the spinach is tender. Place the spinach on a serving dish and top with the tofu.

YIELD: Makes 4 (about 1/2-cup) servings.

NUTRITIONAL ANALYSIS
Each with: **Calories:** 224.85 **Protein:** 23.89 g **Carbs:** 19.95 g **Total Fat:** 5.83 g **Sat Fat:** 0.33 g **Cholesterol:** 0.00 mg **Sodium:** 1492.84 mg **Sugars:** 1.56 g **Fiber:** 10.09 g

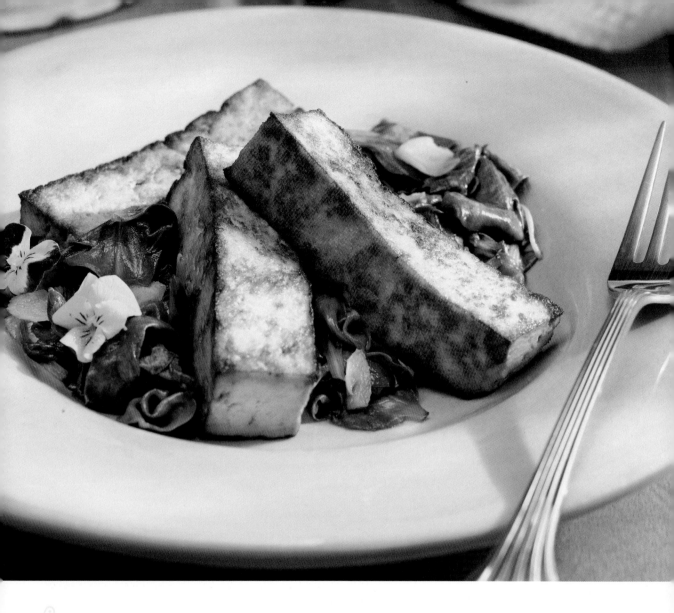

MARGARET'S NOTE

This dish is a bit higher in sodium than normally recommended (usually 700 milligrams or less per meal, for those who are salt-sensitive and/or need to watch sodium intake for blood pressure reasons), but it may be suitable for most people. If sodium is not an issue, you may add a bit of kosher salt to the spinach for added flavor. Also, you can increase the protein content of this dish by adding shredded soy cheese to the spinach. Another option is to toast about $\frac{1}{8}$ to $\frac{1}{4}$ cup (12 to 25 g) of slivered almonds and sprinkle on top. This will add a bit more fat, but no cholesterol, and it will also increase the protein content.

CHAPTER 14

Desserts

Lemon Sorbet

Lemon sorbet is a tasty and refreshing finish to any meal, from a casual barbecue, to your finest dinner.

TEXTURE: Pureed. May also be considered full liquids by some programs.

INGREDIENTS

- 5 large lemons
- 2 limes
- 1³/₄ cups (50 g) sugar substitute, suitable for baking (see page 50)
- 1 tablespoon (5 g) chopped fresh mint leaves
- Sprigs fresh mint

Cut the tops off of 4 of the lemons, about one-fourth of the way down from the top.

With a spoon, scoop out the insides over a bowl to catch the juice and pulp. Reserve the whole lemon peel cups. Zest or grate the lemon peel tops and set the zest aside. Discard the tops. Squeeze all the lemon juice from the pulp and discard the pulp. Cut the remaining lemon in half, juice it, and combine it with the rest of the juice. Zest or grate the outside peel of the fifth lemon, and add it to the juice, along with the zest from the four tops.

Juice the limes and add this to the lemon juice. Add the sugar substitute and mint leaves. Place all the combined juice in a 4-cup (940 ml) measuring container and add water to make 4 cups (940 ml) total liquid. Pour the mixture into ice cube trays and freeze the mixture overnight. Remove from the freezer and place in a food processor fitted with a metal S blade or a blender and blend until smooth. Return the mixture to the freezer until it is firm, but still soft enough to scoop, for 45 minutes to 1 hour. Scoop the sorbet into the reserved lemon cups and freeze until ready to serve. Garnish with the mint sprigs.

YIELD: Makes 4 (6-ounce) servings.

NUTRITIONAL ANALYSIS

Each with: **Calories:** 37.05 **Protein:** 1.85 g **Carbs:** 17.98 g **Total Fat:** 0.47 g **Sat Fat:** 0.06 g **Cholesterol:** 0.00 mg **Sodium:** 4.72 mg **Sugars:** 2.89 g **Fiber:** 7.28 g

Sugar-Free Ginger Applesauce Cake

This is acceptable for diabetic needs, yet oh-so-tasty!

TEXTURE: Soft

INGREDIENTS

- 2 cups (220 g) all-purpose flour
- 1 teaspoon baking powder
- 1 teaspoon baking soda
- 1¹/₂ teaspoons allspice
- ¹/₂ teaspoon salt
- ³/₄ cup (20 g) brown sugar substitute
- 2 eggs
- 2 tablespoons (16 g) fresh grated gingerroot
- 1¹/₂ cups (360 g) unsweetened applesauce
- 1¹/₂ teaspoons vanilla extract

Preheat the oven to 350°F (180°C, or gas mark 4). Spray a 1¹/₂-quart (1.5-L) loaf pan with cooking spray.

In a medium mixing bowl, sift together the flour, baking powder, baking soda, allspice, and salt.

In a separate bowl, mix together the sugar substitute, eggs, ginger, applesauce, and vanilla.

Pour the wet mixture into the dry mixture in thirds, stirring all the while with a wire whisk. Continue mixing until just smooth. (Do not over mix.) Pour the batter into the prepared pan and bake for about 50 minutes, until a toothpick inserted into the center comes out clean. Cool the cake at room temperature for 30 minutes before releasing it from the pan.

YIELD: Makes 12 (about 2-ounce) servings.

NUTRITIONAL ANALYSIS
Each with: **Calories:** 106.71 **Protein:** 3.35 g **Carbs:** 20.23 g **Total Fat:** 1.07 g **Sat Fat:** 0.29 g **Cholesterol:** 40.00 mg **Sodium:** 198.57 mg **Sugars:** 3.64 g **Fiber:** 0.84 g

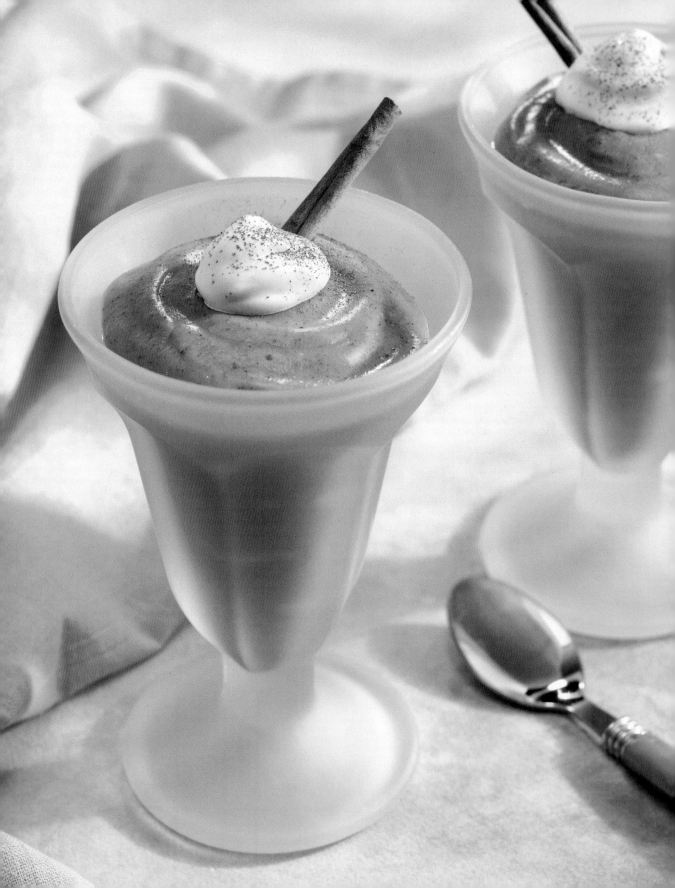

Holiday Pumpkin Parfait

This is a fast, beautiful, low-fat, and delicious dessert for a holiday or any occasion.

TEXTURE: Pureed

INGREDIENTS

- 1 cup (255 g) pumpkin puree
- 1 package (1 ounce, 28 g) sugar-free instant vanilla pudding mix
- 2 cups (475 ml) cold nonfat milk
- 1 teaspoon cinnamon
- 1 teaspoon allspice
- $1/2$ teaspoon vanilla extract
- 6 tablespoons (18 g) nonfat whipped cream topping
- 6 cinnamon sticks
- $1/2$ teaspoon ground nutmeg

In a medium mixing bowl, combine the pumpkin puree, pudding mix, and milk. Add the cinnamon, allspice, and vanilla and mix thoroughly. Evenly spoon the mixture into 6 parfait or martini glasses. Chill in the refrigerator for about 30 minutes, until the mixture sets. Place 1 tablespoon (3 g) whipped cream topping on top of each parfait. Garnish each one with a cinnamon stick and the nutmeg.

YIELD: Makes 6 (about $1/2$-cup) servings.

NUTRITIONAL ANALYSIS
Each with: **Calories:** 55.44 **Protein:** 3.28 g **Carbs:** 9.43 g **Total Fat:** 0.87 g **Sat Fat:** 0.46 g
Cholesterol: 1.63 mg **Sodium:** 99.91 mg **Sugars:** 5.41 g **Fiber:** 1.50 g

Baked Pears with Vanilla Ice Cream

This is a scrumptious and elegant dessert for your finest dinner party.

TEXTURE: Soft

INGREDIENTS

- 1 teaspoon light butter, melted
- 2 teaspoons cream sherry or 1 teaspoon lemon juice mixed with 1 teaspoon sugar-free vanilla syrup
- 1 tablespoon (14 ml) sugar-free maple syrup
- 4 Anjou pears
- 2 cups (270 g) sugar-free, light vanilla ice cream
- 8 cinnamon sticks

Preheat the oven to 375°F (190°C, or gas mark 5).

In a medium mixing bowl, combine the melted butter, cream sherry or lemon juice and syrup, and maple syrup.

Skin, cut in half lengthwise, and core the pears. (Use a spoon to remove the core of the pear, forming a cup in the center.) Place the pears in the bowl with the marinade and gently toss to cover all surface area of the pears. Marinate the pears for about 30 minutes, gently turning them in the marinade three or four times. Place the pears cut sides down in a baking dish large enough to hold the pears and pour the marinade over the top. Bake the pears for about 30 minutes, until caramel begins to form on the outside. Remove the pears from the oven, let cool slightly, and place on dessert dishes, cut sides up. Fill each pear center with a scoop of the ice cream, garnish with a cinnamon stick, and serve warm.

YIELD: Makes 8 (1/2-pear and 1/4-cup ice cream) servings

NUTRITIONAL ANALYSIS

Each with: **Calories:** 104.31 **Protein:** 1.67 g **Carbs:** 20.16 g **Total Fat:** 2.88 g **Sat Fat:** 1.42 g **Cholesterol:** 9.18 mg **Sodium:** 37.29 mg **Sugars:** 10.37 g **Fiber:** 2.81 g

Fat-Free Ricotta with Raspberries and Honey

This simple and elegant dessert is worthy of your finest dinner parties, and it's almost fat-free. It's a small, but super rich and satisfying dessert.

TEXTURE: Soft

INGREDIENTS

- 1 pound (455 g) nonfat ricotta cheese
- 1 cup (125 g) fresh raspberries
- 1 teaspoon sweetened vanilla powder
- 1 tablespoon (14 ml) honey
- 4 sprigs fresh mint
- 8 low-calorie, low-carb gourmet cookies

Divide the cheese among four small custard cups or dessert dishes. Place the raspberries over the top and around the cheese. Using a small sieve, sprinkle the vanilla powder equally over the top of each. Drizzle the honey evenly over each top. Garnish each dessert with a fresh mint sprig and 2 cookies. Use the cookies for spoons.

YIELD: Makes 8 (about ¼-cup) servings

NUTRITIONAL ANALYSIS
Each with: **Calories:** 125.50 **Protein:** 9.18 g **Carbs:** 22.84 g **Total Fat:** 1.10 g **Sat Fat:** 0.00 g **Cholesterol:** 6.00 mg **Sodium:** 90.15 mg **Sugars:** 13.68 g **Fiber:** 1.50 g

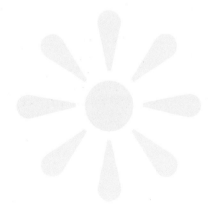

Almond Milk Rice Pudding with Dried Cranberries

Smooth and creamy, this recipe will make a great addition to your fall and winter dessert repertoire.

TEXTURE: Mechanical Soft

INGREDIENTS

- 4 cups (946 ml) unsweetened almond milk
- 2 cups (390 g) cooked brown jasmine rice
- 3 (4-inch, or 10 cm) pieces orange peel, no pith
- 1 teaspoon vanilla extract
- $^1/_4$ teaspoon kosher salt
- 2 tablespoons (30 ml) sugar-free maple syrup, divided
- 3 tablespoons (21 g) unsalted slivered almonds, toasted and divided
- $^1/_4$ cup (30 g) unsweetened dried cranberries, divided

In a saucepan set over medium-low heat, combine the milk, rice, orange peel, vanilla, and salt. Cook, stirring occasionally, for about 30 minutes.

When the rice mixture begins to thicken, stir more frequently. Continue to cook and stir until the mixture is about the thickness of custard, about 10 to 15 minutes. Remove from the heat and let stand for 5 minutes (the mixture will continue to thicken as it cools). Divide the rice mixture between 8 bowls, and top with the maple syrup, almonds, and dried cranberries.

YIELD: Makes 8 (about $^3/_4$-cup) servings.

NUTRITIONAL ANALYSIS
Each with: **Calories:** 152.96 **Protein:** 2.21 g **Carbs:** 29.84 g **Total Fat:** 2.94 g **Sat Fat:** 0.08 g **Cholesterol:** 0.00 mg **Sodium:** 112.77 mg **Sugars:** 11.52 g **Fiber:** 0.70 g

CHAPTER 15

Meal Plans for Various Stages after Your Surgery

The following meal plans are based on recommendations I've given my patients. Follow them depending on your own program's guidelines and your tolerance. This is not meant to be an "end-all be-all" menu, since individual nutritional needs may vary greatly; rather, it's meant as a possible snapshot of what a "regular" meal plan might look like after weight-loss surgery. Many of you won't be hungry at all for several months after your surgery. Some of you, however (especially if you had the gastric band versus bypass or sleeve), may be hungry a week or two later. Meal plans and tolerance are *very* individual and should not be compared to others. Of course, please check in with your surgical center's team, including your dietitian, for your own particular nutrition and texture progression goals. Remember to avoid drinking with meals, or until 30 minutes after meals. Your center may ask you to refrain from drinking fluids 5 to 30 minutes before meals, as well. In most cases, I haven't listed calories, since I encourage my patients to concentrate on fluids, protein, and healthy carbs. Also, fat won't be excessive with these healthy foods.

The First 2 to 4 Weeks Postop: Full Liquids

8:00 A.M.: 8 ounces (235 ml) herbal tea with lemon (artificial sweetener okay)

10:00 A.M.: 1 scoop whey protein isolate powder in 8 ounces (235 ml) soy milk

12:00 P.M.: 6 ounces (173 g) plain nonfat Greek yogurt with pure vanilla extract (artificial sweetener okay)

1:00 P.M.: 8 ounces (235 ml) chicken, beef, or vegetable broth with 1 scoop chicken soup–flavored whey protein isolate powder

3:00 P.M.: 16 ounces (470 ml) calorie-free, noncarbonated, caffeine-free beverage

6:00 P.M.: 8 ounces (235 ml) fat-free cream soup with 1 scoop whey or soy isolate unflavored protein powder

8:00 P.M.: 8 ounces calorie-free, noncarbonated, caffeine-free beverage

TOTAL FOR THE DAY: Fluids: 56 ounces; **Protein:** 84 g; **Carbs:** about 25 g

Weeks 2 through 6 Postop: Puree Texture

8:00 A.M.: 1 serving Frozen Fruit Smoothie (page 72)

10:00 A.M.: 8 ounces (235 m) herbal tea with lemon (artificial sweetener okay)

12:00 P.M.: 1 serving Fall Harvest Pumpkin Soup (page 111)

2:00 P.M.: 8 ounces (235 ml) calorie-free, noncarbonated, caffeine-free beverage

4:00 P.M.: 8 ounces (235 ml) soy, skim, or 1 percent milk with 1 scoop whey or soy protein isolate powder (aim for about 20 grams protein per scoop)

6:00 P.M.: 1 serving Black Bean Soup (page 117)

8:00 P.M.: 8 to 16 ounces (235 to 470 ml) noncaloric, allowed beverages (herbal tea, decaffeinated coffee or tea, or sugar-free beverages, as above)

TOTAL FOR THE DAY: Fluids: 56 to 64 ounces; **Protein:** 72 g; **Carbs:** 90 g

MARGARET'S NOTE

Many of my patients, and other weight-loss surgery patients I've read about online, are downright scared of carbs, but the carbohydrates here are very healthy for you. They provide fiber and lots of vitamins and minerals; they help "spare" protein, to help ensure the protein you *do* eat goes for healing, toward your muscles, and to help you feel more energetic; and they help you feel more energetic for your exercise sessions and overall. I recommend that my patients aim for at least 70 grams of healthy carbohydrates (e.g., about 2 servings of fruit, 2 servings of vegetables, 8 ounces [235 ml] skim, 1 percent, or soy milk, and 1 serving of grain or starch) by 3 months out, 100 grams of carbs by 6 months out, and the Recommended Daily Allowance (RDA) of 130 grams by 1 year out for maximum energy, bowel regularity, protein sparing, nutrient-density, and fat oxidation. Top sports nutritionists I know have cited a great deal of research stating that if you don't have enough carbohydrates in your diet, you won't break down fat stores as well, so remember your (healthy) carbs, please!

Weeks 2 through 8 Postop: Mechanical Soft Texture

The amount of food in this meal plan may be too much for you if it's only 2 weeks after your surgery—and can be too much at even 8 weeks out—so go *slowly* and do the best you can. Please keep in mind that while fluid and protein are key, carbohydrates (healthy ones, of course!) are also important.

8:00 A.M.: 1 serving Greek High-Protein Berry-Licious Milkshake (page 70)

10:00 A.M.: 8 ounces (235 ml) herbal tea or decaffeinated coffee or tea (artificial sweetener okay)

12:00 P.M.: 1 serving Lentil Soup (page 115)

2:00 P.M.: 16 ounces (470 ml) calorie-free, noncarbonated, caffeine-free beverage

4:00 P.M.: 8 ounces (235 ml) soy, skim, or 1 percent milk with half a scoop whey or soy protein isolate powder (aim for about 10 grams of protein per half scoop)

6:00 P.M.: 1 serving Slow-Cooked Bone-In White Chicken Chili (page 252)

8:00 P.M.: 8 to 16 ounces (235 to 470 ml) noncaloric, allowed beverages (herbal tea, decaffeinated coffee or tea, or sugar-free beverages, as above)

TOTAL FOR THE DAY: Fluids: 56 to 64 ounces; **Protein:** 87 g; **Carbs:** 109 g

MARGARET'S NOTE

You'll see that we've cut down the protein powder to half a scoop to wind down protein powders a bit and encourage more whole foods. It should take you at least 30 minutes (chew *very* slowly, until liquid) to eat a meal like the chicken chili. As I tell my patients, "Your teeth and mouth are your new stomach, no matter which weight-loss procedure you had."

Weeks 6 through 12 Postop and Beyond: Regular Texture

As mentioned previously, I don't focus on calories, especially in the first few months postop, since your body takes what it needs, calorie-wise, from your adipose (fat) tissue. Some studies cite the "average" gastric bypass patient is able to get only about 500 to 700 calories a day the first few months (which may vary, of course). I have, however, calculated the approximate calories here since this plan extends far out after surgery. The lower end meets the minimum long-term caloric goal for women and is just under the long-term minimum of about 1500 calories per day for men.

Also, my goal for my patients 1 year and beyond after their procedure is at least 130 grams of carbohydrates per day, a little more than featured here, which could be met by adding a serving of fruit or additional glass of soy or skim milk, to help ensure they have maximum energy and protein sparing.

8:00 A.M.: 8 ounces (235 ml) herbal tea or decaffeinated coffee or tea (artificial sweetener okay)

8:30 A.M.: 1 serving Denver Scramble (page 57), 1 slice wheat or whole-grain toast, ½ large or 1 small banana, and 1 teaspoon butter or margarine (may also choose 50-percent fat varieties, if better tolerated)

10:00 A.M.: 6 ounces (173 g) plain nonfat Greek yogurt and ¾ cup (109 g) berries

11:00 A.M.: 8 to 16 ounces (235 to 470 ml) noncaloric, allowed beverages (herbal tea, decaffeinated coffee or tea, or sugar-free beverages)

12:00 P.M.: 1 Spinach-Turkey Wrap (page 91) and ½ grapefruit or 1 medium orange or apple

2:00 P.M.: 16 ounces (470 ml) calorie-free, noncarbonated, caffeine-free beverage

4:00 P.M.: 8 ounces (235 ml) skim, 1 percent, or soy milk with 1 scoop whey or soy protein isolate powder, if desired (Optional: You may choose a noncaloric beverage here, depending on your tolerance and protein goals. D/S patients may need protein powder indefinitely to meet higher long-term protein needs of 80 to 120 grams per day.)

6:00 P.M.: 1 serving Whole Roasted Chicken with Potatoes and Brussels Sprouts (page 234) and ½ cup (183 g) canned peaches or pears in water

8:00 P.M.: 16 ounces (470 ml) noncaloric, allowed beverages (including herbal tea, decaffeinated coffee or tea, or sugar-free beverages, as above)

TOTAL FOR THE DAY: Fluids: 56 to 64 ounces; **Protein** 84 to 112 g; **Carbs:** 109 to 117 g; **Calories:** 1200 to 1400 (higher end if you choose milk and/or add protein powder to it)

MARGARET'S NOTE

The general protein goal for gastric bypass, sleeve, and band patients is 60 to 80 grams per day; D/S patients, however, may need 80 to 120 grams per day, so this menu is tailored to meet the goal for all four of these procedures. (In rare cases, too, other procedures might require more protein—if, for example, there's a wound infection.) You may not need more than 60 grams of protein per day, however, so please check with your surgical center, including your dietitian, to review your individual protein and other goals.

Vegetarian Considerations

I get more and more requests for lacto-ovo vegetarian meal plans (for people who forego meat, chicken, and fish but eat eggs and dairy products with vegetable protein). I'm delighted to provide a meal plan for this diet; people who are vegan (consuming a diet containing solely vegetable-based protein and free of all animal products) may follow this meal plan as well. Even if you're not a vegetarian, you may decide a "flexitarian" meal plan, whereby you include more meatless meals in your diet, might be right for you. Of course, please always check with your dietitian at your center to ensure all of your nutritional needs are being met, especially if you're new to vegetarian diets. In particular, my main long-term concern for vegetarians who have undergone weight-loss procedures lies with vitamin B_{12} since it's primarily found in animal sources. Vegans must take special care to find well-absorbed supplements. Also, iron may be a concern, since it's not as high in vegetarian/vegan sources. I recommend my vegetarian patients consume soy products (such as soy "hamburgers") in moderation and concentrate on natural soy protein sources, such as edamame.

The First 2 to 4 Weeks Postop: Full Liquids

8:00 A.M.: 8 ounces (235 ml) herbal tea (artificial sweetener okay)

10:00 A.M.: 1 scoop soy protein isolate powder in 8 ounces (235 ml) soy milk

12:00 P.M.: 6 ounces (173 g) plain soy yogurt with vanilla extract (artificial sweetener okay)

1:00 P.M.: 8 ounces (235 ml) vegetable broth with 1 scoop unflavored soy or rice protein powder

3:00 P.M.: 16 ounces (470 ml) calorie-free, noncarbonated, caffeine-free beverage

6:00 P.M.: 8 ounces (235 ml) vegetarian fat-free cream soup with 1 scoop soy protein isolate powder

8:00 P.M.: 8 ounces (235 ml) calorie-free, noncarbonated, caffeine-free beverage

---

TOTAL FOR THE DAY: Fluids: 56 ounces; **Protein:** 84 g; **Carbs:** about 25 g

Weeks 2 through 6 Postop: Puree Texture

8:00 A.M.: 1 serving Frozen Fruit Smoothie, with soy milk (page 72)

10:00 A.M.: 8 ounces (235 ml) herbal tea with lemon (artificial sweetener okay)

12:00 P.M.: 1 serving Fall Harvest Pumpkin Soup, with ¾ cup soy milk in place of ¾ cup nonfat half-and-half (page 111)

2:00 P.M.: 8 ounces (235 ml) calorie-free, noncarbonated, caffeine-free beverage

4:00 P.M.: 1 scoop soy protein isolate powder in 8 ounces (235 ml) soy milk

6:00 P.M.: 1 serving Black Bean Soup, with 1 cup reduced-fat shredded soy cheese in place of cheddar cheese (page 117)

8:00 P.M.: 8 to 16 ounces (235 to 470 ml) calorie-free, noncarbonated, caffeine-free beverage

TOTAL FOR THE DAY: Fluids: 56 to 64 ounces; **Protein:** 78 g; **Carbs:** about 94 g

Weeks 2 through 8 Postop: Mechanical Soft

8:00 A.M.: 1 serving Berry-Mango Breakfast Shake; add 1 scoop soy protein isolate powder or enough to total about 20 grams protein (page 69)

10:00 A.M.: 8 ounces (235 ml) herbal tea with lemon (artificial sweetener okay)

12:00 P.M.: 1 serving Lentil Soup (page 115)

2:00 P.M.: 16 ounces (470 ml) calorie-free, noncarbonated, caffeine-free beverage

4:00 P.M.: 8 ounces (235 ml) soy milk with 1/2 scoop (about 10 g protein) soy protein isolate powder

6:00 P.M.: 1 serving Vegetarian Shepherd's Pie (page 289)

8:00 P.M.: 8 to 16 ounces (235 to 470 ml) calorie-free, noncarbonated, caffeine-free beverage

TOTAL FOR THE DAY: Fluids: 56 to 64 ounces; **Protein:** 75 g; **Carbs:** about 122 g

Weeks 6 through 12 Postop and Beyond: Regular Texture

8:00 A.M.: 8 ounces (235 ml) herbal tea or decaffeinated coffee or tea (artificial sweetener okay)

8:30 A.M.: 1 serving Mushroom and Swiss Cheese Scramble (page 59), 1 slice wheat or whole-grain toast, ½ large or 1 small banana, and 1 teaspoon butter or margarine (may also choose 50-percent fat varieties, if better tolerated)

10:00 A.M.: 6 ounces (173 g) plain nonfat Greek yogurt and ¾ cup (109 g) berries

11:00 P.M.: 8 to 16 ounces (235 to 470 ml) noncaloric, allowed beverages (herbal tea, decaffeinated coffee or tea, or sugar-free beverages, as above)

12:00 P.M.: 1 Fresh Mozzarella Tomato and Tapenade Sandwich (page 96) and ½ grapefruit or 1 medium orange or apple

2:00 P.M.: 16 ounces (470 ml) calorie-free, noncarbonated, caffeine-free beverage

4:00 P.M.: 8 ounces (235 ml) skim, 1 percent, or soy milk with 1 scoop whey or soy protein isolate powder, if desired (Optional: You may choose a noncaloric beverage here, depending on your tolerance and protein goals. D/S patients may need protein powder indefinitely to meet higher long-term protein needs of 80 to 120 grams per day.)

6:00 P.M.: 1 serving Vegetarian Shepherd's Pie (page 289) with ¾ cup (90 g) grated soy cheese or Cheddar cheese for extra protein, 1 serving Greek Salad (page 138) with 1 serving Creamy Lemon Herb Dressing (page 152), and 1 serving Fresh Fruit Salad (page 152)

8:00 P.M.: 16 ounces (470 ml) noncaloric, allowed beverages (herbal tea, decaffeinated coffee or tea, or sugar-free beverages, as above)

TOTAL FOR THE DAY: Fluids: 56 to 64 ounces; **Protein:** 70 to 98 g; **Carbs:** 150 to 158 g; **Calories:** 1200 to 1400 (higher end if you choose milk and/or add protein powder to it)

MARGARET'S NOTE

High-quality, vegan-friendly protein powder includes soy protein isolate and may include enriched rice or hemp protein powder. Hemp protein powder, however, might be absorbed only at about 65 percent rate due to limited amounts of indispensible amino acids, or the building blocks of protein that your body cannot make and that must be obtained through diet.

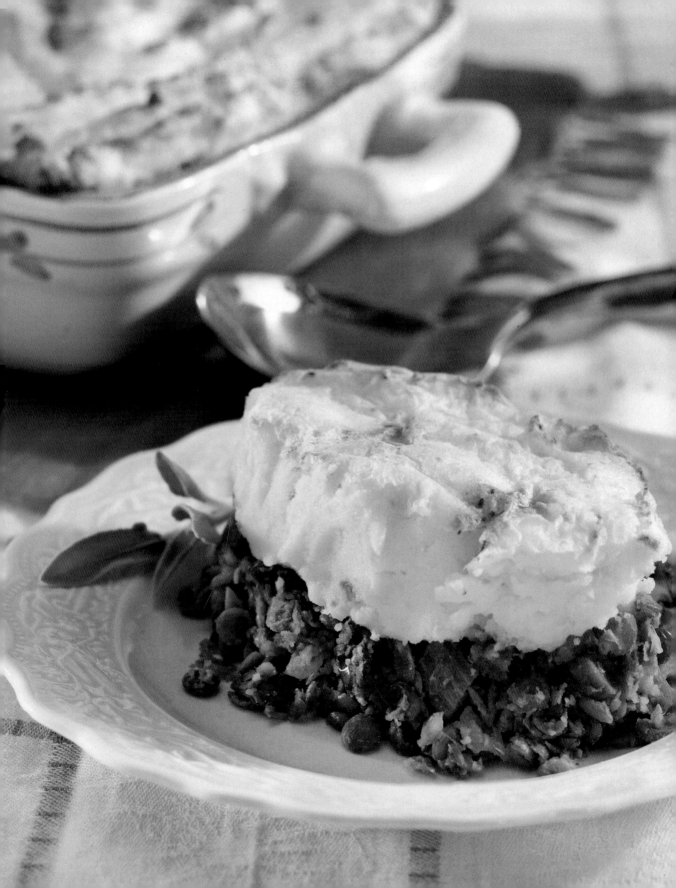

Acknowledgments

Lynette and I would first like to thank the wonderful staff at Fair Winds Press, including our editor, Wendy Gardner, and our marketing and publicity director, Mary Aarons. Without your boundless faith in us, belief in our vision, and endless support and patience, this project could not have happened. We thank you, from the bottom of our hearts, for giving us this opportunity to share and combine our expertise and love of nutrition and the culinary arts to create this book for weight-loss surgery patients. Thank you, also, to Rosalind Wanke and all of the professionals involved in taking such care to photograph our recipes. We really appreciate your attention to detail! Thanks also to our amazing copyeditor, Jennifer Reich.

I'd like to thank my family, including my parents, Ed and Sara, and Maria, Karen, and of course, Zoe, and Bette as well. You're very special to me, and I can't thank you enough for always believing in me and supporting this book. I appreciate the recipes you shared as well! I love you very, very much.

Thank you to my dear friend and coauthor, Lynette, for always being there for me while we developed and tested different recipe ideas and talked about the vision for our book. Although I was in Boston and you in Seattle, the endless phone conversations and e-mails back and forth to tweak the recipes to ensure they were tasty, yet healthy, seemed pretty painless because I knew your heart, as well as mine, was in this project from the start. I can't thank you enough for all of the love you have poured into our book. Molto grazi!

A big thank you to Dr. Scott Shikora, chief of the division of bariatric surgery, at Tufts-New England Medical Center. I've really enjoyed working together at NEMC, as well as on book chapters and speaking at conferences. Your tireless dedication to the field of bariatric surgery is admirable.

Thank you also to Dr. Paulo Pacheco, a successful gastroenterologist in New York City and a dear family friend. I appreciate your introducingthe manuscript to your friend and colleague, Dr. Christine Ren, a prominent bariatric surgeon in New York City, who then took an interest in it and was kind enough to offer to edit it. The comments were very much appreciated, and the insight regarding how your center, among others, may differ with respect to the diet progression after gastric banding, was truly priceless. Thank you, Dr. Ren.

And thank you to Linda Aills, R.D., for her help with our recipe testimonials.

I'd like to give a big thank you to all of my weight-loss surgery patients at NEMC. Although your names aren't mentioned to protect your privacy, please know that you were my inspiration for this book, and I dedicate it to all of you!

Cheers to nourishing the new you!

Margaret Furtado, M.S., R.D., L.D.N.

About the Authors

Margaret Furtado, M.S., R.D., L.D.N., R.Y.T., is a registered and licensed dietitian with over twenty years of clinical experience, including approximately ten years in medical and surgical weight loss, and is also a registered yoga teacher. She is currently seeing patients in the outpatient setting as a clinical dietitian specialist at the Johns Hopkins Center for Bariatric Surgery, in Baltimore, Maryland, including pre- and postop gastric banding, sleeve, gastric bypass and D/S patients. Prior to this position, Ms. Furtado worked at Massachusetts General Hospital's Weight Center and Tufts Medical Center's Weight and Wellness Center. She earned her master's degree in nutrition and dietetics at Florida International University, in Miami, and her bachelor of science degree in nutrition and dietetics from the University of Rhode Island. Ms. Furtado was a coauthor on the American Society for Metabolic and Bariatric Surgery's bariatric nutrition guideline paper, and lectures internationally on issues pertaining to nutrition and weight-loss surgery. In December 2009, her second book, *The Complete Idiot's Guide to Eating Well After Weight Loss Surgery* was released, and she has also authored a mini-ebook on preparing for bariatric surgery.

Lynette Schultz, chef, L.R.C.P., R.T., received her culinary training at various venues around the Seattle area. She currently works as a guest chef at Hedgebrook, a retreat for women writers near her home on Whidbey Island, Washington, and as a licensed respiratory care practitioner at Whidbey General Hospital.

Chef Joseph Ewing, holds a bachelor of science degree in culinary nutrition and an associate of science degree in culinary arts from Johnson & Wales University. He is the coauthor, with Margaret Furtado, M.S., R.D., L.D.N., R.Y.T., of *The Complete Idiot's Guide to Eating Well after Weight Loss Surgery*. Joseph began his culinary career in catering, and then later obtained a cooking position in a restaurant in his hometown of Easton, Maryland. He was awarded first place in the state of Maryland SkillsUSA National Culinary Arts Contest. In nearly a decade of culinary experience ranging from restaurant work, catering, and as a personal chef, Chef Ewing has worked and studied under a number of talented chefs and developed a great deal of knowledge and skill in the craft. He is currently studying to become a registered dietitian through the University of Maryland Eastern Shore Dietetic Internship Program.

Index